D1601279

The New Germany in the East

The New Germany in the East
Policy Agendas and Social Developments since Unification

Edited by
CHRIS FLOCKTON
University of Surrey

EVA KOLINSKY
University of Wolverhampton

ROSALIND PRITCHARD
University of Ulster

FRANK CASS
LONDON • PORTLAND, OR

First published in 2000 in Great Britain by
FRANK CASS PUBLISHERS
Newbury House, 900 Eastern Avenue
London IG2 7HH

and in the United States of America by
FRANK CASS PUBLISHERS
c/o ISBS, 5824 N. E. Hassalo Street
Portland, Oregon 97213-3644

Website http://www.frankcass.com

British Library Cataloguing in Publication Data

The new Germany in the East: policy agendas and social
developments since unification
1. Social change – Germany 2. Germany – History –
Unification, 1990 3. Germany – Social conditions –
1990 – 4. Germany – Politics and government – 1990 –
I. Flockton, Christopher II. Kolinsky, Eva III. Pritchard,
Rosalind M. O.
943′.0879

ISBN 0-7146-5093-5 (cloth)
ISBN 0-7146-8134-2 (paper)

Library of Congress Cataloging-in-Publication Data

The new Germany in the East: policy agendas and social developments
since unification. / edited by Chris Flockton, Eva Kolinsky, Rosalind
Pritchard.
    p. cm.
Includes bibliographical references and index.
ISBN 0-7146-5093-5 (cloth) – ISBN 0-7146-8134-2 (pbk.)
    1. Social change – Germany (East). 2. Germany (East) – Social
conditions. 3. Germany (East) – Economic conditions. 4. Germany
(East) – Politics and government. 5. Germany – Social conditions –
1990–. 6. Germany – Economic conditions – 1990–. I. Flockton,
Christopher. II. Kolinsky, Eva. III. Pritchard, Rosalind M. O.

HN460.5.A8 N48 2000
306′.0943′1–dc21   00-057001

Printed in Great Britain by
MPG Books Ltd, Bodmin, Cornwall

Contents

Part III Social Experiences and Attitude Change

Tables

Figure

Contributors

Vanessa Beck, MPhil (Keele), PhD Student, Institute for German Studies, University of Birmingham.

Mike Dennis, Professor of Modern German History, University of Wolverhampton.

Christopher Flockton, Professor of European Economic Studies, University of Surrey.

Anthony Glees, Reader in Government, Brunel University.

Jonathan Grix, Research Fellow, Institute for German Studies, University of Birmingham.

Ingrid Hölzler, Professor of Sociology, University of Magdeburg.

Dieter Kirchhöfer, Research Professor in Educational Sociology, University of Potsdam.

Eva Kolinsky, Research Professor of German History, University of Wolverhampton.

Steen Mangen, Lecturer in Social Policy and Social Administration, London School of Economics and Political Science.

Hildegard Maria Nickel, Professor of Gender Studies, Humboldt University, Berlin.

Ilona Ostner, Professor of Social Policy, University of Göttingen.

Rosalind Pritchard, Professor of Education, University of Ulster, Coleraine.

Beate Schuster, Research Fellow in Education, University of Potsdam.

Harald Uhlendorff, Research Fellow in Education, Free University of Berlin.

1

The New Germany in the East: An Introduction

Chris Flockton, Eva Kolinsky and Rosalind Pritchard

There have been several new Germanies in the course of the twentieth century, each replacing a political order which was no longer viable. In 1918 and again in 1945, regime collapse and the creation of a 'new Germany' followed military defeat while the destruction of the Weimar Republic and the imposition of a National Socialist 'new Germany' were the product of political forces and their disregard for a democratic constitution and parliamentary government. Compared to these system breaks of the past, the unification of Germany in 1990 was in some respects less far-reaching since it endorsed the west German system by transferring it to the east, and it was therefore only to that part of the country that a new political, economic and social order was introduced. The two post-war German states, however, had moved apart during 40 years of divided politics, and reinventing the former GDR meant entering uncharted waters and embarking on an experiment of transformation. Its outcome has been unexpected in the severity of socio-economic dislocations and in the development of attitudes and behaviour which do not replicate the west. This new Germany in the east is the theme of the present book.

The Federal Republic of Germany (FRG) and the German Democratic Republic (GDR), the two states in which division was institutionalised after World War II, established very different political, economic and social systems although they had not differed much at the outset. The GDR prided itself on constituting a new Germany, a new departure from a tainted past. The FRG had set out to build stable political order based on a democratic constitution, parliamentary government, and commitment to the rule of law in all areas of civil society and human endeavour. No less important for the consolidation of democratic governance and the emergence of a democratic political culture in the FRG was its implementation of the social market economy and its success in generating economic growth, material well-being and unprecedented levels of affluence for all. Legally, the Germany in the West regarded itself as the heir of the Reich – *Rechtsnachfolger* – while its political, economic and social transformation and emergence as a leading European power turned the Bonn Republic into something of a model democracy and a 'new' Germany compared with any of its historical predecessors.

The GDR, by contrast, had redesigned the economic and social order along state socialist principles and made anti-fascism a central tier of state ideology. It purported to have achieved a radical break with the past and to have eliminated from its own territory all traces of Germany's capitalist and nationalist history. In this perspective, eastern Germany, not the one in the West, was truly new and politically better. This self-image was echoed in the name of the state official newspaper, *Neues Deutschland*, and widely endorsed by a public eager to evade the complex issue of facing up to its own Nazi past – *Vergangenheitsbewältigung* – and export responsibility *summa summarum* to the west German state and its inhabitants.[1] Until *Ostpolitik* (the political opening to the East) facilitated contacts and communication across the German–German border, each of the German states used a negative view of the other to help consolidate its own identity, although the Federal Republic proved more successful in gaining acceptance among its own population and also among east Germans. Easterners were reluctant to sever links and proclaim a GDR identity but continued to wish for western affluence and living conditions. Too many facets of everyday life in western Germany looked desirable for eastern Germans, whose economy never functioned efficiently enough to alleviate shortages, whose wages, although sufficient to cover basic living costs, never stretched to luxury goods and quality life-styles and whose dependency on party political conformism and ideological subservience became an irritant to an increasing number of people.[2] The failure to segregate east Germans from west Germans mentally and emotionally, and the failure to deliver the desired life-styles in the GDR played a key role in the system collapse in the east that paved the way for unification.

Unified Germany was spearheaded by the 'peaceful revolution' which brought state socialism to its knees in the autumn of 1989 and by the *Volkskammer* (east German parliament) elections in March 1990, when a majority of east Germans supported the Christian Democratic Party (CDU) and thus cast its vote for unification and against a continuation of an east German state. Taking effect on 3 October 1990, the unified German state abided by the political, economic and social order of its western part and in doing so tried to distance itself from and discard the structures, institutions and orientations that had developed in the east during the 40 years of divided history. When a majority in the Bundestag voted in 1991 to relocate the German capital from Bonn, the symbol of post-war democracy, to Berlin, east German members of the Bundestag hoped to relocate the centre of gravity in an easterly direction and shift policy agendas closer to the concerns and priorities of the new Germany in the east. Although the move to Berlin has now been completed, policy remains indebted to the Bonn spirit.[3]

For the old *Länder*, unification signalled continuity: a confirmation of the institutions, processes, legal frameworks and decision-making processes that had underpinned the west German success story and seemed to deserve the status of a model. In the new *Länder*, by contrast, a transformation of unprecedented scope and intensity was set in motion. The system parameters were detailed in the 1990 Treaties on Social and Economic Union and on German Unity. Resulting from the March elections, these had been discussed and ratified by the east German *Volkskammer*. Once they began to take effect, the regions that had belonged to the GDR were recast and reinvented as political institutions, state administration, local government, trade unions and welfare services; the whole economy, the labour market, housing and all facets of public and private life were remodelled or replaced to implement west German practices.[4] Had this system transfer gone to plan it would have generated a replica western Germany. The transformation of eastern Germany would have been predictable, its outcome measurable and the process itself of limited duration. In the immediate post-war years, it had taken just one decade for the Federal Republic to gain internal stability and external recognition, a success story which prompted Adenauer to choose the slogan 'No Experiments' for the 1957 election campaign, reaping the biggest-ever majority for his party. In 1990, west Germans believed that their post-war success story could be repeated in the east and would unfold even faster than after 1945, given the head start of a consolidated party democracy and a supportive international environment. Unification by system transfer was a bid to obliterate the GDR in all its consequences without entering into the experiment of joint developments such as a confederation, a new constitution or similar ventures in which both east and west German influences would have come to bear. Capitalising, as Adenauer had done 40 years earlier, on system stability and a record of policy success, *Keine Experimente* in the 1990s intended to bring the east into the west and remove relics of the GDR from civil society as well as from people's minds.

This ending was not to be. West German public opinion expected that with the system transfer east Germans would be grateful for their material gains without expecting equality, not least since unification had increased tax burdens and escalated state expenditure. Once the initial flurry of national excitement and goodwill towards easterners had subsided, west Germans also liked to point out that they had created their successful Germany from the rubble through years of hard work while easterners flooded in to claim material rewards without having invested efforts of their own. Unification, then, changed the way in which west Germans looked at east Germans, but did not alter the west German political and economic system or downgrade established forms of behaviour or thought. On all these levels, however, unification unleashed transformation in the east. Despite the seemingly well-ordered system transfer, its impact appeared calamitous to east Germans who saw whole industrial sectors and regions close down, for whom employment became uncertain and unemployment a persistent threat, while the arrival of market principles, cost effectiveness and competition forced transformative changes across civil society and in all facets of daily life. East Germans had to adapt to the unfamiliar structures and institutions and also learn new ways of behaviour and communication. Of course, the influx of consumer goods and the end of shortages that had plagued east Germans throughout the existence of their state, met long-held desires for less hardship and a more affluent standard of living. The sheen of a mini-miracle, however, wore off as employment uncertainties mounted, as prices followed the market rather than state doctrine and as unification did not appear to meet the – admittedly unrealistic and inflated – hopes and expectations invested in it. A decade on, there is no east German sense of *Wir sind wieder wer* – 'we are somebody again' – which had buoyed west Germans in the mid-1950s in their bid for normalisation. Although the system of institutions, laws and political structures was in place within four years or so, convergence of living conditions, socio-economic circumstances and patterns of social participation has yet to set in. Indeed, the negative impact on east Germans of the new norms and institutions in their region resulted in a 'problematic normalisation' where individuals find it impossible to construct or rebuild their lives in a predictable and secure manner. Although transformation has been accomplished at the macro level of institutions and policy formulation, this normalisation has not filtered down to the micro level of social environments and personal life-plans where unfamiliar risks persist and adaptation to uncertainties has become part of everyday reality itself.[5]

The new Germany in the east bears the imprint of two processes of transformation. The first of these arises from 40 years of state socialist control in eastern Germany and its impact on the region and its people. Some of the distinctive developments that set the new Germany in the east apart from western Germany are post-communist and can be traced to the former GDR and its social or economic order. This applies, for instance to the high employment motivation among east German men and women or the positive views held generally about the effects of institutional care on the well-being of the child. The second process of transformation does not originate from the challenges of post-communist reconstruction but from changed policy agendas at state level. When unification began to impact on the east, west German society had already ceased to offer the secure environment of the economic miracle years. It had turned into a risk society where improved avenues of social participation through education, employment or income as well as threats of social exclusion through unemployment, poverty or homelessness had become endemic.[6] By 1990, employment biographies in west Germany were increasingly fragmented while welfare safety nets were less secure than in the past. In addition, globalisation had added a new volatility to economic development in Germany and Europe, and intensified the pressures on government to cut costs and reduce the role of the state in the protection of its citizens from social risk.

While west Germany had become such a risk society well before unification, east Germans had been shielded from these uncertainties by a state-administered employment society. Although the primacy of political conformism impeded quality, achievement and individuality in such a social order, it did guarantee education up to the age of 16, vocational or occupational training and, most importantly, full-time employment for all men and women up to retirement age. Part-time working needed special permission and, in any case, normally amounted to over 30 hours in a society where standard weekly working time was just over 43 hours. In none of its components – education, training, life-time employment until retirement – could the state-socialist 'employment society' survive. Yet, in their dislike of the *Sozialistische Einheitspartei Deutschlands* (Socialist Unity Party of Germany (SED)) government in 1989 or their calls for western conditions and finally unification, east Germans did not look for a change in these core components of their lives or declare themselves dissatisfied with the centrality of employment in the social policy agendas of the GDR. The collapse of these 'normal' dimensions of everyday life made it easier for individuals with drive, ability and ambition to gain recognition and advancement; the majority of east Germans, however, experienced the changes negatively as multiple uncertainties and as unwarranted disregard for their abilities and their personal qualities.

The new Germany in the east is facing the sudden and full impact of risk society development and of redrawn policy agendas. While the German government has attempted to cushion the blow by devising special aid programmes for the east, the majority of targeted programmes ran out in the mid-1990s although massive financial support continues to flow from central funds into the region. The second tier of transformation has begun to leave distinctive marks as east Germans develop strategies of career planning and risk management including a reduced commitment to

marriage-based families and a postponement (or even avoidance) of child
bearing. Specific to the experiences of transformation since unity, these
strategies and responses are also specific to the new Germany in the east.

Looking back over the 1990s, the chapters in this volume attempt to
draw a balance sheet in a range of policy areas and delineate the
distinctiveness of attitudes, behaviour and performance in the east. The
ready dismissal of such distinctiveness as a 'wall in the head',[7] a doomed
remnant from the past, overlooks that since unification, an 'eastern
identity'[8] has gained ground which bears the hallmarks of both processes
of transformation: the persistence despite post-communist reconstruction
of attitudes and practices from the GDR era and the impact of
employment uncertainties, diluted welfare provisions and risk society on
the new Germany in the east and its inhabitants.

This study seeks, therefore, to explain and elucidate the kind of civil
society which has emerged in east Germany since the *Wende* (the fall of the
Wall), and to assess how it has fared in the process of transformation to a
social market economy and liberal democracy of the federal German type.
In the first of three parts, it builds on the notion of a 'dual transformation'
by looking at the process of post-communist transformation in east
Germany, at the macro levels of the economy and the welfare state: in
parallel, it elucidates those processes acting on Germany and Europe as a
whole, which are felt in most advanced industrial societies. In its second
part, contributors address the question of what kind of civil society has
emerged in the new *Länder*, by assessing developments in key areas of east
German society. Here they assess the policy agenda and policy regime put
in place and, by reviewing personal and public opinion responses to these
policies, seek to highlight whether state-socialist legacies continue to
influence the policy debate and continue to inform the social values held
by the population. In a third section, at the micro level of system
transformation, contributors seek to trace personal experiences and
attitude changes among the eastern population since 1990, over a range of
key social, family and educational policy questions. Ranging from the
larger-scale macro policy debate to the micro level of personal experience
and personal values, the book seeks therefore to capture the dual
transformation which is changing Germany and redrawing the notion of
social citizenship, even as east Germany is in transformation, and to make
clear how, in a broad range of societal areas, a problematic normalisation
continues to define the condition for many east Germans.

SYSTEM TRANSFORMATION AND THE ECONOMIC AND SOCIAL POLICY AGENDAS

Post-communist transformation in the new *Länder* involves not simply the transfer of western institutional structures and policy agendas, and the east German behavioural reactions in this new setting; it involves also changes at the macro level of economy and 'social state' under the mounting pressures of globalisation and European integration. The transferred western regime itself is in a state of deep change. Here, the openness of the economy channels European and global competitive and deregulatory forces and, linked in part with this, there is the interplay of factors which lead inexorably to long-term welfare state reform. This posits a restructuring of welfare provision based on a renegotiation of the implicit contract between citizen and state, sometimes called a redrawing of 'social citizenship'. There has therefore been in the Federal Republic, both in practice and at the level of proposals for further fundamental change, a reformulation of the commitment of the state to its citizens. This has occurred at the same time as the east German population has had to come to terms with the narrower and qualitatively different coverage of social welfare benefits in a unified Germany, after the all-encompassing provision, at an albeit modest level, of the GDR regime. Such a narrower coverage of the social safety net and social provision (even if the purchasing power value of many federal German income-related benefits is far higher than in GDR days), reinforces the fact that the east German workforce and its families have now entered a 'risk society', different in so many regards from the security and solidarity offered by the 'employment society' which they had known in the GDR.

Throughout the developed world, welfare arrangements have come under increasing financial strain and their effectiveness has been the focus of a searching critique. In most western European countries there have been proposals during the 1980s and 1990s for a long-term reform of welfare provision. Historically, over the post-war decades, welfare states had typically exercised a legitimating function, so gaining loyalty of the population to liberal democracy and social democracy, incorporating social classes to the system. However, this function had progressively lost effectiveness and had come to be seen even as counter-productive. While heavy social expenditure had earlier been justified as investment in human capital (where income support measures reduced risks, facilitated mobility and training), with the oil shocks, falling productivity growth and reduced profit share in national income, it later came to be perceived as a contributory factor in long-term structural unemployment, rather than helping promote a solution. The panoply of measures, and the unresponsiveness of the bureaucracies, failed also to respond to an increasing differentiation of needs. As Steen Mangen demonstrates in Chapter 2, a reordering of functions between the state, markets and the family in the sphere of social support came under discussion, especially in the areas of health and pension insurance, where long-term pressures (the 'demographic crisis') were greatest. Writers such as Esping-Andersen posed the question of whether the aim of equality is still viable, when the negative effects of the social state in its pursuit of greater egalitarianism are acknowledged.[9] A renegotiation of the contract implicit in social citizenship therefore had to be countenanced.

The all-encompassing social state came to be seen in the west as ineffective (and certainly in New Right political discourse) from the ways in which it appeared to foster dependency and 'moral hazard' (inducing unintended and undesirable responses), to produce insider–outsider effects, and in failing to reduce the blight of long-term structural unemployment. 'Passive' measures, particularly in the labour market, which gave income maintenance to the unemployed and promoted early retirement on a large scale, appeared to generate a dependency culture rather than one of taking personal initiative. The 'moral hazard' character of the benefit system, working through poverty and unemployment traps, reinforced this dependency. The continuation of long-term unemployment clearly also burdened the social insurance contribution costs of the productive sector, weighing down on future growth by depressing investment levels. Under a revised 'social citizenship', contractual rights would be renegotiated to offer a changed role for welfare, but a role which nevertheless would continue to provide risk management to citizens over their more volatile life-cycles.

A reordering of benefit systems is underway (particularly for pensions, health and nursing care). This will particularly affect countries such as Germany since, to complement provision through social insurance schemes of the Bismarckian type (where employer and employee contribute equally to nationally organised schemes), there would be a new emphasis on company schemes and personal indemnity: these would assume a greater role and so relieve the state schemes. There would also be a fundamental revision in the form and levels of benefit, of the tax and social security systems, which would stress 'employability', labour market participation and the eradication of the unemployment and poverty traps which so harm the return of the unemployed to active labour market participation. In short, a move to an 'active' social welfare system. This is the 're-commodification' of labour in the sense used by Ilona Ostner in Chapter 3. Such a revision of the European Social Model is in prospect which nevertheless continues to guarantee social minima, even if there remain differences in the model between the UK and European continental countries. However, as stressed by both Ilona Ostner and Steen Mangen in their contributions, labour market instruments and benefit schemes which stress 'employability' and participation may be built on unsafe foundations if there is a large-scale shortage of employment in the east, and if employment insecurity more generally is so prevalent that discontinuous employment histories are the norm. One may therefore question their suitability for an east Germany which continues to suffer from mass unemployment and deep labour market uncertainty.

Transition to the west German 'social state' also wrought fundamental changes in terms of income support, gainers and losers, and exposure to the 'risk society'. In GDR days, the east German population had enjoyed an all-encompassing social policy and welfare system, from heavily subsidised rents, foodstuffs, energy and travel, through favourable child allowances, crèches and child-support systems for working mothers, to a right to employment and (officially, at least) to an absence of unemployment. For them, the advanced and comprehensive welfare system, together with job security and very limited income differentiation, were the prime advantages of socialist central planning: the regime used such welfare policies as a deliberate tool to legitimate the regime in the eyes of the population. An exhaustive social security system came to be seen by the population as a right, and equally a right under a democratic system such as that of the Federal Republic.

At unification, the transfer of the west German social welfare system to the east brought fundamental changes in institutions, coverage and real level of benefits. Significant changes involved the downgrading of child-support provision for working mothers and a very marked rise in the relative value of pensions, but it was the income-support provisions for the unemployed, those on short-time working, those in retraining and early retirement, that represented the key innovation for the broad mass of the working population, given the way in which unemployment scarred the eastern workforce and particularly the female cohort. In such a huge labour market upheaval, easterners came rapidly to depend upon the western social security system which guaranteed the value of benefits linked to rising wages, even as unemployment intensified. Effectively, it sustained incomes and living standards for the 30 per cent of the workforce who were unemployed or on special labour market programmes. Naturally, for a population which had grown up to assume a right to employment and which valued social equity and limited social differentiation, the mass unemployment, the increased income disparities and the less all-embracing social welfare coverage meant that these costs of transformation had to be set alongside the gains of a democratic order and civil society.

This process of dual transformation is equally evident at the level of the economy more generally, whether at the macro-economic levels of growth and public finance or more micro-economically in terms of branch- and firm-specific developments. The financial burdens imposed by the east and the difficulties of sustaining transformation in a socially acceptable manner have left their mark on the western economy and have led to certain distortions in the application of its policy instruments. Thus, driven to a considerable degree by the costs of income support for those affected by mass unemployment, net financial transfers from west to east reached a total of DM888 billion over the first seven years following unification. Within this huge amount, the high levels of social spending indicate that, to a considerable degree, the so-called 'crisis' of the west German welfare state in the 1990s was heavily influenced by these costs of the east.[10] However, notwithstanding these macro-economic burdens, it is in the realm of industrial aid and competition policy that distortions have attracted the most attention, particularly from the EU Competition Directorate, as Chris Flockton shows in Chapter 4. Germany has become by far the largest subsidiser in the EU and special regimes in agriculture, housing and electrical power in the east continue to offer protection in a range of ways. As quite long-running departures from the social market model, this type and degree of intervention in the east attracts criticism from those particularly of market liberal persuasion.

It is, however, the scale of unemployment, employment uncertainty and the prevalence of disrupted career histories (*Bastelbiographien*) which shows the greatest divergence from GDR realities and which provides new challenges for coping with risk and transformation. Taking together those registered as unemployed and those benefiting from second labour market measures, consistently 30 per cent of the workforce has been affected by unemployment at any time. Women have fared particularly badly in this painful transition and only one-fifth of employees have retained their original jobs after unification: such statistics point to the scale of the changes which have hit the eastern working population. And, while average gross effective wages in the east reached 79 per cent of the western level by 1998, wage disparities have risen markedly and the uncertainty of household incomes has given rise to deep discontent. Important differences with the west also lie in the fact that east Germany is moving towards the status of a 'tariff wage-free zone'. In contrast with the west, the force of the imperative to cut the scale of financial losses has led firms to break free from the regional or branch-based bargaining structures. The consequence has been a rapid fall in union membership and the free setting in many companies of wage levels outside of any collective wage agreement. This, together with the prevalence of small- and medium-sized companies in its enterprise structure lead to the question of whether the new *Länder* are the German economy's 'new frontier'.

WHAT KIND OF CIVIL SOCIETY HAS EMERGED IN THE EAST?

Over the past ten years, east German society has, in a sense, been reinvented, and a new society, a 'new Germany' in the east has taken form. One could approach this, as Offe[11] does, in terms of an 'experiment', where contemporary east German society is neither that which preceded it, nor is comparable with the west German model which provided both the framework and the policy direction. It may share many key social attributes, norms and values with the western *Länder*, but retain nevertheless certain significant distinguishing characteristics which would allow one to speak of an 'eastern identity'. This would clearly be the fruit of a long historical regional identity, of the systematic induction into 40 years of state socialism and would bear the impress of the deep and painful restructuring of the recent past. East German society today can be seen as unfolding under the interplay of the relations between citizen and the state (whereby east Germans have come to learn and exercise their rights in a liberal democracy), under the interplay of the policy agendas and social developments during the transition, and as a result of the discrepancy between the evolving attitudes, expectations, practices and the requirements of the system change itself. Eastern German society retains specificity; but is it evolving in close conformity to that of the west, and will generation change and an eventual economic prosperity eradicate these differences? Are there any aspects of east German society which deserve to be perpetuated and even copied in west Germany?

It would be scarcely surprising if after ten years, differing values and attitudes between the east and west German populations did not show great resilience, given the socialisation processes in the GDR and the depth of the economic and social transformation which has since taken place. There is considerable evidence that psychological unity and the forging of a common social identity between the two parts of Germany has still not been achieved and that an east–west mental divide continues. Of course, a fundamental question concerns the problematic nature of the creation of a German national identity, given the barbarism and tyranny which has occurred in the twentieth century. Both western and eastern German regimes alike expressed ambivalent attitudes and divergent approaches to this national question. However, there is plentiful evidence of common values, traditions and a shared experience of the GDR past which are strongly felt and to which the east Germans subscribe; these lead one to postulate the existence of an eastern identity. Very few east Germans wish to see a return of the GDR and most recognise the gains of political freedom and pluralism. However, among the cherished values of the population are many born of GDR times, namely, social justice, security and solidarity. As Michael Dennis shows in Chapter 5, attitudes in favour of the right to employment, fixed rents, generous pre-school child-care provision and opportunities for women are strongly and widely held. The *Ostalgie* or nostalgia for an imagined, rather than a real GDR past sees the losses outweighing the gains of unification in many fields, particularly those related to social provision, equity, equal opportunities for women and personal safety. In part this helps explain the continuing support for the *Partei des Demokratischen Sozialismus* (Party of Democratic Socialism (PDS)) as successor party to the SED. The widespread antagonism generated by what is perceived as western arrogance also fuels a certain 'otherness' in the east. Economic growth, generational change and political participation can be expected over time to foster convergence between the old and the new *Länder*, but there will remain for many years a set of social values which will continue to form part of an *Ostidentität*.

Posing the question of how civil society has emerged simultaneously raises the issue of what is the measure of civil society under state socialism, as well as during social transformation towards a western model? A key aspect of civil society can be found in dense networks of voluntary associational behaviour which demonstrates active participation by citizens in organisations, whether trade associations, political parties, trade unions, clubs, charities, etc. In a democracy-based model of civil society, such formal associations can be expected to flourish: they build social capital and social trust. In contrast, under state socialism as practised in the GDR, the state sought to incorporate associations under direct party influence and control. In a situation inimical to the growth of free formal associations, much associational activity flourished on an informal basis, both to escape the ideological and political channelling of activity and to meet basic needs common in a shortage economy: such was the *Laubengesellschaft* ('dacha' society) of vegetable garden smallholders in the GDR, or informal neighbourhood and workplace networks. Given that formal associational behaviour has been highly developed in West Germany, one might expect convergence between east and west to be exhibited in the form of a marked rise in associational behaviour in the east. Furthermore, the spontaneous, oppositional groupings which flourished in the pre-*Wende* period as vehicles for protest, had the capacity to mobilise the eastern population into more formal associational activity, principally political membership and action. However, both the GDR inheritance and the profound restructuring of the post-unification transformation have obstructed formal, voluntary participation and these oppositional groups of the *Wende* and pre-*Wende* periods proved incapable of playing a significant role in the future institutional structure which was adopted very largely from the west. As Jonathan Grix shows in Chapter 15, the informal networks common in GDR times continue to predominate, with little evidence of the *Verein* (voluntary association) phenomenon so typical of the west. The economic upheavals, deep restructuring and uncertainties of the 1990s have harmed the growth of trade union and trade association representation, and have continued the informal relationships typical of the GDR period, as the population seeks to overcome the deep uncertainties which they have experienced.

Post-communist transformation put an end to secure employment in east Germany and challenged the working population to adjust to unfamiliar practices and unexpected social risks. While unemployment, early retirement and other forms of labour market exclusion became shared experiences in the new *Länder* after unification, the old *Länder* had already been exposed to risks of modernisation including employment uncertainties before unification transferred the western model to the east. This dual transformation has been the hallmark of economic and social development in eastern Germany after the collapse of the GDR.

In her chapter 'Employment, Gender and the Dual Transformation in Germany', Hildegard Nickel examines the impact of this dual transformation on the employment opportunities of women in three key areas of the service industry: retailing, financial services and the German railway company Deutsche Bahn AG. At the time of unification, the breadwinner model of male employment and a female homemaker role had been modified in western Germany but remained valid; in the east women were normally employed and breadwinners in their own right. As unification unleashed a competition for jobs, women were hit harder than men by the fallout of economic restructuring and de-industrialisation. Rejecting the notion that women were losers of unification, Nickel shows that some ten years after unification, more east German than west German women were employed (66 per cent and 45 per cent respectively) and more east German than west German women with small children were employed. Female employment has changed in the course of economic restructuring and also become newly differentiated. In the GDR, retailing and financial services had been virtually all-female areas of employment. This changed somewhat after unification as young men, usually from outside the sector and often from western Germany, were appointed to middle or higher management positions, particularly in retailing. While women were not excluded altogether, their chances of advancement were limited. In the financial sector, matters developed differently. Here, corporate training offensives enabled women employees to upgrade their qualifications, remain in post and rise to managerial posts which would have been out of reach for them in GDR times. Recent pressures on the sector, however, to downsize, reduce customer services and curtail middle-management have eroded this 'home advantage' and begun to threaten ex-GDR women who had rebuilt and accelerated their careers.

In the Deutsche Bahn pressures on women have assumed a different profile: here, the high staffing levels of the east German railway system remained visible as a relatively high employment of women in the eastern section of the merged company. In the transformation, women had been more affected by redundancies than men: in the consolidation after merger, new rules of flexible working, geographic mobility and constant pressures or threats to reduce staff have again hit women harder than men. In her study of the sector, however, Hildegard Nickel found that women were judged by their qualifications, not by their status as mothers or their family duties. Women who coped with change management had excellent chances of employment and advancement. The age group between 30 and 40 was particularly motivated to succeed and had gained a foothold in management. Nickel concludes that women's employment opportunities are differentiated and that, increasingly, processes of company change determine prospects of labour market participation. Path dependency seems to determine employment opportunities for east Germans generally, not merely for women. For women, opportunities and experiences of employment vary; there is no such thing as a good or a bad female labour market scenario in the new *Länder*.

In the social policy area, there is no field that better illustrates the changed objectives and changed policy agendas than that of education. Objectives and structures embody intimately the social organisation of society itself. With the *Wende*, we can see how the direct transfer of the prime elements of the western system imported a marked change in educational objectives and provision. The relative emphasis afforded to individualisation and achievement among educational goals contrasts with the collective socialisation and equity goals of the GDR regime. Equally, the structures and differences in provision transferred from the west are evidence once more of a quite different notion of social citizenship: the new structures of provision, the changed relationships between teacher and pupil, the shift in educational objectives, all required an adjustment and adaptation by east German parents and children which, in certain respects, led to disappointment and dissatisfaction with the new provision.

In pre-school education and childcare, there is an excellent example of how the transferred western system was in some respects inferior to the all-embracing provision offered in the GDR. The *Krippe* (crèche) for infants aged up to 3 years, the kindergarten for 3 to 6-year-olds, and the *Hort* which offered after-school childcare for children of working parents, were viewed as signal achievements of GDR social policy. Their objectives were ones of collectivist integration of children into the group, promotion of the emancipation of women, establishment of equality of opportunity between children of different backgrounds at an early age and, of course, transmission of the rudiments of political socialisation. Notwithstanding shortcomings in its model of childcare, the GDR state fully accepted responsibility for providing pre-school childcare, and the vast majority of children and infants took advantage of it. In this, the contrast with FRG practice was pronounced: provision there was much lower, and there was a certain antagonism to the objectives of the *Hort*, since employment roles were more gendered and female labour market participation much lower. At the *Wende*, primary legislation took the form of the October 1990 *Kinder- und Jugendhilfegesetz* (Child and Youth Support Law) which established the western system and essentially continued western practice. Its pedagogical and social emphasis stressed more the concepts of participation and individualisation, as would be expected, but, critically, there was only a legal responsibility for the provision by local authorities of kindergartens, not of *Krippen* or *Horte*. Provision is far lower than under the GDR and, in response to the collapse in the birthrate in the new *Länder* during the early 1990s, there have been widespread closures and redundancies among trained childcare staff. The legal requirement to offer kindergarten places (therefore at the expense of the *Krippen* and *Horte*) has also created distortions in provision. The cost, the limited opening hours, the greater travelling distances, all compare unfavourably with GDR provision and represent a signal loss in the eyes of the regional population, as Rosalind Pritchard demonstrates in her study in Chapter 7 of this volume. Yet, the example of the east has helped impress upon the west the notion that child-rearing and the care of the young are not just an individual matter: they are of importance to the whole of society. If that society wants children for the future, and desires as equal a relationship as possible between men and women, then the rearing of children should not be predominantly at the cost of women's self-fulfilment. Late, but in earnest, the west is beginning to follow the example of the east by increasing its childcare provision and adopting a more positive attitude towards daycare and kindergartens.

The test of a civil society can also be found in its attitudes to foreigners and to the incorporation of immigrants and asylum seekers. The growth in the cultural and ethnic diversity of a society which results is both a gain and a test of the fine mesh of formal rights, of self-expression, of possibilities for association and participation which are contained within the notion of social citizenship. Immigration is an area where legislation and policy since unification has forced some reorientation in attitudes and created dissatisfaction among at least part of the population in the east: it has revealed among part of the eastern population illiberal and rather xenophobic attitudes to foreign immigrants. GDR society was largely homogeneous in terms of its overwhelmingly German population: the SED regime had sealed borders, and migration was not a feature of socialist state policy. Commonly, temporary foreign workers were contract workers (*Vertragsarbeiter*) from COMECON and other socialist countries, brought in to meet manpower shortages. Overall, the population had little experience of the otherness of foreign cultures. The Unification Treaty, however, not only opened the borders to legal migrants, extending work permits to EU citizens, but it imposed on eastern *Länder* the west German commitment to receive asylum seekers. Their numbers were rising rapidly during the early 1990s, and this led to opposition among both west and east Germans alike. For the previous contract workers, a restrictive *Bleiberecht* had been agreed from 1990, which allowed them temporary residence until the expiry of their contracts. The number seeking asylum has fallen markedly since the passing of new legislation in 1993, and the numbers of non-Germans in east German cities remains low, though they are growing rapidly from a small base. As Eva Kolinsky shows in her study in Chapter 8, hostility among the east German population to the presence of foreign workers, while perhaps less overt than in the early years of the decade, continues as east Germans perceive here a threat to their employment, and a challenge to the homogeneity of the east German society. The opportunity for migrants to contribute to their host societies by innovation and cultural diversity remains an essential element in a civil society and this issue will continue to put east German society to the test for some time to come.

Another area to reveal the unacceptable face of the GDR concerns the treatment of dissenters and the human rights abuses perpetrated by the GDR authorities. The GDR government did not subscribe to the rule of law, nor did it guarantee human rights to its citizens and to everyone within its borders. After the use of Stalinist terror in the 1940s to eliminate remaining 'war criminals' and to defeat political opponents in other parties opposed to the leading role of the Socialist Unity Party, the SED continued to operate human rights abuses against its perceived opponents to 1989. Even if the brutality of the methods used by the Stasi secret police in their defence of this young communist state became progressively less severe, nevertheless the psychological torture, denunciation, subversion, imprisonment and loss of livelihood that they enforced remain deeply repugnant and grossly offensive in any civilised society. The Stasi remained to the end the 'sword and shield' of the GDR state and its terror was a prime instrument of state power. In such a system, how can civil society grow, when elementary rights, freedom of association and personal trust, even between intimates, are absent or inadequate? The peace movement in its development through the 1980s, and in its progressively growing emphasis on the necessary link between human rights and peaceful coexistence, came to challenge the SED order directly, by its very insistence that the SED regime hold to the principles of peace and individual rights enshrined in the GDR constitution and constantly reiterated as official doctrine.

Such uneasy opponents were difficult for the SED state to suppress brutally and, as Anthony Glees demonstrates in his contribution in Chapter 9, the SED went to great lengths to subvert the movement and its UK contacts. Among such oppositional groups who sought a peaceful socialism which would live up to its expressed ideals, one can find the origins of a civil society founded in formal rights and free association. However, the limited discussion since unification of the injustices perpetrated by the Stasi, and of their victims' histories and ideals, recalls the 'amnesia' shown by many in west Germany in the decades after the defeat of Nazism. In becoming the new Germany, the regions in the east will have to face up to this history of terror and wrongdoing, perpetrated by the Stasi and its state, and commit themselves to the rights and principles of civil society and social citizenship, as they are enshrined and promised in Germany's democratic constitution and ultimately in all democracies. Peace is not so much the absence of conflict as the presence of justice, and the transformation will only be complete when the evaluation of injustice is complete. Victim testimony is a very important part of the inheritance from the GDR; there was indeed a worthwhile civic tradition in the GDR and this is a resource which deserves to be exploited in the new Germany.

PERSONAL EXPERIENCES AND ATTITUDE CHANGE IN THE EAST SINCE UNIFICATION

The debates over a 'wall in the head', over a 'battle for moral supremacy between two collective identities',[12] the slowness of eastern adjustment to western behavioural patterns, 'anomie' among the population, and concern over the 'lost generation of youngsters'[13] show that there has been no linear convergence or direct transformation in social attitudes with the adoption of the western system. Such debates contain a considerable element of exaggeration but they do point to the fact that, in a multi-dimensional way, eastern attitudes and behaviours are not simply converging on those of the west, but may continue to show specificities for decades to come. Inherited beliefs, values and patterns from the 40 years of state socialism have not been thoroughly transformed, in spite of the political and civil freedoms, the individualism, the economic relationships and social agendas introduced from the west.

The question of how east Germans have coped with mass unemployment and whether they have experienced the psychological transition found in much research is investigated by Vanessa Beck in her contribution in Chapter 13. The psychological transition findings point to a four-phase process ranging from optimism to depression, withdrawal and, finally, apathy. Given the scale of unemployment in the east, the fact that the GDR was a 'work society' which aspired to offer women equality of opportunity in the workplace and society at large, and given that east German women's work motivation remains extremely high, one could expect profound dissatisfaction and despair among the many who have suffered truncated or very disjointed employment histories over the last decade. This might be particularly so in view of the fact that working women can be counted among the losers of the transformation, as the western male breadwinner model became imposed on the east and as the highly developed GDR network of support for working mothers was cut away. The family-based social security system was replaced by a greater individualisation in the new 'risk society' and the nuclear family pattern declined faster in response to the unemployment crisis. In interviews, however, east German women with poor chances of full-time re-employment manifested considerable ability to cope: they did not show the withdrawal and apathy of earlier studies. Rather, they displayed a resilience and determination, a *Durchhalte-Ideologie*, and a high level of activity, maintaining networks and contacts, particularly as a substitute for the lost societal function which working relationships offer. In many ways, this resilience and capacity to cope fitted them excellently to meet the demands of a 'risk society'.

Familial relations can also be expected to have been substantially influenced by unification: the question arises whether mother–child interactions, which had differed between east and west, were now in a process of convergence. The shaping by the unification process of east German parents' educational ideas and their behaviour towards their children, is the subject of Harald Uhlendorff's study in Chapter 11. The changed daily working conditions with greater performance pressure, the loss of prestige attached to certain posts under the old regime, the wider consumer choice and blandishments of the advertisers, the changed relations between teacher and pupils, all affect and strain parent–child relationships. Parents in particular missed the formerly intensive teacher–student group relation and missed alike the societal pressure on educator and school class (*Kollektiv*) to raise the performance of the weaker children. Whereas, in the GDR years, the school took an active role in the sport and hobby activities of children and oversaw the transition later to higher study or training, this has been replaced by much greater individual responsibility on the part of schoolchild and parents. It is now up to them to seek out appropriate clubs and groups. The expense and uncertainty about quality render this a somewhat stressful exercise for eastern parents unused to negotiating through a system with far more possibilities in theory, but financial limitations in practice; fewer fixed rules and channels now, but bewilderment as to the best direction to take. Tensions with children over their demands for expensive, often branded, toys and sports goods raised parents' dissatisfaction over the pervasive materialism of the new system. Uhlendorff's study also demonstrates the counterpoint between the clear moral values characteristic of the GDR and a post-*Wende* tendency to lie in order to save face; a family in his study no longer criticises its son for egotistical behaviour because 'in this society, a sheep can't do anything against wolves: he must be a wolf himself'. Such forms of adaptation to capitalism hold the mirror up to western society in a way that is not particularly flattering.

In her Chapter 10 study of mother–child interactions during the passage from childhood to youth, Beate Schuster compares inter-personal negotiations of eastern and western mother–child pairs playing a cleverly designed game. Earlier studies had pointed to differences in upbringing beliefs between the Old and New *Bundesländer* and those studies were broadly confirmed by the Schuster study. Differences in child-rearing styles are passed down through the generations, in spite of changes common to both parts of Germany. West German parenting had been characterised by greater liberalisation – after all, today's parents emanate from the 1960s generation with its widespread cult of anti-authoritarian education. Liberalisation was both external in the form of the decline of the nuclear family, common to both east and west, but also internal, whereby a greater equality was sought in parent–child relations. Schuster found a substantial degree of commonality in child-rearing styles between east and west German mothers: in both east and west, the children expressed their individuality by demonstrating their competence. Mothers in the New *Bundesländer* dealt more confidently with their role as authority persons, which had the effect of making the children challenge their parents more openly by criticising their attitudes. Contrary to what might have been expected, this did not alienate the east German mothers; rather, they supported this challenging attitude on the part of their children, and were more oriented than their western counterparts towards *explaining* their concepts of educational values in interaction with their children. The east German children were by no means cowed and were not afraid to challenge. Their mothers had more traditional views than western counterparts, whereby they controlled more, inculcated a range of educational values, and attached more importance to duties and obedience. Typical of GDR days was the approach that children had to be 'kept on a tight rein'. Mothers from the Old *Bundesländer*, by contrast, were less secure in their role as authority persons. They had to try to achieve a mutually acceptable solution, and aimed to make their children understanding and cooperative, but sometimes their offspring disregarded the basic rules of the interaction, and used their knowledge of their mothers' insecurities to manipulate them. It is possible, however, that this cooperative, negotiating approach of western mothers may prepare the children effectively to be able to find their way in a western social system with no clear options or guarantees in adult life. These differences seem to indicate the perseveration of a clear-cut values model on the part of the easterners compared with a more agnostic one on the part of the westerners. In the former GDR, the values code associated with Marxism-Leninism was clearly articulated; after the *Wende*, freedom and democracy were introduced into the east, but they were disseminated in a much more diffuse form and there were many conflicting messages within the transformed society. It became more difficult for young people to work out which boundaries to respect, and difficult for their parents to know where to draw those boundaries.

The role of time, with its disciplining effects, its importance in the sequencing and interlocking of activities within the family and in a child's daytime activity can be expected to show modification with the transition to a western model. In the GDR, time as an organising and disciplining force was heavily utilised and taught widely at all levels, sometimes in the form of the Law of the Economy of Time. Children in particular always had a full curriculum and organised free time, such that they suffered 'time shortage'. The use of free time had to be purposeful: unstructured activities such as relaxing or day-dreaming were seen in a very negative light. Dieter Kirchhöfer (Chapter 12), in his contribution on the changed relation to time in children's activities, shows that there have been signal changes since 1990. Owing to the discontinuity of employment and the greater irregularity of working hours, the family organisation of time (family mealtimes, play hours) has lost much of its significance and children's activities through time have become more fragmented, less sequential and less sustained. Children tend to switch more among activities such as computer games, surfing and TV, when in GDR days a hobby activity sustained over several days at a time was more common. These changes are not a direct, linear result of the social transformation but result from the multi-dimensional interplay of several factors.

Sexual violence against women and sexual abuse of children is the focus of Ingrid Hölzler's Chapter 14 study, drawing on her research for the *Land* Saxony-Anhalt. While male violence of this type can be expected to have existed in both parts of Germany historically, nevertheless a case can be made that it could have increased as a result of social transformation, even though the data coverage is wholly insufficient. Such violence can be traced to gender inequality, to the uneven power positions of men and women, to the image of maleness in society and the media, and as a compensation for male inadequacy. In GDR times, such forms of sexual violence were given low levels of recognition by the authorities and researchers alike, primarily because of the ideology of female emancipation and equality of opportunity for women. The argument in favour of the proposition that such violence will have increased since 1990 focuses on the rise in unemployment, the increasing dependency of a woman on her husband, stronger media images of male violence, and a more gendered labour market.

In a united Germany, the Law of 26 January 1998 to combat sexual offences and other dangerous acts of violence amended earlier legislation by placing rape inside marriage as a criminal act on a par with rape generally. Since 1990 the approach of the Saxony-Anhalt authorities to these forms of sexual violence has been to establish refuges for women and their children, and to create help networks, including helplines for children at risk. Although this response has to be assessed against a background of earlier lack of recognition of the problems, nevertheless there remain widespread inadequacies of provision, inadequate staffing and poor coordination among social workers, help agencies and the police. Closer interaction of authorities responsible and in particular greater educational efforts among the population would help redress these often hidden or disguised acts of violence.

This discussion of the social transformation in east Germany over the past decade, the policy agendas and practices pursued in key areas, the personal experiences and responses to these fundamental changes, reveals the complexity of system transfer and system transformation. Even as policy makers and the population in east Germany at large seek to accommodate to the thoroughgoing changes involved in system transfer, so the west German system itself, its economic regulation and its welfare state have been evolving, impelled by globalisation pressures and by the problems inherent in welfare state provision, challenges which all of developed western Europe is having to meet. This dynamic evolution, or dual transformation, reflects in part the impact on the west German economy and polity of the imperatives of accommodating the east, and it certainly sharpens the tensions involved in the problematic normalisation which is occurring in east Germany. The depth of the economic and social restructuring, the mass unemployment and employment uncertainty in the east which have accompanied the transition to the western 'risk society' for the easterners, have involved equally an adjustment to a welfare system which is far less comprehensive than that of the GDR, and which is itself in transition. Advanced western states are having to renegotiate the relations of social provision between state and citizen, relations implicit in the notion of social citizenship. This social citizenship, extended more broadly to include educational goals and educational provision, free association and participation in political parties and trade union activities, the rights of minorities and of immigrants, has been transformed since unification and is in a state of dynamic change as the relations between authorities and individual change in evolving western societies. This question of what sort of civil society is emerging in the east, whether it is distinctively different from that of west Germany and whether it retains attributes from the GDR state socialist period, is investigated in detail here: where is east Germany heading? The contributions in this volume point to much that remains specifically east German in terms of experiences, behaviours and attitudes, as the region continues its problematic normalisation to the western system, and as it adjusts to the risks and opportunities which that poses. There are clearly good as well as less good elements in this distinctiveness.

NOTES

1. M. Thompson, 'Reluctant Revolutionaries: Anti-Fascism and the East German Opposition', in *German Politics*, 8, 1 (1999), pp. 40ff. Also D. Pollack and D. Rink, *Zwischen Verweigerung und Opposition: Politischer Protest in der DDR 1970–1989* (Frankfurt am Main: Campus, 1997).
2. For a detailed discussion see R. Geissler, *Die Sozialstruktur der Bundesrepublik*, 2nd edn (Opladen: Westdeutscher Verlag, 1996); W. Weidenfeld and H. Zimmermann (eds), *Deutschland-Handbuch*. (Munich: Hanser 1989); and I. Ostner *et al.* (eds), *Sozialer Wandel in Ostdeutschland* (Opladen: Leske und Budrich, 1999).
3. W. E. Paterson, 'Between the Bonn and the Berlin Republics', in *Discussion Papers in German Studies*, 99/5 (University of Birmingham: Institute for German Studies, 1999).
4. C. Flockton and E. Kolinsky (eds), *Recasting East Germany: Social Transformation after the GDR* (London: Cass, 1999).
5. For the term 'problematische Normalisierung' see A. Segert and I. Zierke, *Sozialstruktur und*

Milieuerfahrung: Aspekte des alltagskulturellen Wandels in Ostdeutschland (Opladen: Westdeutscher Verlag, 1997), p. 48.

6. U. Beck, *Risikogesellschaft* (Frankfurt am Main: Suhrkamp, 1986) first introduced the concept of a 'two-thirds-society'; manifestations of social exclusion are analysed in W. Hanesch *et al.*, *Armut in Deutschland* (Reinbek: Rowohlt, 1994) and M. M. Zwick (ed.), *Einmal arm, immer arm? Neue Befunde zur Armut in Deutschland* (Frankfurt am Main: Campus, 1994).

7. 'Erst vereint, nun entzweit', *Der Spiegel* (8 January 1993), p. 170; also C. Zelle, 'Socialist Heritage or Current Unemployment: Why do the Evaluations of Democracy and Socialism Differ between East and West Germany?', in *German Politics*, 8, 1 (1999), pp. 1ff.

8. For a detailed discussion see Chapter 5 by Mike Dennis in this volume.

9. G. Esping-Andersen, 'After the Golden Age? Welfare State Dilemmas in a Global Economy', in G. Esping-Andersen (ed.), *Welfare States in Transition* (London: Sage, 1996).

10. Deutsches Institut für Wirtschaft (DIW), 'Vereinigungskosten belasten Sozialversicherung', *Wochenbericht*, 40 (1997).

11. C. Offe, 'German Reunification as a "Natural Experiment"', *German Politics*, 1, 1 (1992), pp. 1–14.

12. L. Ensel, 'Warum wir uns nicht leiden mögen: was Ossis und Wessis voneinander halten' (Münster: Agenda Verlag, 1993), p. 115.

13. A. Hessel *et al.*, 'Psychische Befindlichkeiten in Ost- und Westdeutschland im siebten Jahr nach der Wende', in *Aus Politik und Zeitgeschichte*, B13 (1997).

Part I

The New Germany in Europe

2

Political Transition, Social Transformation and the Welfare Agenda

Steen Mangen

Since the 1970s western European countries have been exposed to the exigencies of deep-seated social and economic transformations which have progressively stimulated a certain convergence of views on future welfare objectives. This has occurred because the pace and irreversibility of change in the economic base, associated with structural de-industrialisation, has exposed the mounting inadequacies of policies devised in the economic 'miracle years' of the 1960s. Reliance on *ad hoc* cost containment measures in the 1970s has given way to a common search for stable strategic reformulations. The resolutions identified incur fundamental renegotiation of the distribution of major responsibilites for action among state institutions, markets and the various manifestations of civil society.[1] It is a framework that involves public agencies in managing a changing balance of regulation and deregulation, economic efficiency and social effectiveness and a review of needs, contingencies and claims on collective provisions.

Policy pressures, then, are uniquely extensive and permeate gender, family and demographic change, new formations of life-cycles, the conjunctural uncertainties of current labour markets which have reinforced insider–outsider effects, and so forth. What we are witnessing is a revision of popular expectations of intimate support over a lifetime. Although it is easy to overstate the case, taking western Europe as a whole, a second phase in the dissolution of familial bonds can be perceived. After the weakening of commitments to the extended family, contemporally there are manifestations of the dissipation of the bonds of the dual parent nuclear family. European trends do vary substantially, but are everywhere associated with secular individualism and changing gender relations, not least with regard to labour market status. (The strength of family bonds diverges internationally on a number of key indicators – extended dependence of young adults on the parental home, the number of elderly persons living with their children, and so on. Divorce rates are also an important indicator: in 1996, after a rapid fall in the early years of unification, the divorce rate in the new *Länder* had once again risen to 21 per cent. In the old FRG (including. east Berlin) it was 35 per cent.) To these trends must be added a loosening of wider social networks which may prove to be a less reliable resource over time. In parallel, too, macro-economic changes have produced across-the-board labour market restructuring to meet the rigours of globalisation or, at least, a 'Europeanisation' of the economy. These processes for Rhodes[2] have advanced what he terms 'subversive liberalism', relegating long-term welfare objectives to the immediate concerns of growth and competition (see also Wilding[3] and Flockton in this volume).

Social transformation is naturally linked to social policy in an intricate mosaic of cause and effect and, since their inception, state welfare provisions have had to accommodate the exigencies imposed by sometimes profound upheavals. However, there is the argument that (at least at the institutional level which itself is an expression of cultural preferences) welfare, as a complex set of sub-systems, tends to respond rather laggardly to new social demands thrown up by transformation.[4] Recent survey evidence, discussed later, suggests that this has particularly acute implications for the development of a unified welfare system in Germany, where west and east had such divergent traditions and, with them, popular expectations.

In order to cast the interaction of social transformation and political transition in the former GDR over a wider arena, comparative reference will primarily be made to the evolution of the Spanish social state in the quarter of a century since the re-establishment of democracy. (Spain has been a reference point for central and eastern European countries seeking means of accelerating democratisation. Greece and Portugal, which had different political trajectories, have proved less of a benchmark. But there are key differences in the experiences of the two European regions. The secularisation effects redolent of southern Europe are absent in the east. Critically, in Spain democratisation can be depicted as 'reform from above' with, initially, a reliance on the political economy of pactism[5] while in the GDR, after the groundswell of bottom-up pressures for democracy, unification imposed a 'reform from outside' involving an externally dictated timetable for its assimilation into mature west German institutions. Nonetheless, there are also important gains deriving from the southern European experiences at the conceptual level, not least in stimulating a re-examination of functionalist approaches to modernisation and transition theories.) It goes without saying that every transition has essential specificity in time and location; but some broad comparisons between southern and eastern European experiences can profitably be drawn. Echoing somewhat the GDR, although with more immediacy, the Spanish Transition had been preceded by 'miracle years' that had come to an abrupt end. Growth, however, had not substantially alleviated the ill effects of uneven development, a trend noted generally in eastern Europe.[6]

Transitional costs in both southern and eastern Europe have been borne by the growing number of excluded workers. High unemployment has been the result, depressing the legitimation of the new political order. The dilemma for Spain, as for other democratising states, has been how to balance the short-term and long-term economic and social policy effects; in brief, whether to grasp the nettle or hope for the best by muddling through. Political elites were well aware of the legitimising value of welfare and employment. On establishing democracy, the rhetoric was to revolve around short-term sacrifice in the interests of economic growth; this would provide a panacea through the ideal of convergence with western European standards of living. It was, in many ways, a rehearsal of the '*Aufschwung Ost*' argument to be put forward 15 years later in the case of the economic convergence of the new *Länder* with the former FRG. However, what transpired in Spain was 'jobless growth, since economic modernisation was achieved by the dismantling of heavily protected labour markets and its replacement by capital intensive production, coexisting with a profusion of low-skills, services-related employment located in 'precarious' labour markets and unemployment rates which have consistently been much higher than the EU average.

Thus, convergence continues to be elusive and a more expensive enterprise than originally envisaged; Spanish per capita GDP stands at the same percentage of the European average as it was at the time of the death of Franco in 1975. The greater inequalities of income distribution and, more generally, the winners and losers in the southern transitions are mirrored in the east. In the former GDR pensioners have been among the winners, with benefit levels in 1996 achieving 82 per cent of those in west Germany. On the other hand, the gross earnings of industrial and commercial workers in 1995 were still 73 per cent of the western equivalent;[7] since then, Berger and colleagues[8] cite evidence of a deceleration in salary convergence. Crucially, eastern registered unemployment in May 1999, at 17 per cent, remained practically double that of the west.

Pre-transition developments can be decisive in moulding path dependencies in the transition process in both the south and east.[9] Lanzaro[10] identifies 'pockets of modernity' – local community groups with social, gender and environmental ambitions – which gradually form more extensive pragmatic alliances with elements in the political establishment. Similar to events in the GDR before the fall of the Wall, modernisation pressures had started in Spain a decade before Franco's death, helping reshape political forces there before being themselves partially absorbed.[11] But many pathways linking the past with the present regime constrained the flourishing of democracy.

Reorganisation within the democratic state – administrative decentralisation and regional devolution, for example, proceeded at a faster pace than the spontaneous evolution of an extensive civil society and its contribution to neo-corporatist welfare arrangements. In any case, institutional renewal was being made at a time of disillusion with the functioning of many sectors of the post-war democratic accommodation and the principal actors it had fostered. In Spain in the initial period of the socialist government there was a deep-seated mistrust of voluntarism. Similar echoes were found in the former GDR where suspicion of collaboration with the former regime together with a lack of preparation for engagement in *Verbändepolitik* (special interest group lobbying) only reinforced their exposure to west German colonisation.[12]

For these sorts of reasons, Castles[13] is right to point out that the social and economic effects of the southern transitions can be perceived over a longer period than the formal completion of the erection of democratic institutions. This is because democratic consolidation requires much broader social engagement and support than the initial phase of regime transition which is typically managed by elites.[14] For McDonough[15] consolidation matures at the point where the expectations of democracy move beyond political liberalisation towards the centrality of notions of social equity. Consolidation effects in the new *Länder* are more complex. Roller[16] examines legimation effects both 'from above' (principally perceived as guaranteed rights under law) and 'below' (derived from the quality of public services). She argues that the role of social policy in the GDR, as a mechanism of ideological competition with the FRG, makes east Germany a special case. The results of her survey show a predominant 'bottom-up' effect: respondents in the east associated the ideal of generous social provisions with democracy more frequently than those in the west. Two-thirds of easterners judged their welfare status to have deteriorated since unification and this was statistically correlated with negative views of (west) German democracy. In contradistinction to the situation analysed by McDonough, Roller judges her data to indicate that pressures for social equity, in the ex-GDR, constrain the consolidation of support for liberal democracy rather than being a manifestation of it.

TRANSFORMATION AND THE REVALUATION OF WELFARE

About 25 years ago, critical evolving events set the tone for a comprehensive reassessment of what had largely been a functionalist analysis of the mass state welfare, whatever its formation in western Europe. From different interpretations, both liberal and neo-Marxist analysis elaborated a legitimation crisis in terms of welfare's fiscal demands which acted as a drag on capitalist accumulation. A collective social system that had been appraised as an investment in human capital lubricating the economic miracle years of the 1960s collided with the twin pressures of the oil crises, which were a defining break and, secondly, the longer-term evolution of increasing claims arising from maturity and enhanced coverage. The result was heavier financial burdens threatening European competitiveness and accelerating de-industrialisation. In summary, as evidenced in the 'Standort Deutschland' argument, a high cost welfare system contained inbuilt and strong pressures for continued expansion and stymied innovation and modernisation. Moreover, the sustainability of what was a heavily regulated system was placed in question. Thus, the changing economy and associated political values required a renegotiation of the contract which existed between the individual and the state.

Welfare services, then, were increasingly seen as out of kilter with rapid social and demographic transformations which required a review of implicit gender and generational contracts. There were also specific critiques about heavy bureaucracy that had lost its capacity to plan over space, time and speciality; uniform, massified services which had no mechanisms of responding to the highly differentiated needs associated with social fragmentation; a lack of consumer involvement; and the fostering of passivity and welfare dependency.[17] To these concerns were added worries about the ecological dimensions of welfare investment expressed from the early 1980s by Scandinavian and west German Greens which were to have a progressive impact on the way mainstream parties approached policy.

Thus, a view gaining widespread currency was that the welfare state constructed in the Fordist era was exacting its nemesis, manifest in its contradictions on all fronts. Sluggish economic performance contributed to new and chronic social and spatial cleavages, the flourishing of an unregulated, submerged economy, and tax resistance and evasion.[18] Esping-Andersen[19] locates the contemporary discourse in arguments about the continued relevance of the varying European post-war notions of egalitarianism: was the pursuit of equality through extending social citizenship compatible with the intensifying demands of economic efficiency and employment generation? Reporting on the Spanish situation, O'Donnell[20] records that greater equality of provision has not necessarily been conducive to promoting greater levels of citizen participation, but rather has run the risk of passivity, dependency and institutionalised clientelism, all of which exhibit strong spatial dimensions – the so-called 'Mezzogiorno effect'. The product is intensifying inter-regional resentments among more prosperous areas and a lower collective self-esteem in recipient areas: this *Geringschätzung* has, for example, been reported in the case of the former GDR.[21] At issue, then, was the traditional function of social policy as an adaptive engine for system integration, building political consensus, social stability and popular trust in the state.[22]

Of course, analyses defending the welfare state were not unforthcoming. Espousing the benefits of social democratic neo-corporatism, Mishra,[23] for example, alluded to the partial explanations of antagonistic macro-critiques for their signal underestimation of the dynamic flexibility of capitalist production to respond to new social and political pressures. Gradually the focus on 'crisis', typical of the 1970s and early 1980s, gave way to a more speculative and longer-term evaluation of 'transformation'. And, although the New Right had been indicted for failing to formulate a consistent theory for an alternative to welfare,[24] parties of that persuasion incidentally assisted the transformation process by infusing elements of privatisation and a range of process efficiency techniques collectively known as 'new public management'.

Part of the reinvigoration of theoretical effort lay in the gradual reconstruction of the European centre-left in the major northern EU states along 'modernising' revisionist lines, arguably mirroring the agenda pursued after 1979 by the Spanish socialists.[25] Contextual support for a reformed but extensive welfare system received considerable impetus during the Delors presidency of the European Commission during which agreement was progressively achieved on the need to retain the welfare *acquis* as a social asset quintessential for the goal of a European leading edge economy, despite the fact that no formula for its funding was devised. Part of the revisionism was pragmatic and deeply expropriatory: self-help, beloved of Kohl and Thatcher, in a growing number of countries has been transmuted into a hand-up, 'stakeholder' society. Responses to post-Fordist pressures on welfare states have sought to supplement collectively subsidised individual risk-taking with policy options for coping with contingencies that are close to centre-right preferences for private sector solutions. In its turn, a discernible outcome in many countries in the late 1990s, as addressed by Ilona Ostner in this volume, is the enforced response of the centre-right which represents a new welfare consensus revolving around a three-tier social protection model integrating state, occupational and private indemnity.

The scene was set for a renewed intellectual and political effort addressing the matter of how to adapt the traditional positive functions of social policy – as collective investments in time, space and social groups – to meet both the constraints and opportunities of contemporary economies: in short, how a modernised welfare policy could assist new accumulation processes. Authors like Vobruba[26] approached afresh the long-held defence of social security – its functions in promoting risk-taking, labour market mobility and flexibility, social adaptation and stability and the maintenance of the consumption function, and so forth. His conclusion is that democratic and social transformations are highly reliant on social policy which offsets transitional costs of the minority without threatening newly acquired rights of the majority. This fresh analytical approach took as a given that continued political legitimacy required a renegotiation of the principles of solidarity and equity based on the evolving 'new citizenship', outlined below. This involves a critical analysis of how state institutions have determined an individual's risk profile[27] and how in the future states could arrive at popularly acceptable means of supervising the management of emerging and highly differential risks, as well as accumulated claims, over a now much more unpredictable life cycle.[28]

Accordingly, Vobruba elaborates a political economy of time, speculating on widened temporal horizons which offer mechanisms to assuage the uncertainties and threats of change and which, therefore, permit rational actors to be prepared to defer any benefits of economic and social transformation that might accrue. In a later essay, he extends his ideas on the political management of time by challenging the idea that, in the wake of pressures of a globalising economy, less state welfare would render more economic prosperity, faced as western states are with highly mobile capital fleeing from regulation. Vobruba and Mabbett and Bolderson[29] are critical of the underlying convergence assumptions of globalisation theory which tend to minimise cross-national differences. Instead, Vobruba insists that globalisation must be contextualised: although he concedes that its effects inevitably impact on labour market expenditures, the major impulses for social expenditure derive from domestic pressures on health care and pensions. In this environment there are positive opportunities offered by a robust social policy, not least in offering differentiated compensatory support to guarantee the compliance of both short-term and longer-term losers in the process.[30]

WELFARE INCORPORATION AND 'NEW' SOCIAL CITIZENSHIP

The accumulation of policy reform and profound social transformations which have created highly differentiated social structures are fundamentally reshaping our understanding of solidarity, reciprocity and dependency. The effect is to render problematic consensual welfare settlements on trade-offs between equality, equity and efficiency. The growing divergence of interests between winners and losers in the east German transformation is a case in point.

The reaction to perverse effects of welfarism has stimulated a stable of current policies designed to engender a new sense of social citizenship which prioritises the active, the consumerist and the entrepreneurial. What is being inculcated is a greater sense of personal liability for managing and anticipating contingencies over lifespan: in short, a new sense of rights, responsibilities and loyalties among citizens and between citizens and the state which *inter alia* have vital gender, generation, labour market, ethnic and spatial dimensions. But whatever the dimension it is personal initiative and adaptability that are prized. In significant ways this policy line is being pursued as an antidote to the relaxation since the 1980s of concern with what Germans term 'social symmetry'. There is an argument that this has been replaced by a new moral economy of self-satisfaction on the part of those in the labour market core who have voted for lower taxation, support greater inequality and tolerate 'two-tier' welfare rights.[31]

The crucial benchmark of this new citizenship is social incorporation or, more euphemistically, 'inclusion' and, essentially, this is measured in terms of labour market participation. Levitas[32] warns us of the underlying conservatism behind this reformulation. The voguish currency of 'social exclusion' should not blind us to the fact that it entails largely top-down, state-directed attempts to manage risk by dictating an agenda which is naive to the functions of the social periphery for the capitalist core and, moreover, obscures the deep inequalities and exclusions that parts of the labour market perpetuate.

In response to emerging policy exigencies, some governments are redoubling efforts at redesigning welfare delivery systems through new forms of private and third sector engagement, mainstreaming as well as embracing more explicit developmental and, in some states, environmental agendas. In terms of social protection there are attempts to reconcile principles of equity and transparency with measures revising universalism and more refined targeting. The anchoring of Bismarckian social insurance in the contributory principle has been dented by these innovations and by the institionalisation of partial fiscalisation after *ad hoc* state subsidies in the 1970s and 1980s. How compatible new policy lines will be is one of the themes taken up by Ilona Ostner. All carry risks: greater targeting, for example, may threaten social efficiency if middle class detachment from welfare entitlements to which they previously had access reduces their political support for extensive social policies and may well not avoid process inefficiencies if poverty traps cannot be eradicated.[33]

What follows is a brief analysis of interventions to enhance the possibilities of social incorporation in certain key inter-related areas, together with an assessment of present risks and the outstanding task.

INCORPORATION AND COMMUNITY

Building on the positive impacts from the late 1960s onwards of the spontaneous evolution of new issue-driven associationism, the local community, prized for harbouring informal supportive networks, has been invested as a principal means forward for engendering civic engagement in the exploitation of social capital. It has almost become an article of faith that the extensive immanence of civil society and its exploitable asset of social capital is critical for the resolution of socio-economic problems at the local level and, moreover, aids new forms of accumulation. Indeed, the varying level of associationism has been taken as a cross-national indication of modernity.[34] Although such indicators are not unproblematic, on most standards Spain, in common with other southern countries, has a relatively low rate. (Wessels[35] presents persuasive data that there is an intimate link between the pervasiveness of social capital and modernity. He is critical of the contention that an erosion of social capital is associated with 'modernising' secular individualism. Using World Value Surveys of 1990/91 he calculates that in Spain only 18 per cent of respondents claimed membership of informal groups compared to about 55 per cent in west Germany, and as many as 80 per cent in Sweden and in the Netherlands. Wessels concludes that the longer states had afforded citizens the experience of guaranteed democratic participation pathways, the more productive this is of associationism.) Yet no account of the Spanish transition would be complete without an analysis of the impact of these new social movements.[36] Therein lies a caution: for greater reliance on a social capital strategy is not universally without risks. As discussed earlier, the Spanish case demonstrates the volatility of informal resources and how they can be subverted. Many of these movements were soon colonised by the newly established political parties, particularly the socialists, and were either marginalised or formally incorporated into the political process. Similar observations have been made of the social movements arising in the last throes of the GDR and, more recently, of smaller associations in west Germany. (In the former Federal Republic the number of self-help groups rose from 25,000 in 1985 to 60,000 in 1995. Kettler and von Ferber[37] record that there is a strong pressure for their incorporation by the established voluntary organisations.)

There is evidence that these 'bottom-up' tactics may not displace expectations of the state in certain electorates' minds. Kaase and Bauer-Kaase[38] identify a constraining effect delaying more 'contemporary' expectations in developmental relations between citizens and state: their survey indicated that respondents in the new *Länder* were more sceptical of the positive benefits accruing from greater reliance on informal supports and the deeper social inequality it implied and sought state-led socio–economic planning solutions, indicating a considerable east–west German cleft. Similar attitudes have been expressed in Spain.[39]

INCORPORATION AND THE GENDER CONTRACT

Despite considerable policy effort, the full incorporation of women in European welfare systems remains problematic on three critical, inter-connected counts: recognition of family responsibilities; participation in labour markets; and the reconciliation of social and fiscal welfare. Assumptions about reproduction roles in traditional family structures and growing demands for female participation in the diversified production processes reinforce women's continued occupation of the social periphery.

The greater differentiation of roles fulfilled by women has been played out against the background of a proliferation of recognised household forms, not only in the growth of lone parenthood which is, in part, associated with the decreasing value of long-term partnership with males who have poor prospects of labour market inclusion, but also with the small but growing number of countries (including Spain) that are making statutory revisions to accommodate same-sex partnerships which provide each partner with access to the other's welfare entitlements.

The implications of full female incorporation were raised during the first phase of 'second wave' feminism from the late 1960s onwards which witnessed reforms of fertility control and marital dissolution, elements of which are not uncontroversial, as events in Spain and unified Germany with regard to abortion testify. In fact, family policy remains one of the principal areas of social policy in which there is a considerable divergence of priority among EU states, rendering an effective EU-level policy problematic. Fundamentally, the issue revolves around the full contribution of female labour in the economy, much of which is unpaid and which is imposing increasingly contradictory demands, given the larger numbers of women who have obtained formal employment. The outcome is felt in low fertility rates, which in the EU by 1996 amounted to only 1.44 children per woman, and are a direct source of the pensions crisis (see later). Both Spain and the new *Länder* have experienced an even more intense plummeting of rates since their transitions, falling to 1.15 and 0.95 respectively.

Formal policy responses so far have been modest – child-rearing leave, 'baby year' pension credits, and so forth, introduced in Scandinavia, Germany and elsewhere. On the other hand, international evidence is scarcely reassuring that we have substantially arrived at a reconciliation of domestic and employment duties through a greater sharing of responsibilities in the home.[40] Survey evidence is strongly suggestive that this was also the case in the former GDR, where women were highly integrated into labour markets.[41] Until the problem of unpaid work is resolved more effectively, social protection systems will be deficient in the face of women's specific attachments to labour markets and the way social entitlement accrues through employment in those markets. Since it appears that European men, even in liberal Scandinavia, cannot, or care not to, do a fair share in the home and that women are increasingly contributing to household income, the principle of equal citizenship and incorporation would demand serious consideration of a comprehensive valuation of home duties in determining the value of welfare benefits.

Until there is some action in this regard the argument that female labour market participation imposes a double burden on women is incontrovertible. The gradual erosion of the concept of the 'family wage' has more or less dragooned women into employment, irrespective of volition. There is a perfectly valid argument expressed in the social catholic concept of '*neue Mütterlichkeit*' ('new motherhood') arguing that current developments have undermined the institution of marriage or life-long partnership by exacting too heavy an economic and psychological price, including, at least by implication, a devaluation of full-time motherhood. Moreover, those who entertain reservations about formal employment can point to intransigent occupational segmentation, marginalisation through over-representation in part-time and short-term contracts and, despite EU and national legislative provisions, the less favourable profile of women's salaries when compared to those of men in comparable employment.

This situation in Germany is reinforced by the continued lower female participation in tertiary education. One-third of female employees in Spain work part-time, a similar proportion for Germany. In relation to men, women's representation in higher education in Germany in 1993/94 was only 73 per cent, while in Spain it was 104 per cent. The EU average was 99 per cent.[42] However, there is also evidence that educational attainment is not sufficient to eradicate wage differentials.[43] German data, in respect of the gross annual income of full-time workers in industry and commerce, demonstrate that, in 1995, western women earned 67 per cent of the male level, and in the east 76 per cent.[44]

There is, then, an outstanding task in reconciling social, fiscal and labour market policies for alignment with an acceleration in the transformation of gender roles. Peripheralisation of women in social security systems consigns many to means-tested, discretionary 'assistential' benefits which in no small measure contributes to the feminisation of poverty. In many cases tax systems provide a strong disincentive for married women to engage in full-time work. This has classically been the outcome of (west) German 'tax splitting' provisions in situations where the wife would earn substantially less than the husband. In these typical cases, it is highly advantageous to exploit the possibility of dividing the tax liability of the usually higher earning husband between the spouses.[45] Nor have more recent innovations in individual taxation necessarily eradicated these constraints: in Spain, for example, joint assessment is normally still advantageous.[46]

INCORPORATION AND THE GENERATION CONTRACT

Although by no means immune to the effects of economic transformation, pension schemes have been among the most protected from budgetary retrenchment. The major concessions to pensioners as represented in the Spanish Toledo Pact of 1995, the granting of a social supplement to east German pensioners during the Transition and the continuing delay in long-term reform of the all-German PAYGO pensions formula attest to the political influence of the grey vote in deferring unpopular funding decisions. The outcome is that today's recipients are cushioned at the cost of tomorrow's. In the face of policy accretion, the conventional argument originating in the late 1970s is that, if left unabated, deteriorating fiscal burdens will stretch into the middle of the new century. The generation contract implied in pensions policy is, in many ways, the most explicit in relation to reciprocity – expressed via the 'dependency'-ratio. That this has become a source of major concern about equity is to do with demography: in fact, over 60 years ago, German social catholic theorists such as Nell Breuning insisted that the generation contract – trust and cooperation over time – could only be sustained through the maintenance of cohorts of broadly equal size, something that is now not in prospect for several generations.

UN projections of dependency ratios to 2025, based on 1984 data, do indicate that German unification moderately eased the adverse demographic profile, although the subsequent fall in the eastern birth rate represented a deterioration. Recent OECD simulations of pension expenditure for all Germany are strongly suggestive that, *ceteris paribus*, outlays would have to more or less double by 2040 to maintain real value. In addition, as spending on those over 80 years old would rise as a result of their need for heavier health and social services investment, sharply increased social protection funding via debt is in serious prospect. The problems vary internationally. On the whole, EU countries heavily reliant on the PAYGO system as opposed to capitalisation are most disadvantaged; although Germany is outpaced by Italy, which is particularly exposed.[47]

This sort of analysis, typical of the 'demo-crisis' literature from the late 1970s onwards, has progressively given way to more measured analysis of demographic and social transformations which stress the varying prognoses of EU states, and attempt evaluation of potential solutions through, for example, curbing early retirement, raising pension ages and female activity rates, and so on.[48] Nonetheless, many future options do imply that without much higher levies a reduction in the quality of entitlements in the state system over the long run is in prospect. New models of incorporation through income maintenance in old age are therefore being formulated and revolve around a three-tier schema embracing state, compulsory occupational and private voluntary schemes, the latter two principally funded via capitalisation. Currently, there is marked variation in capitalised funds, which are most significant in the United Kingdom and the Netherlands where they represent about 90 per cent of GDP, compared to a mere 5 per cent in Germany. But the single European market, with the deregulation of the private pension market, and the introduction of the Euro are critical events, permitting pension funds to cover liabilities anywhere in the EU and, thereby, stimulating a massive change in asset allocation. ·

That such models, while helping to guarantee adequate social protection for increasing numbers, will impose at least middle-term transitional costs in terms of exacerbating inequities of treatment is undeniable. Pensioners have never formed a homogeneous population in terms of their incorporation into statutory schemes. Reforms enacted in the past quarter of a century have only partly alleviated inequities and, in some ways, have institutionalised a cleavage which is strongly gendered. Early retirement strategies, which were much favoured in the earlier phase of economic transformation in Germany no less than elsewhere in continental systems, have been a critical indicator of such inequality. For the privileged, largely male core worker, it has been an attractive means of exiting from the labour market, but for the less favoured, including many of those on average incomes, it has led to an imposed impoverishment in relation to their original expectations. (A German survey shows that early retirement at 60 years of age, if it incurred a reduction in pension entitlement of 10 per cent, would be tolerated by only 13 per cent of respondents, although almost 70 per cent were willing to forgo a slight reduction in lifetime earnings to offset costs.)[49] Nor did one of the justifications of such schemes – the releasing of jobs for younger workers – largely transpire since employers' immediate interests in the project lay in job shedding, a prime example being that of Spain where high rates of early retirement in the 1980s and 1990s coexisted with high rates of youth unemployment. Some other contemporary innovations such as the universalisation of non-contributory pensions, although extending benefits to groups without entitlement, could have a negative long-term impact in deepening social divisions of welfare. These would be most acutely felt along contributory-assistential cleavages, especially if women remain tangentially incorporated or high rates of long-term unemployment persist, without imaginative means of flexibilising the way in which contribution records can be calculated.

INCORPORATION, SOCIAL EXCLUSION AND THE LABOUR MARKET

A primary driving force of post-war European welfare states was the incorporation of the 'core' working class while retaining the support of the middle classes. This legitimising and integrative function of the welfare state has been increasingly challenged through a multi-dimensional phenomenon now termed 'social exclusion': a fourfold marginalisation of diverse groups in society through deficits of civic, economic, social and inter-personal integration[50] as a result of global economic change, the failure of state bureaucracy and cultural changes.

Central to comprehension of these processes are new regulatory functions of the state and civil society which interact with markets to delimit the boundaries of social exclusion. Paugam[51] sees this multivariate manifestation of deprivation as something new, distinct from older 'traditional' forms of poverty. Its impact is a form of moral and social detachment – 'disqualification' as Paugam terms it – which provokes a double fragility in terms of distributional and relational vulnerability.[52] Recent German analyses have reinvested effort in the 1920s concept of *Lebenslagen* (how a person's biography reveals structural patterns which determine their fluctuating adhesion to the labour market).[53]

All evidence points to the relative permanence of both social and spatial core-periphery effects. As stated earlier, economic growth has proved a dubious exit route for marginalised populations. Spain has enjoyed above-average growth rates in the last 20 years, but has consistently recorded one of the highest rates of poverty in Europe, one which evidences a noticeable concentration in fewer households. By 1996, 15 per cent of households with an adult of working age contained no employed person.[54] The impact of short-term and part-time work on the former GDR labour market is such that the proportion of households in which only the woman is working is more than double that of the former Federal Republic.[55] Predictably, 'non-German' households are most disadvantaged: the relevant poverty rate in west Germany in 1995, at nearly 23 per cent, being more than twice the rate for the host population.[56]

These manifestations are, in large measure, general to western Europe, especially with regard to the increasing tendency for the poorest to oscillate between unemployment benefit and various forms of minimum social income.[57] European economic transformation costs have been expropriated from those exposed to the increasing labour market marginalisation of women and ethnic minorities, as evidenced in higher rates of unemployment. Trends in youth unemployment are more varied, although much of the economic activity for this group derives from the panoply of training and placement schemes. Thus, in 1997, youth unemployment rates in Spain were almost 40 per cent and those for women were 28 per cent at a time when the general rate was 20 per cent.[58] Disaggregated data for the new *Länder* show that women's unemployment rates are higher than the general rate in all the five states, though the youth rate is below the average. Baldwin Edwards[59] notes that in most countries the ethnic minority unemployment rate is between two and three times that of the host population. In 1995, foreigners' unemployment was almost double that of west Germans, although in the former GDR it amounted to only 1 per cent.[60] The effect is to restrict female labour mobility (as discussed earlier) but there is also an under-investment in the socialisation of youth, at least in southern Europe where there is a growing dependence on the parental home which extends well into their twenties. Critically, such reliance on the family is an essential prop for the welfare state and a source of social stability: a 1980s study cited in Programa 2000[61] shows that, at 26 years of age, less than a half of males and about two-thirds of females are economically independent and, as already stated, high proportions continue to live at home. On the other hand, in the new *Länder* the percentage of ageing 'Nesthocker' (young adults reluctant to leave home) is lower than in the west, due in part to more youthful age at family formation.[62]

Labour market instruments have been the major – sometimes the sole – mechanism adopted for combating social exclusion. But the question remains as to whether the labour market can continue to be the mainstay for the transmission of welfare rights, given the exclusion of large numbers from its core. Nonetheless, 'employability' has gained common currency, principally through supply-side measures. This implies a continuing personal commitment to investment in human capital. Despite the agreement achieved in the Employment Chapter of the Amsterdam Treaty, there persists a disagreement between those European political actors arguing for the focus of investment in the 'leading edge' of European labour markets and those arguing the moral value of any sort of job. These viewpoints, which revolve around tactical and strategic employment decisions, have immediate implications for the accumulation of welfare rights. Precarious jobs may solve some short-term problems, but if the employment conditions they offer are below the threshold for social insurance they can store up problems for future entitlements, compromising the very form of personal entrepreneurial investment in life that is advocated. Part-time and temporary work can therefore be a mixed blessing, reinforcing insider–outsider effects without affording avenues for upward mobility[63] or, where state regulation is imposed, failing to create much additional net employment.[64]

Both flexibility and (re-)training are not without risk. At the end of the day, it is the quality of local vacancies that determines status in the labour market: a retrained middle-aged worker in a deprived area has not necessarily improved employment chances. One person's opportunity provided by flexibility might for another potentially threaten long-term precariousness. In both cases rational survival choices might involve entry into the unregulated 'submerged' economy or resort to *pluriempleo*. Survey evidence quoted by Springer[65] estimates that the submerged economy could account for as much as 10 per cent of employment opportunities in the Mediterranean EU states. Recent data for Germany suggest a rapid growth, amounting to 15 per cent of GDP.[66] These forms of flexibility, evolving outside the umbrella of social insurance, only serve to reduce its continuing fiscal feasibility.[67] Even within the regulated sector, Timmins[68] questions whether this new contractarianism has necessarily low current cost implications. For example, workfare in the United States, which embodies a long-term commitment on the part of public authorities, is expensive to operate and could require sustained high levels of public funding, since there is a moral commitment to permanent engagement with the world of work, rather than the temporary contact typical of most European measures.

TRANSFORMATION AND WELFARE STATE INSTITUTIONS: TOWARDS FLEXIBLE INTEGRATION?

The discussion so far suggests an ongoing need for accommodation at the institutional level to the effects of social transformation. As Ilona Ostner demonstrates in Chapter 3, there has been renewed interest in institutional processes and how they act, constrain or could be exploited so as to assist flexible systemic adjustment in the interests of social incorporation.

Mann[69] has investigated how welfare regimes regulate different levels of social integration. Regulatory pressures for conservation are strong. Sweden offers a prime example: despite some inroads into its model, the coalition of neo-corporatist institutional interests among suppliers and recipients makes it difficult to generate majorities for comprehensive reform.[70] There are familiar echoes here with recriminations over policy immobilism inherent in the German federal model. It is, then, the essentially national confine of welfare systems that is a critical constraint, one which is increasingly challenged by high rates of international mobility in a globalising economy that produces growing numbers of people with varying marginal statuses.[71]

The issue of how states and forms of citizenship interact has been expanded by Halfmann.[72] Traditionally, the state has conferred rights of institutional inclusion through full citizenship. Modernisation has been associated with a range of state-mediated inclusion mechanisms at the level of sub-systems such as welfare, giving rise to what Hammar[73] terms a large population of 'denizens' who obtain certain welfare rights, and obligations, principally through labour market participation while being denied full state protection and political participation. EU states now contain a highly differentiated 'denizenship': EU citizens, third country nationals and growing numbers of asylum seekers and refugees. Pressures of social transformation oriented to a Europeanisation of rights will demand that the denizen problem be resolved – an issue long resisted at EU level in the case of third-country nationals – if effective incorporation is to be extended to these ever larger groups occupying the social periphery.

This study, then, has sought to examine the interactions among social transformations, political transition and the changing recent conceptions of the role of the welfare state, within a wider arena. It is clear that both the example of the Spanish Transition and the recent evolution in western Europe have considerable relevance in any study of transformation in eastern Germany. In the GDR, social policy was used explicitly to legitimise the SED regime and this preference among the eastern population for an advanced and encompassing state-supported welfare provision remains quite marked. In social provision and the reform debates, west Germany and the new *Länder* have experienced divergent traditions, with a resultant division in popular expectations. East Germans perceive democracy and generous social provision to be closely linked: therefore the perceived attack on social equity associated with the rigours of market transition has constrained easterners' support for a liberal democratic order. The divergence of fortunes between winners and losers in the transformation has weakened faith in democracy.

The much discussed 'crisis' of the welfare state in Germany, which constitutes a significant element in the 'Standort Deutschland' discussion (of excessive production costs there) has, as elsewhere, led to a succession of reform plans from the Kohl government and recently from the Red–Green coalition of Chancellor Schröder. Although little more than timid incremental reforms have so far been introduced, nevertheless proposals within Germany follow the broad principles set out above: these prioritise social incorporation via the labour market and seek a three-tier protection model (including occupational and private indemnity certainly for pensions, in addition to compulsory social insurance schemes). In east

Germany, the precariousness of employment status of a very significant proportion of the working population and, in particular, of females and the older male worker poses particular dangers under any new welfare order, where labour market participation is a source of rights and entitlements. The precariousness, marginalisation and the fact that so many are employed on subsidised job-creation programmes make labour market participation an unsound basis for the reform of welfare provision.

NOTES

1. P. Abrahamson, 'Welfare Pluralism: Towards a new Consensus for European Social Policy', in L. Hantrais, M. O'Brien and S. Mangen (eds), 'The Mixed Economy of Welfare', *Cross-National Research Papers*, 2nd Series (1992), pp. 5–22.
2. M. Rhodes, '"Subversive Liberalism": Market Integration, Globalisation and the European Welfare State', *Journal of European Public Policy*, 2 (1995), pp. 384–406.
3. P. Wilding, 'Globalization, Regionalism and Social Policy', *Social Policy & Administration*, Vol. 31, 4 (1997), pp. 410–28.
4. S. Bislev, 'European Welfare States: Mechanisms of Convergence and Divergence', *European University Institute Working Papers, Robert Schumann Centre*, No. 97/24 (1997).
5. J-M. Maravall, 'Politics and Policy: Economic Reforms in Southern Europe', in L. Bresser Pereira, J-M. Maravall and A. Przeworksi (eds), *Economic Reforms in New Democracies: A Social-Democratic Approach* (Cambridge: Cambridge University Press, 1993).
6. A. Smith and J. Pickles, 'Introduction: Theorising Transition and the Political Economy of Transformation', in J. Pickles and A. Smith (eds), *Theorising Transition: The Political Economy of Post-Communist Transformations* (London: Routledge, 1998); J-M. Maravall, 'Politics and Policy: Economic Reforms in Southern Europe', in L. Bresser Pereira, J-M. Maravall and A. Przeworksi (eds), *Economic Reforms in New Democracies: A Social-Democratic Approach* (Cambridge: Cambridge University Press, 1993).
7. Statistisches Bundesamt, *Datenreport: Zahlen und Fakten über die Bundesrepublik Deutschland* (Bonn, 1997).
8. H. Berger, W. Hinrich, E. Priller and A. Schultz, *Privathaushalte im Vereinigungsprozess – Ihre soziale Lage in Ost und Westdeutschland* (Frankfurt: Campus, 1999).
9. G. Pridham, 'Political Actors, Linkages and Interactions: Democratic Consolidation in Southern Europe', *West European Politics*, Vol. 13 (1990), pp. 103–17; A. Smith and J. Pickles, 'Introduction: Theorising Transition and the Political Economy of Transformation', in J. Pickles and A. Smith (eds), *Theorising Transition: The Political Economy of Post-Communist Transformations* (London: Routledge, 1998).
10. J. Lanzaro, 'Transition in Transition: Parties, State and Politics in Uruguay, 1985–1993', *Working Paper* No. 90, Institut de Ciencès Politiques i Socials, Barcelona (1994).
11. G. Pridham, 'Political Actors, Linkages and Interactions: Democratic Consolidation in Southern Europe', *West European Politics*, Vol. 13 (1990), pp. 103–17.
12. S. Mangen, 'German Welfare and Social Citizenship', in G. Smith, W. Paterson and S. Padgett (eds), *Developments in German Politics: 2* (Basingstoke: Macmillan, 1996).
13. F. Castles, 'Social Security in Southern Europe: A Comparative Overview', *Australian National University Public Policy Programme Discussion Papers*, No. 33 (1993).
14. G. Pridham, 'Political Actors, Linkages and Interactions: Democratic Consolidation in Southern Europe', *West European Politics*, Vol. 13 (1990), pp. 103–17.
15. P. McDonough, S. Barbes and A. Lopez Pina, 'The Growth of Democratic Legitimacy in Spain', *American Political Science Review*, 80 (1986), pp. 735–60.

16. E. Roller, 'Sozialpolitik und demokratische Konsolidierung – eine empirische Analyse für die neuen Bundesländer', in F. Plasser, O. Gabriel, J. Falter and P. Ulram (eds), *Wahlen und Politische Einstellung in Deutschland und Österreich* (Frankfurt: Peter Lang, 1999).

17. P. Rosanvallon, 'Beyond the Welfare State', *Politics & Society*, 18 (1988), pp. 533–43; P. Rosanvallon, *La Nouvelle Question Sociale: Repenser l'Etat Providence* (Paris: Seuil, 1995); A. de Swaan, 'A Perspective for Transnational Social Policy', *Government and Opposition*, 27 (1992), pp. 33–51.

18. OECD, 'New Orientations for Social Policy', *Social Policy Studies*, No. 12 (Paris: OECD, 1994).

19. G. Esping-Andersen, 'After the Golden Age? Welfare State Dilemmas in a Global Economy', in G. Esping-Andersen (ed.), *Welfare States in Transition* (London: Sage, 1996).

20. G. O'Donnell and P. Schmitter, *Transitions from Authoritarian Rule: Tentative Conclusions about Uncertain Democracies* (Baltimore: Johns Hopkins University Press, 1986).

21. M. Kaase and P. Bauer-Kaase, 'German Unification 1990–1997: The Long, Long Road', *Estudios/Working Papers*, No. 1998/119, Instituto Juan March, Madrid (1998).

22. J. Alber, 'Is there a Crisis in the Welfare State?', *European Sociological Review*, Vol. 4 (1988), pp. 181–207.

23. R. Mishra, *The Welfare State in Crisis: Social Thought and Social Change* (Brighton: Wheatsheaf Books, 1984).

24. C. Offe, 'Some Contradictions of the Modern Welfare State', *Critical Social Policy*, 2 (1982), pp. 7–16.

25. S. Mangen, 'The Welfare State and the Spanish Socialists', *Social Policy Review*, 9 (1997), pp. 337–58.

26. G. Vobruba, *Politik mit dem Wohlfahrtsstaat* (Frankfurt: Suhrkamp, 1983); G. Vobruba, *Jenseits der sozialen Fragen* (Frankfurt: Suhrkamp, 1991).

27. Y. Kazepov, 'Citizenship and Poverty: The Role of Institutions in the Structuring of Social Exclusion', *Working Papers*, No. 98/1, European University Institute, Florence (1998).

28. U. Beck, *Politik in der Risikogesellschaft: Essays und Analysen* (Frankfurt: Suhrkamp, 1991); G. Esping-Andersen, 'After the Golden Age? Welfare State Dilemmas in a Global Economy', in G. Esping-Andersen (ed.), *Welfare States in Transition* (London: Sage, 1996).

29. G. Vobruba, *Jenseits der sozialen Fragen* (Frankfurt: Suhrkamp, 1991); D. Mabbett and H. Bolderson, 'Theories and Methods in Comparative Social Policy', in J. Clasen (ed.), *Comparative Social Policy* (Oxford: Blackwell, 1999).

30. G. Vobruba, 'Das Globalisierungsdilemma: Analyse und Lösungsmöglichkeit', in D. Messner and G. Vobruba, 'Die sozialen Dimensionen der Globalisierung', *Working Paper*, No. 28, Institut für Entwicklung und Frieden, Duisburg (1998).

31. K. Galbraith, *The Culture of Contentment* (Harmondsworth: Penguin, 1993).

32. R. Levitas, 'The Concept of Social Exclusion and the New Durkheimian Hegemony', *Critical Social Policy*, 16, 1 (1997), pp. 5–20.

33. G. Esping-Andersen, 'Positive-Sum Solutions in a World of Trade-offs', in G. Esping-Andersen (ed.), *Welfare States in Transition* (London: Sage, 1996).

34. D. Messner, 'Stärkung internationaler Wettbewerbsfähigkeit und die soziale Dimension von Entwicklung? Wirkungszusammenhänge und Spannungsfelder aus entwicklungspolitischer Perspektive', in D. Messner and G. Vobruba, 'Die sozialen Dimensionen der Globalisierung', *Working Paper*, No. 28, Institut für Entwicklung und Frieden, Duisburg (1998).

35. B. Wessels, 'Organising Capacity of Societies and Modernity', in J. van Deth (ed.), *Private Groups and Public Life* (London: Routledge, 1997).

36. A. Brassloff, 'The Church and Post-Franco Society', in C. Abel (ed.), *Spain: Conditional Democracy* (London: Croom Helm, 1984).

37. U. Kettler and C. von Ferber, 'Selbsthilfeförderung: Ein wirkungsvoller Beitrag zur Reform des Sozial- und Gesundheitswesens', *Sozialer Fortschritt*, Vol. 46 (1997), pp. 226–31.

38. M. Kaase and P. Bauer-Kaase, 'German Unification 1990–1997: The Long, Long Road', *Estudios/Working Papers*, No. 1998/119, Instituto Juan March, Madrid (1998).

39. J-M. Maravall, 'Politics and Policy: Economic Reforms in Southern Europe', in L. Bresser Pereira, J-M. Maravall and A. Przeworksi (eds), *Economic Reforms in New Democracies: A Social-Democratic Approach* (Cambridge: Cambridge University Press, 1993).

40. L. Hantrais, 'Interactions between Socio-Demographic Trends, Social and Economic Policies', *Cross-National Research Papers*, 5th Series, No. 1 (1999).

41. H-M. Nickel, 'Women and Women's Policies in East and West Germany, 1945–1990', in E.

Kolinsky (ed.), *Social Transformation and the Family in Post-Communist Germany* (Basingstoke: Macmillan, 1998).

42. Eurostat, 'Education in the EU', *Statistics in Focus: Population and Social Conditions Series,* No. 4/97 (1997).

43. Eurostat, 'How Evenly are Earnings Distributed?', *Statistics in Focus: Population and Social Conditions Series,* No. 15/97 (1997).

44. Statistisches Bundesamt, *Datenreport: Zahlen und Fakten über die Bundesrepublik Deutschland* (Bonn: 1997).

45. K. Zimmerman, 'Labour Responses to Taxes and Benefits in Germany', in A. Atkinson and A. Mogensen (eds), *Welfare and Work Incentives: A North European Perspective* (Oxford: Clarendon, 1993).

46. OECD, *The Tax-Benefit Position of Employees: 1995/6* (Paris: OECD, 1997).

47. OECD, 'Ageing Populations, Pension Systems and Government Budgets', *Working Papers,* No. 168 (Paris: OECD, 1996).

48. OECD, 'Ageing Populations, Pension Systems and Government Budgets', *Working Papers,* No. 168 (Paris: OECD, 1996); P. Besseling and R. Zeeuw, *The Financing of Pensions in Europe* (The Hague: Central Planning Bureau, Memo III, 1993); J. Falkingham and P. Johnson, 'Funding Pensions over the Life Cycle', in J. Falkingham and J. Hills (eds), *The Dynamics of Welfare* (Hemel Hempstead: Harvester Wheatsheaf, 1995); P. Johnson and J. Falkingham (eds), *Ageing and Economic Welfare* (London: Sage, 1992).

49. *Der Spiegel,* 'Der Abschied der Alten', No. 47 (1998), pp. 86–8.

50. J. Berghman, 'Social Exclusion in Europe: Policy Context and Analytical Framework', in G. Room (ed.), *Beyond the Threshold: Measurement and Analysis of Social Exclusion* (Bristol: Polity Press, 1995).

51. S. Paugam, 'Poverty and Social Disqualification: A Comparative Analysis of Cumulative Social Disadvantage in Europe', *Journal of European Social Policy,* Vol. 6, 4 (1996), pp. 287–303.

52. R. Castel, *Les Metamorphoses de la Question Sociale* (Paris: Ed. Fayard, 1995).

53. S. Leibfried, L. Leisering and P. Buhr, *Zeit der Armut: Lebensläufe im Sozialstaat* (Frankfurt: Suhrkamp, 1995).

54. European Commission, *Social Protection in Europe: 1997* (Brussels: European Commission, 1997).

55. H. Berger, W. Hinrich, E. Priller, and A. Schultz, *Privathaushalte in Vereinigungsprozess – Ihre soziale Lage in Ost und Westdeutschland* (Frankfurt: Campus, 1999).

56. Statistisches Bundesamt, *Datenreport: Zahlen und Fakten über die Bundesrepublik Deutschland* (Bonn: 1997).

57. EAPN, 'Spotlight on Minimum Income: The Final Safety Net of Social Protection', *Network News,* 64 (Brussels: European Anti-Poverty Network, 1999), pp. 2–3.

58. European Commission, *Employment in Europe: 1998* (Brussels: European Commission, COM/98/666 Final, 1999).

59. M. Baldwin Edwards, 'Immigrants and the Welfare State in Europe', in E. Taylor and J. Arango (eds), *Migration at Century's End* (Oxford: Oxford University Press, 1999).

60. Statistisches Bundesamt, *Datenreport: Zahlen und Fakten über die Bundesrepublik Deutschland* (Bonn, 1997).

61. Programa 2000, *Sociedad en Transición* (Madrid: Ed. Sistema, 1987).

62. M. Härtl, 'Auszug aus dem Elternhaus – "Nesthocker" und "Nestflüchter"', in W. Bien (ed.), *Familie an der Schwelle zum neuen Jahrtausend* (Opladen: Leske and Budrich, 1996).

63. S. Bentolila and J. Dolado, 'The Spanish Labour Market', *Economic Policy (*April 1994), pp. 55–99.

64. G. Esping-Andersen, 'Welfare without Work: the Impasse of Labour Shedding and Familialism in Continental European Social Policy', in G. Esping-Andersen (ed.), *Welfare States in Transition* (London: Sage, 1996).

65. D. Springer, *The Social Dimension of 1992* (New York: Praeger, 1992).

66. *Financial Times,* 23 February 1998.

67. G. Esping-Andersen, 'Welfare without Work: the Impasse of Labour Shedding and Familialism in Continental European Social Policy', in G. Esping-Andersen (ed.), *Welfare States in Transition* (London: Sage, 1996).

68. N. Timmins, 'America's Great Experiment', *Financial Times,* 28 November 1997, p. 23.

69. S. Mann, 'Ungleichheit und Gerechtigkeit', *Mitteilungen,* No. 79, Wissenschaftszentrum Berlin (1998), pp. 26–8.

70. J. Stephens, 'The Scandinavian Welfare States: Achievements, Crisis and Prospects', in G. Esping-Andersen (ed.), *Welfare States in Transition* (London: Sage, 1996).
71. A. de Swaan, 'A Perspective for Transnational Social Policy', *Government and Opposition*, 27 (1992), pp. 33–51.
72. J. Halfmann, 'Immigration and Citizenship in Germany: Contemporary Dilemmas', *Political Studies*, XLV (1997), pp. 260–74.
73. T. Hammar, *Democracy and the Nation State: Aliens, Denizens and Citizens in a World of International Migration* (Oxford: Berg, 1990).

3

Towards a New Deal? Recasting Social Policy in Germany and Europe

Ilona Ostner

DILEMMAS OF TRANSFORMATION

During the first years after German unification debates of all colours concentrated on issues of economic transformation, e.g. on wages and their relation to productivity, or on labour market trends on the one hand, and on financial burdens on the other. These concerns have remained significant up to the present and will continue to be salient also in the next few years.[1]

The pace at which the east German economy is catching up to west German levels has been said to be decisive not only for the German economy as a whole but is critical also for the legitimacy of the considerable financial transfers from better-off *Länder* to economic laggards, the majority of them in the east. Economic transformation has put continuous and increasing pressure on German *Länder* as well as on citizens' willingness to put ideas of social inclusion and the integration of German society first and not to defect in times of decreasing resources and sharpening competition for scarce resources, be they revenue, jobs or, more generally, opportunities. German unification can increasingly be analysed in terms of such dilemmas. The objective of this chapter is to discuss the background to this trend.

The dilemma sketched above is a typical collective action problem: a situation where all involved in an action would be better off if they cooperated than if they all defected, but where it is not in each person's, party's or group's individual interest to cooperate.[2] Why should the individual agree to forgo resources (money or opportunities) and thereby also sacrifice improvements of his or her position in a competitive setting? Will the other party use these resources in a way that all would end up in a comparable or even better position? As is well known, 'pessimists' defect, which sooner or later will increase overall pessimism.[3] They do so more readily if repeated sacrifices do not lead to expected outcomes. A collective action framework can explain part of the nature of the dilemmas which

German unification posed for all parties involved; it also gives support to those who maintain that economics should reasonably be at the heart of transformation politics and policies. Finally, such a framework hints at the possible exhaustion of resources of solidarity and thereby highlights salient questions of fairness, reciprocity and responsibility.

'RESHUFFLING THE CARDS': TWOFOLD TRANSFORMATION AS ·COMPARATIVE ADVANTAGE FOR EAST GERMANS?

The sociologist Karl Ulrich Mayer[4] criticised the narrowly economic focus of the transformation debate. He maintains that the process of unification is complex and entails a multitude of diverse aspects – among them economic ones. Transformation, Mayer argues, has so far included the adjustment of the legal system, an issue which was solved through the transfer of west German institutions, the still unfinished agenda of equalising educational and occupational opportunities and – even more difficult to achieve – the creation of shared beliefs and collective identities.[5] In sum, Mayer's approach to transformation includes: (1) institution building; (2) social transformation in a strictly sociological sense: changing patterns of social inequality; the elimination of old and the creation of new positions; (re-)allocation of individuals or resources to positions as well as the redefinition of rules for allocation; and (3) an encompassing cultural change, for example, the transformation of deeply rooted mentalities. His structural analysis focuses on the second aspect of transformation – the re-allocation of positions and resources – according to Mayer a lasting and arduous problem.

Difficulties in promoting faster social change, Mayer's second aspect of transformation, may be due to the stubbornness of social structures and related strategies which unification inherited from socialist east Germany. But this explanation can only partly convince. It neglects the wider German and EU-European context and connected collective action problems. Traditional forms and rules of allocating positions and resources to individuals or groups have been questioned in west Germany too. A broad range of institutions has been scrutinised, for example, social security or labour market institutions, with regard to eligibility rules, particularisms and selectivity. As a consequence, east Germany is experiencing what Hildegard Maria Nickel coined in her writings a 'twofold transformation':[6] it has had to adapt to the west German way while unified Germany has been exposed to a whole set of new challenges which in turn require vital structural and institutional changes.

In the longer run, some of the presumed 'socialist' liabilities may turn out to be valuable assets for overcoming competitive disadvantages: the tradition of full-time, life-long employment and the blurred boundaries between work and social life, both of which explain the readiness of today's east Germans, especially women, flexibly to take whatever job and work under equally flexible schedules; the familiarity with universal minimum provisions of cash and services, which meanwhile have reached the German and EU-European policy agenda – all of these can be discussed under the heading of east German comparative advantages. In sum, a west German model for east German social transformation – transformation of allocation patterns and rules – no longer exists.

'TWOFOLD' TRANSFORMATION

The concept and reality of a 'twofold' transformation process make up the backdrop of this chapter. The discussion below focuses mainly on the changing context and connected challenges to national welfare states and labour markets, which have brought into question existing institutions while increasing intrastate and interstate collective action problems, such as those within Germany and between *Länder*, or those within EU-Europe and among EU member states.

The chapter first delineates shifts in discourses on the future of welfare states and their respective social policies. Secondly, it distinguishes 'endogenous' institutional inefficiencies which have resulted from welfare states' respective institutional logics and which have been aggravated by exogenous pressure, for example, changes in the global economic environment. These inefficiencies (if not contradictions) can be assessed with regard to welfare production, legitimation and market regulation. They constitute the framework for new political (mostly social democratic) strategies of welfare reform. National policies aimed at a restructuring of the welfare state have been mainly concerned with addressing such inefficiencies. Minimum income schemes and basic social provisions have gained a strategic role in this process. The largest section of the chapter compares institutions and institutional restructuring in three countries: the UK, Denmark and Germany. But why make a comparison and why a comparison of these countries?

The comparative approach complies with basic rules for sociological inquiry: it should not generalise trends on the basis of one country (welfare state); it should be aware of the peculiarity of each case and its setting (which necessitates comparison) and therefore aware of the limits of 'regime-shopping'; it should take into account the international context, identify actors (one may add: institutional leverage and policy feedbacks) in a comparative perspective in order to avoid a linear or functionalist–evolutionist argument. Finally, it should consider institutional legacies in a long-term perspective.

The cases under consideration fit a simple Beveridgean versus Bismarckian distinction which juxtaposes pan-universal and pan-professional welfare systems. A more sophisticated assessment would distinguish austere versus generous universal systems, for example, Scandinavian versus British ones, on the one hand, and institutional versus clientelist systems, for example, Germanic versus southern European ones, on the other. Hybrids, such as Ireland, France or the Netherlands, exist also. The choice is a pragmatic one: the United Kingdom and Denmark have recently and, as is said, successfully fought their institutional inefficiencies.

FROM DE-COMMODIFICATION TO RE-COMMODIFICATION

As a consequence of Maastricht, EU member states' policy logics moved from de-commodification to re-commodification, from – as it was coined – passive to active (or activating) measures or in-work benefits and provision (familiar to east Germans). Social policies were accused of paying-off passive, non-working but employable adults. Consequently, they have increasingly abandoned the redistribution needed for compensating those unemployed and turned instead towards financing employability, stressing (again) the obligations which correspond to the individual's rights.

Arguments put forward stressed the right *and* obligation to self-reliance through paid work and individual contributions to social security funds. In turn, policies are designed to and actually do grant job seekers initial endowments in order to improve starting conditions, remove existing barriers towards men's and women's labour market participation, and combat those forms of discrimination which have hindered employability. As regards the other side of the same coin, any employment-intensive growth strategy has to rely on the creation of all sorts of jobs, many of them low paid and low standard. A recent estimate forecasts that 700,000 full-time jobs have to be created in Germany in order to bring social assistance recipients of working age (excluding lone mothers) back into employment. This number has to be added to jobs required for the roughly 4,000,000 unemployed. Problems of job creation explain the social partners' and member states' reluctance fully to regulate flexible jobs. In sum, equal opportunities have gained a new meaning as 'equality of employability'.

There are many reasons for the shift towards equal employability in the EU and, consequently, in Germany: macro-structural ones, like the defeat of socialism; global economic challenges to both member states' competitiveness and to that of the EU itself which constitute a major strain on political choices. Micro-level changes have added to the changing political landscape: individualistic attitudes and values, the emphasis on rights at the expense of obligations have strained solidarity and boosted moral hazard and free-riding in the welfare state. These, in turn, lowered the acceptability of redistributive policies and provided problems of justification. At the end of the day, EU member states are finally bound to come to terms with the market and with governance through the market.

Two reservations have to be made. First, it is not argued here that economic – macro- and structural-economic – factors do not matter. Growing internationalisation and globalisation, the rise of new technologies, and what Bob Jessop and others[7] call the paradigm shift from Fordism to post-Fordism are *push factors* for welfare state restructuring. But western welfare states have been struck by their success and have become weighed down by inefficiencies and strategic dilemmas. These are *pull factors* for shifting welfare state logics. More research is needed which is capable of establishing the relative and combined effect of economic push and socio-political pull factors.[8]

The second point concerns the issue of path dependency: welfare state reform does not automatically imply cut-backs or the termination of programmes. Drawing upon Ditch and Oldfield,[9] one can distinguish welfare states which consolidate and/or preserve their institutional setting through reform (the Danish case); others are *extenders* (Portugal); some operate at the same time as consolidators as well as *extenders*; others may do away with traditional programmes (leave their path), or at least with some of them. Ditch and Oldfield call the latter 'innovators'. Again, combinations are likely and vary over time. Institutional legacies predict to some extent the type and scope of reforms; at least, they may tell us something about the range of available choices (choices compatible with existing institutional logics). They do not fully determine, however, the path to be taken. German unification can be interpreted in terms of a critical juncture which may be decisive for the continuation along or deviation from a trodden path. Solutions to social problems, buried or forgotten alternatives which were defeated years or even decades ago may re-emerge and be put on the policy agenda again. The changing institutional configuration and new coalitions may help them to succeed.

INSTITUTIONAL INEFFICIENCIES OF EUROPEAN WELFARE
STATES IN A COMPARATIVE PERSPECTIVE

Torfing has recently recalled that welfare states consist of a mix of macro-economic and structural-economic policies combined with a mix of social welfare (de-commodifying) and workfare (re-commodifying) policies.[10] In his view, both the discourse of structural competitiveness and that of structural unemployment, the first to be enhanced, the latter overcome, have strengthened the relative importance of welfare policies *vis-à-vis* traditional social policies.

It has now become a truism that welfare state measures while pursuing their intended social, political and economic goals – equality, equalisation and inclusion, loyalty and entitlement, efficiency and competitiveness – inevitably produce unintended effects: new inequalities/social divides and exclusion, defection and disentitlement, inefficiencies and sclerosis. While fighting first-order problems, the welfare state creates second-order ones.[11] Earlier theoretical writing was pretty aware of the dialectic that citizenship is itself becoming the architect of social inequality.[12]

A good deal of registered poverty (cross-sectional data on people on social assistance) in Germany is institutional – caused by administrative failure. Many social assistance recipients are just bridging the pension or unemployment benefits which are overdue. Generous benefits for average risks of people who are unknown to each other increase moral hazard and free-riding and erode inter-generational solidarity. This may lead to a legitimation crisis and harm efficiency. Needless to say, these dialectics – how and to what extent they occur – depend on respective institutional settings.

One can roughly distinguish three types of inefficiencies which result from the various institutional logics that constitute the respective welfare states: poverty and unemployment traps; moral hazard and free-riding; vested rights or interests. The three types of welfare state inefficiency nicely fit Esping-Andersen's three worlds of welfare capitalism.[13] A fourth type results from post-socialist transformation. They can be identified as undesirable and/or contradictory effects of welfare state intervention in three areas: welfare production, legitimation, market regulation. The latter define the central social, political and economic functions of the welfare state.

Poverty and Unemployment Traps

Poverty and unemployment traps (mainly of low-skilled individuals and households) result from the polarised protection offered by a welfare state in a deregulated low-wage/low-skill economy, from the austerity of tax-financed minimum income schemes and options for better-off strata to exit from state schemes. These in turn initiate a vicious circle of further eroding mimima. With respect to the first function – welfare production – the welfare state has effectively failed to fight poverty and is facing rising numbers of welfare dependants despite increased and growing expenditures for the poor. The legitimation problem can be coined in terms of a 'fairness gap' between working poor (families) and non-working poor, rather than in terms of diminishing overall poverty and inequality.

The typical case for this scenario is the UK. Welfare reform policies set out in the 1998 Green Paper 'A New Contract for Welfare' are not 'about a few benefits paid to the most needy' (Blair), but intend 'to rebuild the system around work and security' (income security tied more closely to work). Building on reforms and initiatives of the Conservatives, the Contract aims especially at the unskilled and low-skilled, including lone mothers with children older than 5 years. The main objective is to assist in short-term intensive job search (through cash and services) rather than to raise skill levels. Critics who argued that to help lone parents into unrewarding, low-paid employment with little or no skills development is not enough were let down by the Secretary of State for Social Security. She made it clear that to ensure that 'children are not brought up in workless households ... is part of our programme for tackling social exclusion'.[14]

At the same time tax credit policies for families and children (child-care) were significantly extended and a notable redistribution of resources from childless couples to families with children, especially poorer ones, put into force. The negative side to this is that care provided within the family and home is no longer counted as work and a valuable contribution to society: this renders the family a mere function of the labour market and of employability. The devaluation of family care is also apparent in the low value attached to child-minding which is treated (through a child-minding benefit) as an unskilled activity. Further, the new redistributive measures will be partly paid by women's disentitlement to their husbands' basic pensions (SERPS) notwithstanding the already existing high poverty risks facing elderly women.

Moral Hazard/Free Riding

The second endogenous challenge to modern welfare states results from the generosity of provisions (such as wage replacements, but also services) which may be due to the inclusion of the middle classes into public social security. Generosity of income replacement and high quality of services are a *conditio sine qua non* for the loyalty of the middle classes and their readiness to pay taxes (legitimation). On the other hand, generosity very much depends on the assumption that only a few people make use of the schemes on a long-term basis or, put differently, that the majority of citizens of working age participate in the labour market (is 'commodified' or 'active'). In cases of defection, the 'fairness gap' relates to rights which are not matched by obligations. Typical cases are the Scandinavian countries, but also continental European ones which run generous schemes, and which are in their essentials close to universal schemes, for instance, the Netherlands, Germany or Austria.

Torfing[15] elaborates on the Danish welfare reforms, speaking of 'reforms of the Danish economy' – as a move from the Keynesian welfare to a Schumpeterian workfare state (from standard to flexible employment, from passive welfare to active workfare). Denmark has attached activation plans to unemployment benefits and social assistance; it has also restricted the number of years of entitlement, but benefits have not been reduced. Torfing argues that, due to constitutive factors in Danish society and its welfare state, Denmark has been capable of preserving its generous provisions while at the same time successfully fighting its institutional inefficiencies.

Factors here are a strong political consensus that the existing welfare state should be preserved, plus support for high taxes, wage equality and redistribution. This has so far prevented any race to the bottom. Support also comes from the middle classes and the elites, including employers (in contrast to UK or US). The political climate has been hostile towards neo-liberal workfare strategies – Torfing[16] calls these 'defensive' (mostly disciplining) – that they violate Danish civil liberal principles. However, seemingly Danes appreciated 'offensive' – truly activating – workfare policies. Welfare reforms have also been advanced by longer-term social-democratic rule and economic growth.

Vested Interests

The issue at stake here with vested rights or the interests of labour market insiders is that they operate at the expense of the labour market outsiders, mainly the younger generations, and of the majority of women. Vested interests have resulted from the focus of social protection on standard employment, which privileged again the middle classes and the better-off – better qualified – strata, mostly full-time employed men and male breadwinners who could hence afford a wife and mother at home.

The serious erosion of both standard employment and male breadwinning which has resulted in the growing number of non-standard forms of employment reduced the legitimacy of this kind of institutional particularism. Fairness problems have come to the fore: between labour market insiders and outsiders, between women and men, although a growing proportion of women have managed to become insiders, while many men, especially young ones, have been losing out; also there are fairness problems between generations. Typical cases of countries with such vested interests are Germany, Austria, France, but also Italy and Spain.

Germany is well known for privileging full-time skilled (mostly male) standard employment through labour legislation, social policy and collective bargaining agreements at the expense of non-standard employment. With the increase in the latter, the social security system has been challenged. Structural unemployment and the insider–outsider problem have added to this challenge. In Germany, structural unemployment often results from the disappearance of low-skilled industrial work in combination with decommodifying social policies and very relaxed eligibility rules for unemployment benefit (reduced obligations to accept jobs and incentives for firms to place their ageing workers on early retirement schemes). The problem of long-term unemployment or early retirement has been intensified by the principle of status maintenance: in the case of lay-offs, employees were not expected to accept jobs of a lesser status or significantly lower incomes. The previous government seriously eroded this principle.

The problem of German unemployment and, consequently, of the German welfare state, has recently been reformulated in terms of the transition from industrialism to post-industrialism with Germany being a laggard in this process.[17] The strength of the German economy, its competitive advantage, still lies in the highly skilled and competitive industrial production sector and, if in services, then in production-related ones which in turn – as is commonly argued – do not provide sufficient job opportunities for the less skilled or for those whose skills no longer match expected standards. Therefore, in contrast to the UK or Denmark, skilling does not constitute a solution – rather a number of measures are said to be needed in order to reduce unit labour costs and to change consumption patterns of households.[18]

Negative income tax schemes, citizens' wage subsidies, the exemption of employers from social insurance contributions and various tax credits have been proposed as solutions. The new government has announced further restrictions in entitlements to benefits and eligibility rules. The previous government had already started measures intended to accelerate the transition from one-earner to two-earner households. Women of working age and also mothers of school-children are expected to be at least part-time employed and thereby contribute to social security schemes.

Part-time work has been enhanced by the legal right to (part-time) child-care for children older than 3 years. The social-democratic Minister for the Family is drafting new parental leave legislation which tries to reverse de-commodification (mothers' exit from employment) by prioritising part-time leave for both parents.

Obviously, the situation in east Germany differs significantly from that in west Germany: unification has led to a rapid and radical de-industrialisation of east Germany, new competitive industries have rarely and only slowly emerged while consumption patterns have not significantly boosted the number of service jobs which could have compensated for the loss of industrial employment opportunities, women's higher labour market participation notwithstanding. Too often, women's income is needed to raise the household's standard of living to a decent level which allows it to buy goods that could not have been bought on the basis of one-earner income. However, since women dominated the service sector in the GDR (even in those occupations that in the west were gender neutral or monopolised by men, such as in banking and insurance) and since women usually worked full-time, they have become catalysts and forerunners of post-industrial employment and a model for a west German transition to the two-earner household.

Slipping Anchors and Torn Safety Nets

This heading hints roughly at problems faced by the emerging welfare states in central and eastern Europe – some of which are applicants to become EU members. The issue at stake is a very different one. The introduction of shock therapy policies as advised by the IMF and World Bank in order to transform the comprehensive socialist social safety net into a market-friendly, basic one has led to an enormous increase in all sorts of inequalities in central and eastern Europe which has left the poorer strata constantly losing benefits and wage incomes. One means of adaptation was to let the level of statutory minimum wage drop to incredibly low levels. The latter, although paid to only a small number of workers, has continued to determine the pay of many workers and, even more importantly, to define thresholds for a wide range of social benefits. Holding down minimum pay soon became a convenient means of reducing money wage inflation and social spending totals.[19]

East German transformation has deviated crucially from the east European path, not only with regard to its input, the nearly unmodified transfer of west German welfare state institutions, but also with regard to some outcomes, such as the degree of income security and equality. Although the distribution of market income has become more unequal in east Germany, net household income equality has increased to a greater extent in east than in west Germany due to transfers during the 1990s. Looked at from the perspective of the outcome, one can at least conclude that transfers have worked for east Germany. The final section looks more closely at the east German case.

PECULIARITIES OF THE EAST GERMAN CASE SUMMARISED

The west–east transfer of institutions implied a transfer of typical German institutional inefficiencies. Rules of eligibility, particularism and selectivity which are at the heart of the institution of standard employment and which often privileged one gender or generation at the expense of the other were put into force in east Germany. In a short-term perspective, that helped to mitigate the transition.

Women and men above the age of 50 who had been laid off mostly due to the ongoing closing down of old or non-profitable industries were treated as standard early retirees. Pensions were dealt with according to west German rules and raised to west German levels – a measure from which especially east German full-time working women profited. Since it was granted without corresponding previous east German contributions and was predominantly borne by the west German old age social insurance funds, this soon led to objections from the west. Complaints have also been put forward from a west German women's perspective: for instance, it has been argued that the institutional configuration, related rules and the performance of the west German welfare state (for example, its emphasis on cash benefits at the expense of public service provision) have restricted mothers' full-time and/or continuous employment in contrast to their east German counterparts.

In sum, the transfer of standard employment to east Germany induced the emergence of connected vested interests on the one hand and of inefficient allocation of resources and opportunities on the other. It does not come as a surprise therefore, that more east than west Germans defend the scope and scale of social benefits and provisions with the exception of those for asylum seekers and migrants. However, the transfer advantaged mostly those east Germans, women and men, who had worked full-time, life-long in socialist times, neutralising the standard employment particularism for this group. But it did not tackle income security, nor the status maintenance problems of younger cohorts who had either an insufficient employment record or lacked one. In the latter case, the transfer of standard employment, the related forms of collective bargaining and of social security added to their disadvantaged position or to the already existing moral hazard and unemployment traps.

The ongoing de-commodification of labour via the welfare state reduced labour supply, especially of older workers, but many of those who had newly entered or remained in the labour market enjoyed standard employment, among them many women. Contrary to eastern European post-communist countries, east German poverty rates do not exceed west German rates and, as was said above, equality of post-transfer real income has even slightly increased in the second half of the 1990s. At the same time, the numbers of self-employed and of marginally employed people have grown, together with the rate of those who are unemployed. The east German labour market seems to be more flexible than the west German one. However, as many argue, it is still too inflexible, especially with regard to wages, to attempt to fight unemployment with any degree of success. Not surprisingly, it is east German employers who insist on ending west German-style standard employment, and ask for an exemption from social security contributions and collective bargaining agreements (provided they had been party to such an agreement) in order to secure jobs not solely for unskilled labour – turning thereby into prime supporters of OECD or EU employment strategies.

Since many east German households can rely on two earners, at least part-time ones, unemployment notwithstanding, they will presumably be better equipped to cope with declining wages and a move towards basic social security than west German households. While east German peculiarities might impact upon west Germany and add to the existing politics and policies of boosting employability, west Germany – the *Länder* as well as individuals – might in turn increasingly defect to self-interested strategies and at least implicitly reduce or even terminate cooperation. This scenario will come closer to reality if the mismatch between financial transfers and outcomes – both objective and perceived ones – continues to exist.

NOTES

1. See the chapter by Flockton in this volume.
2. M. Olson, *The Logic of Collective Action: Public Goods and the Theory of Goods*, 2nd edn (Cambridge: Harvard University Press, 1971).
3. J. de Deken and C. Offe, 'Working, Time, and Social Participation', Mimeo (Berlin: Institut für Sozialwissenschaften, Humboldt University, 1999).
4. K. U. Mayer, 'Vereinigung soziologisch: Die soziale Ordnung der DDR und ihre Folgen', *Berliner Journal für Soziologie*, Vol. 4/3 (1994), pp. 307–21.
5. For these latter points see D. Pollack and G. Pickel, 'Die ostdeutsche Identität – Erbe des DDR-Sozialismus oder Produkt der Wiederveinigung? Die Einstellung der Ostdeutschen zu sozialer Ungleichheit und Demokratie', *Aus Politik und Zeitgeschichte*, B 41–2/98 (1998), pp. 9–23; and C. Zelle, 'Soziale und liberale Wertorientierungen: Versuch einer situativen Erklärung der

Unterschiede zwischen Ost- und Westdeutschen', *Aus Politik und Zeitgeschichte,* B 41–2/98 (1998), pp. 24–36.

6. H. M. Nickel, 'Lebenschancen von Frauen in Ostdeutschland', in W .Glatzer and I. Ostner (eds), *Deutschland im Wandel. Sozialstrukturelle Analysen* (Opladen: Leske & Budrich, 1999), pp. 255–64.

7. B. Jessop, 'Towards a Schumpeterian Workfare Regime in Britain? Reflections on Regulation, Governance, and Welfare State', *Environment and Planning,* Vol. 27/11 (1995), pp. 1613–26. See also J. Torfing, 'Workfare with Welfare: Recent Reforms of the Danish Welfare State', *Journal of European Social Policy,* Vol. 9/1 (1999), pp. 5–28.

8. J.Torfing, 'Workfare with Welfare'.

9. J. Ditch and N. Oldfield, 'Social Assistance: Recent Trends and Themes', *Journal of European Social Policy,* Vol. 9/1 (1999), pp. 65–76.

10. J. Torfing, 'Workfare with Welfare'.

11. F-X. Kaufmann, *Herausforderungen des Sozialstaates* (Frankfurt am Main: Suhrkamp, 1997); S. Lessenich, 'Soziologische Erklärungsansätze zu Entstehung und Funktion des Sozialstaats', in J. Allmendinger and W. Ludwig-Mayerhofer (eds), *Soziologie des Sozialstaates* (Weinheim: Juventa (forthcoming)).

12. L. Mead, 'Citizenship and Social Policy: T. H. Marshall and Poverty', in Ellen Frankel Paul *et al.* (eds), *The Welfare State* (Cambridge: Harvard University Press, 1997), pp. 197–230.

13. G. Esping-Andersen, *Social Foundations of Postindustrial Economies* (Oxford: Oxford University Press, 1999).

14. *Guardian,* various issues. For the USA, see L. Mead, 'Citizenship and Social Policy: T. H. Marshall and Poverty', in E. Frankel Paul *et al.* (eds), *The Welfare State,* pp. 197–230. For the UK, see H. Land, 'New Labour, New Families?', in *Social Policy Review,* 11; H. Dean and R. Woods (eds), *Social Policy Association* (Luton, 1999), pp. 127–44

15. J. Torfing, 'Workfare with Welfare'.

16. J. Torfing, 'Workfare with Welfare'.

17. G. Esping-Andersen, *Social Foundations.*

18. K-H. Paqué, 'Unemployment and the Crisis of the German Model: A Long-Term Interpretation', in Herbert Giersch (ed.), *Fighting Europe's Unemployment in the 1990s* (Berlin: Springer, 1996), pp. 119–55.

19. G .Standing, 'Social Protection in Central and Eastern Europe: A Tale of Slipping Anchors and Torn Safety Nets', in G. Esping-Andersen (ed.), *Welfare States in Transition: National Adaptations to Global Economies* (London: Sage, 1996), pp. 225–55.

4

Policy Agendas and the Economy in Germany and Europe

Christopher Flockton

GERMAN ECONOMIC UNIFICATION IN AN INTEGRATING EUROPE

German unification has of course presented great challenges for European integration, and it is commonly accepted that the drive for deepening, in the form of the Maastricht Treaty path to European Monetary Union (EMU), and widening, in the form of the Europe Agreements and accession negotiations for central European countries, have been a conscious response. These bind the larger Germany into a deeper form of EU integration, while providing part of the architecture for a wider Europe, following the end of the Iron Curtain. Specific arrangements and levels of EU assistance were also agreed at breakneck speed, for the admission of east Germany itself to the EU.[1] The economic strains of unification within Germany have also been felt in Europe as a whole, whether through German interest rate policy and its effect on the European Monetary System (EMS), or the financial strains on public budgets, as evidenced in the close constraints imposed by the Maastricht Treaty convergence criteria for public budgets, their extension in the form of the Stability and Growth Pact for eurozone members and in Germany's desire to reduce its EU budgetary contributions.[2] However, it is not at the macro-economic level, but at the micro-economic level of economic constitutions upon which the present discussion focuses, for German economic unification has posed a range of challenges to Germany's social market order, which economic liberals believe has led to distortions in that order, and so have generated tensions with Brussels.[3] Germany was for much of the period since the signing of the Treaty of Rome the model of a social market order, the country which ensured that the economically liberal principles of trade inter-penetration underpinned integration in the Common Market (outside the agricultural sector of course).[4] It was Germany that insisted on rigorous application of competition policy rules and restrictions on state industrial aid and regional assistance to ensure that trade flows were not distorted.[5] It is, therefore, only since unification and a consequent large increase in German aid to its industry and labour market in the east, that the Federal Republic has come to find Brussel's competition policy frustrating and irksome. It is these very distortions to Germany's social market order arising from integrating the east that are the core of the present investigation: the disputes with the EU Commission over subsidies and special regimes are one test of such departures from the social market prescriptions.

As will be seen in the next section, Germany appears to have been well ahead of many EU member states in the liberalisation current of the 1990s. It remains the case, however, that the policy regime established to promote market transition in east Germany has produced some deviation from the social market model. Of course, the prospect of mass unemployment had to be addressed. Support mechanisms had to be put in place as crutches to underpin the ex-GDR monopolistic combines, which were collapsing under world competition at Deutschmark prices translated at the newly established Ostmark:DM exchange rate. However, the very scale of social welfare assistance, the scale of unemployment and second labour market measures, the privatisation strategies of the Treuhandanstalt, particularly in respect of the older industrial cores, the levels of regional assistance, the special regimes in sectors such as agriculture, energy or housing – all these represent a degree of intervention and support not experienced in earlier times in the old Federal Republic. It is scarcely surprising that such interventions have led in a range of cases to conflict with the Brussels Competition Directorate. This notwithstanding, it is difficult to imagine how else, in practice, the federal government could have acted, once the terms for unification had been set, given the very low productivity of east German industry and the push for wage harmonisation.

In the following discussion, after a brief survey of Germany's response to the Single Market Programme liberalisation currents, the economic evolution in eastern Germany and the accompanying federal development policy will be examined, particularly with a view to establishing how the policy regime and decisions taken differed from practice in west Germany. It will be seen that the economic evolution in the east, in addition to the obvious economic slump and high unemployment, also demonstrates significant structural differences compared with that in the west. Additionally, special sectoral regimes remain in place, almost ten years after unification. Distortions to the social market regime which have attracted criticism from the Brussels Competition Directorate are then addressed, and, finally, conclusions from this development experience in the east are drawn as lessons for EMU and the EU enlargement to the east. For, while in many aspects the eastern experience is unique, there are nevertheless significant features in relation to exchange rate, labour market, industrial and welfare policy issues, which must be avoided in an EMU, if aspects of the east German condition are not to be reproduced in lower productivity regions in the eurozone currency area.

Germany and the Single Market Programme: The Liberalisation Challenge

The Single Market Programme encapsulated in the Cockfield Report of 1985, and the later Brussels liberalisation directives in the areas of financial services, energy supply, air transport and telecommunications, appeared driven much more by a British, Thatcherite agenda than by any Federal Republic leadership. Rather, the FRG appeared reactive and restrictive towards the new proposals emanating from Brussels. In part, this reflected the fact that the services and utilities areas of the federal German economy had remained quite tightly regulated since the Weimar Republic, that competitive market pressures were permitted only in manufacturing. It is as well to recall that one of the key principles underlying the Single Market Programme, the mutual recognition of norms and standards, was established by the European Court of Justice in its rulings against Germany over the Cassis de Dijon and the German beer *Reinheitsgebot* cases. Likewise, the Court's ruling on the Schleicher case concerning the closed nature of the German insurance market in the early 1980s, established market opening for the insurance of larger commercial risks.[6] Of course, even in manufacturing, German opinion was far from wholly in favour of free trade. Views were strongly held over the impact of recognition of other countries' norms and standards on the quality, safety and environmental impact of goods traded, over the loosening of the relatively closed world of German public procurement, particularly in telecommunications and medical equipment, over 'social dumping' and tax competition.[7] To a German understanding, the social market order comprised social regulation aspects as well as market relations.

The Brussels liberalisation directives in the fields of financial services, electricity, air transport and telecoms were all regarded at first as an unwelcome challenge in Germany,[8] but it can be argued that in each area, Germany is now among the first, at the forefront of liberalisation. In all of these areas, the markets remained heavily cartelised at the beginning of the 1990s: Lufthansa and the Bundespost (Deutsche Telekom) were in state hands, power generation was largely in the hands of the four big generating companies, and banking and stock exchange reforms were only just in progress, in response to the EU Investment Services Directive.[9] Whereas European liberalisation of the air transport market came into full force only in early 1997, the opening of EU telecoms markets in January 1998, and the opening of the EU electricity markets to up to 25 per cent of their demand commenced only in February 1999, Germany was already well ahead in each of these areas. Lufthansa AG was privatised in mid-decade and the partly privatised Deutsche Telekom faces ferocious price competition in what must be the most open telecoms market in the world. Electricity competition has already forced savings in Germany of 25 per cent for larger users, with the establishment of an energy futures market in April 1999.[10] Reforms in the organisation and operation of the railways and postal services also follow Brussels agreements.

FEDERAL GERMAN DEVELOPMENT POLICY FOR THE EAST

The terms for economic and monetary unification and for national unification, as set out in the State Treaty on Economic, Monetary and Social Unification and in the Unification Treaty, have been analysed in detail in many texts.[11] Suffice it to say then that the exchange rate adopted led to a fourfold overvaluation of the Ostmark, which crippled the east German traded goods sector, soon to be hit also by the demise of COMECON. The very low productivity of the capital stock, its obsolescent and often polluting character, when allied to the rapid harmonisation of eastern wages on western levels, meant that eastern output was rendered almost wholly uncompetitive, with unit costs of production far in excess of those of the already high costs in the west. In a sense, in insisting on the adoption of the Deutschmark at parity and on rapid wage alignment, east Germans unknowingly had gained rapid rises in purchasing power for those still in work, at the expense of the productive assets (which had thereby become worthless), and at the cost of mass unemployment. The angry complaint, commonly heard later, that eastern assets had been given away for nothing to the west, at least pointed to the reality that the assets had become worthless under the prevailing cost conditions: only western finance, and the support of the western social insurance funds, could prop up and turn around the collapsed economy.

The State Treaty and the Unification Treaty introduced the federal German economic constitution in full to the east, including its labour market, social welfare and health systems, its regional aid and infrastructure development mechanisms, its distribution of functions among territorial authorities, and its system of tax revenue equalisation among the *Länder*, (although this had delayed application in the east). In addition, the treaties took over from the very late GDR period the Treuhandanstalt institution, as the manager and disposer of all productive public GDR assets. At that time, the Treuhand was said to be the world's largest property owner, and the Unification Treaty took over the formulation from the GDR legislation that the role of the Treuhand was one of 'privatisation, careful restructuring and cautious closure of assets unprofitable over the long-term'. In the eyes of the Kohl government, which had allocated only DM45bn for unification costs in the first year, unification would largely pay for itself by asset sales. Fundamentally, therefore, in the early period of unification, there was great confidence that east Germany would adopt market relations quickly, would flourish under the social market constitution and would catch up with the west within a span of perhaps four years. However, given the unimagined severity of the shock to the eastern economy, and the damage caused by wage harmonisation, it was inevitable that the newly transferred instruments of labour market and welfare support, heavy capital transfers in the form of infrastructure spending and regional aid and, finally, enormous liquidity credits by the Treuhandanstalt to its haemorrhaging firms, would be expenditure props to keep the collapsed regional economy afloat. An alternative approach, which would have paid wage subsidies to Treuhand firms (subject to their maintaining tight control of wage costs), and restructuring of Treuhand firms while in state hands (again subject to tight wage control), was in such circumstances scarcely possible.[12] Instead, the federal government and its agents faced huge unemployment costs, and the Treuhand sought desperately to find buyers for bankrupt enterprises.

In brief, in addition to the labour market, welfare and Treuhand measures referred to above, there were five main sources of assistance to the east. The DM115bn German Unity Fund helped pump-prime the social insurance funds in the new *Länder*, and it gave infrastructural and property modernisation aid to local authorities. The federal regional development programme, the *Gemeinschaftsaufgabe* or Joint Task, offered the highest level of investment subsidy and low-interest loans, while the KfW (*Kreditanstalt für Wiederaufbau*) offered low interest loans for the establishment and expansion of small- and medium-sized enterprises (SMEs). The Bundesbahn and Bundespost each allocated DM 100bn over a ten-year period for the upgrading of rail and telecommunications infrastructures in the east and the ERP (European Recovery Programme) offered modernisation loans for housing. Finally, the *Erblastentilgungsfonds* took over the inherited housing debt from the GDR state.[13] Overall, gross federal transfers to the east have continued to run at DM140bn (DM90bn net), with gross social transfers alone continuing at DM85bn annually. To the end of 1996, DM1 trillion of public and private funds had been transferred. Thus, instead of German unification paying for itself, federal transfers have been running at 4.5 per cent of GDP annually, and the present scale of expenditure is to continue under the spending plans of both the Kohl and Schröder governments until at least 2004. At that stage, the federal regional aid programme and the States Revenue Equalisation Fund are to be reconsidered. However, the long time-scale indicates the continuing dependence of the new *Länder* on large-scale transfers.

The Debate over the Treuhand's Privatisation Strategy

One can scarcely do justice here to the ferocious debate over the Treuhand's strategy of 'privatisation first'. Following the assassination of the Treuhand's president, Detlev Rohwedder, in early 1992 by the Red Army Fraktion (against a background, let it be said, of deep public dismay over the closure of flagship companies of the east German economy) his successor, Birgit Breuel, took the firm view that privatisation was the best form of restructuring. In the eyes of much of the east German public, the Treuhand played the role of 'die grosse Plattmacherin' (the great bankrupter), transferring public productive assets into private western hands at risible prices.[14] In addition, there was public anger over the transfer of prestige real estate and of *Filetstücke*, the prize assets from state enterprises, at what seemed very low prices. One example concerns the sale of a 50 per cent share of Carl Zeiss Jena to its western sister in Oberkochen for DM1, after the Treuhand and the *Land* of Thüringen had injected DM1bn in investments and running cost liquidity into the firm. It is clear that the sales revenues achieved by the Treuhand reflected largely the negative profit flows achieved in firms whose business had haemorrhaged away. How else can one explain the fact that the total property valuation at Ostmark 1 trillion in March 1990 and at DM600bn by Treuhand President Rohwedder should have melted away to a loss of DM275bn by the time the Treuhand closed its doors in December 1994? Of course, these valuations were over-optimistic and based on very faulty accounting (GDR exchange rate coefficients, long historic amortisation periods, commercial contracts with COMECON, etc.) Also, the very desire of the Treuhand to sell quickly placed it at a marked disadvantage in relation to prospective purchasers.

There can be little doubt that the Treuhand was overwhelmed by the burden of supporting the running costs of failing enterprises, in the form of liquidity credits, and this explains the fact that so much of its expenditure took this form, rather than in new investment: in 1992, DM8bn was spent in liquidity credits to support running costs and only DM2bn in investments. Critics on the left who favoured the retention of ex-GDR enterprises in Treuhand ownership while they were being restructured,[15] who called for an industrial strategy to preserve the industrial core in the east, understate seriously the costs in terms of running cost subsidies which would have been required to maintain enterprises in being, until new investments came on stream. The reality has been that unimagined amounts of money have been spent in subsidy and public investment in the old industrial core of steel, shipbuilding, rolling-stock and chemicals: further examples are given below. Furthermore, the employment and investment commitments which new owners of privatised firms made in their purchase contracts with the Treuhand, reflected these huge continuing costs, which therefore depressed the sale price. The ex-Treuhand enterprises are now a rump of the east German economy, employing only 656,000, or only one in nine of east German employees, compared with a total of 3 millions in 1989.[16]

The scale of state aid to the east

The Sixteenth Subsidy Report of the federal government[17]makes clear how aid to the east has been the prime factor driving the rise in subsidies and tax allowances to the economy, and how the east has come to take an ever larger share. In the period 1991–97, the volume of total public subsidies (direct financial aid and tax allowances) rose from DM102.3bn to DM115.2bn annually, with the eastern share rising from 24.1 per cent to 33.5 per cent. The federal government in particular succeeded in driving down the levels of assistance to the west, although ever-rising coal subsidies (particularly after the ending of the *Kohlepfennig* levy on electricity consumption to fund coal usage and the miners' strike in 1997), have tended to thwart government attempts at restraint. Given that east Germany has only 20 per cent of the German population and 9.3 per cent of the total output, its one-third share of total assistance is therefore highly favourable. Furthermore, while total aid per head of population in the east reached DM2,517 against DM1,211 in the west in 1997, the subsidy levels per employee in manufacturing stood at DM16,000 in the east and at DM887 in the west in 1995 and 1996.[18] This data discloses the huge transfer from the west into the eastern productive sector.

A breakdown of total subsidy expenditure in the east shows that 14 per cent of the total was devoted to tax allowances for the amortisation of one-half of investment costs, and an equal proportion was devoted to interest charge subsidisation by means of ERP credits: 7 per cent of the total subsidy level was devoted to investment grants and 3 per cent to aid for primarily small- and medium-sized enterprises under the *Gemeinschaftsaufgabe* regional aid programme. Under this last heading, a total of DM18.15bn in assistance, shared jointly by the federal government and the *Länder*, was given to the east during the years 1991–96, under the special statute for regional aid to the new *Länder*. This was subsequently replaced consequent upon the integration of the eastern *Länder* into the States Finance Equalisation Fund arrangements, whereby they came under the normal *Gemeinschaftsaufgabe* regime.[19] Outside of the aid to industry itself, the federal railways received 14 per cent of eastern aid in 1996, and agriculture and housing (tax reliefs and interest subsidies for new building and modernisation) gained 12 per cent each. From the foregoing, it is clear then that, within a only moderately rising total level of federal subsidy, there have been huge shifts of support to the east, primarily in favour of manufacturing there. Much has been spent to help keep alive the old industrial core left until recently in Treuhand hands, since there were no ready buyers for the obsolete technology and products.

MANUFACTURING RECOVERY IN THE EAST

The details of the slump in activity following economic union are well known and have been discussed in detail elsewhere.[20] In brief, at the depth of the slump in mid-1992, industrial output in the east had fallen to 60 per cent of its June 1990 level, and up to 2 million workers were benefiting from short-time working pay and other second labour market measures, as means to avoid mass unemployment. In 1998, average unemployment reached a peak of 18 per cent, but if one were to take together, for the intervening years, the numbers on both special labour market measures and in unemployment benefit, then this approximated consistently 30 per cent of the labour force. The workforce, as a result of the profound upheavals, had shrunk from 10 million to 7 million, and only one in five employees had continued to hold on to their job throughout the transition. However, from late 1992, rapid rates of GDP growth were achieved of the order of 8 per cent to 9 per cent annually, and the new *Länder* were said to be the most rapidly growing regions in Europe.[21] This continued until the end of 1996, since when a divergent path between east and west Germany has been experienced. In practice, a significant part of the east's recovery was due to a boom in construction, fuelled by tax allowances worth in aggregate DM30bn, and when these allowances ceased in 1996, a deep slump in the construction sector ensued.[22]

   The position of the manufacturing sector in the east has been partly disguised by the boom and subsequent recession in the construction sector. Yet the sustained rapid growth in manufacturing since the depth of the trough in 1992 has created the basis for a strong regional economy, even if the sector remains too small and continues to suffer from key problems affecting its profitability. Growing at rates of between 9 per cent and 18 per cent annually, manufacturing in the east grew at 10.9 per cent in 1997 and at 10 per cent in the first half of 1998. Thus, while the region as a whole continues to depend on large-scale transfers from the west, there is a dynamic to the industrial transformation in the east which gives optimism that self-sustaining growth may be possible in the medium term. As will be seen, there remain severe problems of unit costs and profitability, with the burden of the ex-Treuhand firms still readily detectable. Employment in manufacturing in the east appears to have stabilised in 1998, but the sector remains too small for its rapid growth to have a determinant impact on employment evolution and incomes in the region as a whole.[23]

In 1997, there were just 1 million employed in eastern manufacturing, of whom two-fifths worked in small companies of fewer than 20 employees. In the industrial sector, meaning firms of more than 20 employees, only 540,000 employees remained, or one-tenth of total east German employment; such has been the shrinkage since 1990. It is scarcely surprising therefore that manufacturing contributes only 16 per cent to eastern GDP, and only 3 per cent of total German exports. In terms of firm structure, the pattern reflects both the privatisation strategy of the Treuhandanstalt and the rate of new firm creation by west German and foreign investors, and by east Germans themselves. There are now almost no firms left in the hands of the Treuhand successor organisation, the BvS (*Bundesanstalt für vereinigungsbedingte Sonderaufgaben*), although approximately 6,800 privatised firms remain.[24] These represent two-fifths of the manufacturing firms and at the beginning of 1998 accounted for 66 per cent of the industrial workforce.[25] One-half of firms in the sector were established after 1990, and 40 per cent of these are relatively small, subject still to a ruthless selection process.

Of course, it was always a central tenet of the transformation model that a raft of SMEs would offer the best hope for the future in terms of net job growth, entrepreneurial dynamism and structural change. The Treuhand itself had explicitly sought to create such a sector in its small privatisations policy, of selling small enterprises at fixed prices to east German entrepreneurs. Likewise, it also favoured the MBO (management buy-out) of medium-sized companies. In cities such as Leipzig, therefore, in a manufacturing sector dominated by large publicly owned enterprises in 1989, six years later 83 per cent of companies in the sector had fewer than 20 employees. If one were also to include the construction and services sectors, then clearly the city's firm structure is dominated by SMEs.[26] These are subject to considerable financial risk and the majority tend not to survive more than a few years. Further, the east German founders of such companies often have inadequate management training and development policy tends to be poorly targeted on such companies, in spite of official rhetoric.

In terms of the branch structure of these manufacturing enterprises, it is apparent that there have been structural shifts which reinforce differences between the old and the new *Länder*. Of course, the kernel of west German industry, the metalworking, electrical engineering, chemical and food-processing industries, are all well represented in the east. However, there are significant differences, such as that the chemical industry has only one-half the proportionate share of that in the west, while the food and metalworking industries have a representation twice as strong. The deviations in branch structure between west and east have increased significantly since 1990 (such that the sum of the deviations from the average was 50 per cent greater in 1997 than in 1990).[27] This reflects the federal policy of high levels of support to consumption and construction activity in the east, as well as the politically induced support by the Treuhandanstalt for the heavy industrial core. Thus branches such as food-processing, printing and building materials, which serve a regional market, are over-represented, as are steel, rolling-stock, shipbuilding and machine tools industries, all of which received extremely high levels of liquidity support when they were in Treuhand ownership.

The competitiveness of the manufacturing sector has grown rapidly, with a narrowing of productivity and unit cost differentials with the west, induced partly by new capacity coming on stream, and also by a better control of wage costs in recent years. Productivity in the east has risen fourfold over the period 1991–97, under the influence of very severe labour shedding and replacement of moribund industrial capacity. The very heavy investments in car and computer equipment manufacture have generated rapid productivity growth in these branches, and this applies to a lesser extent in instruments technologies. Low productivity growth has been experienced in food processing, textiles and leather goods, as well as branches such as rolling-stock and shipbuilding, so long under Treuhand control. Overall, manufacturing productivity in the east lay at 30 per cent below western levels in 1998.[28]

These improvements reflect in part the heavy investment undertaken in the region since 1990, even if there have been marked fluctuations by branch and through time. Thus the high growth rates in investment of the years 1992 and 1993 (of 25 per cent and 10 per cent, respectively) could not be sustained in later years, and in fact investment volumes have fallen with the low GDP growth since 1997. However, by the end of 1996, the stock of manufacturing investment per employee reached DM143,000 in the east, compared with DM255,000 in the old *Länder*.[29] There were, however, important differences according to the origin of the firm: in 1997, firms owned by west Germans or foreigners invested DM35,000 per employee, while east German-owned firms invested DM21,500 and ex-Treuhand firms DM24,300 (or only DM5,000 in 1996). This reflects the fact that locally owned firms tend to be smaller, and that there remain significant restructuring and profitability problems among ex-Treuhand firms. 'Greenfield' investments from scratch appear to have presented far fewer problems. Overall, the structure of investment in eastern manufacturing displays a greater concentration in the more capital intensive branches than does west German investment, which may reflect the high levels of investment offered as regional assistance.

Firms in east Germany report that they have retired old plant and that they achieve satisfactory levels of capacity utilisation. The fact that only one-half of manufacturing firms achieved a profit in 1997, and that one-quarter continued to suffer losses requires further investigation. Overall, the sector incurred losses equal to −1.8 per cent of turnover in 1997, compared with profits of 1.2 per cent in the west. It appears that smaller firms, with a turnover of less than DM5 million, have been enjoying good returns, while larger firms, with a turnover of more than DM10 million, have suffered losses. This reflects once again the fact that there are far too few high performance medium and large firms: in this size category, the ex-Treuhand enterprises depress the results such that 30 per cent of this group incurred losses in 1997, while only 15 per cent of firms established since 1990 did. We return then to the question of wage costs, since, although the effective wage cost level (including non-wage labour costs) in manufacturing lies at 80 per cent of the western level, the unit labour costs, taking account of productivity remain 25 per cent higher than in the west. The wage cost burden is particularly high in ex-Treuhand firms of the old 'industrial core', namely, the chemicals, shipbuilding and engineering branches: in chemicals, for example, unit wage costs in 1997 were twice as high as net value-added in the industry.[30] As will be seen below, smaller firms have more easily escaped the crushing pressures of wage harmonisation in the east, by leaving the industrial relations machinery, while ex-Treuhand firms and subsidiaries of large western companies have struggled to contain the costs of rapidly rising wage levels.

Studies, such as that of the Institut für Arbeitsmarkt-und Berufs-forschung (IAB; Research Institute for Labour Market and Occupational Questions) in 1999,[31] take the view that it will in future be more difficult for east German companies to narrow the productivity gap with the west, since such companies already operate largely with post-1990 machinery and near or at full-capacity working. Rather, what this indicates is a focus in the east on goods of lower R&D intensity, and on products which are lower in the price/quality range. The IAB noted, for example, that although investments per head in east German firms between 1993 and 1996 ran at levels twice as high as in the west, nevertheless investments in research intensive and high value-added areas of manufacturing represented only 50 per cent of investment, compared with 55 per cent in the west. However, the employment levels in east German firms appeared to have stabilised in total in 1997–98. While in 1996–97, employment levels in 400,000 east German firms fell by 150,000 persons, they stabilised in the later period at 5.9 million employees.[32] Overall, it is clear that the east German manufacturing sector displays very significant differences when compared with that of the west, and that in terms of branch structure, these differences have widened since unification. In spite of the shrinkage in the relative weight of ex-Treuhand firms, it remains the case that the lower investment rates, the high unit labour costs and the continuing poor profitability of many of these ex-state firms act to depress overall performance of the manufacturing sector in the east.

'NICHT NACH WESTMODELL': INCOMPLETE TRANSFORMATION OR FACETS OF AN 'EASTERN' MODEL?

The above discussion illuminates the point that, in the deeply painful process of transition to the market, to which the east German economy was exposed overnight on 1 July 1990 with the introduction of economic, monetary and social union, the fundamental changes wrought have in certain important respects continued to maintain a regional economy different from that of the west. In an obvious sense, the continuing very high unemployment, the all-pervasive second labour market measures, the shrunken size of the manufacturing sector, the heavy reliance on financial transfers, accounting still for over 30 per cent of regional income, all denote the dependence which arises when a low productivity region is rapidly absorbed into an advanced industrial economy. The discussion above of the contemporary manufacturing structure of east Germany shows that there are not only important quantitative, but also qualitative differences with the west. Structurally, the inherited burden of the Treuhand enterprises in the old industrial sectors is still felt: as stated, these tend to be more loss-making and have lower investment rates. The many new firms tend, of course, to be smaller and to serve local markets. They are financially very insecure, but tend to make a profit, which reflects in part the fact that they often lie outside the tariff wage negotiating machinery. The subsidiaries of west German or international firms have invested heavily in the most up-to-date technology and represent a core for the reconstructed manufacturing sector: however, their profitability at present is uncertain. Again, a key influence here is the extent to which firms take part in the national wage negotiating machinery, or whether firms have left their employers' association to escape the pressures of wage harmonisation (*Tarifflucht*). As will be seen, two-thirds of east German firms, and almost 40 per cent of employees now lie outside the German wage bargaining system, such have been the pressures to reduce wage costs.

The distortion of the west German social market model can be found in the operation of the labour market in the east, with for example, the all-pervasive second labour market measures representing a high level of subsidisation. In the shape of the so-called '*Beschäftigungsgesellschaften*' (essentially firms consisting of job creation places, designed as an instrument to ameliorate large-scale lay-offs from labour-shedding Treuhand firms) there was a direct and heavily subsidised competitive challenge to the small-scale, newly established private firms in the east. The erosion of collective bargaining, assessed in some detail below, is a further major departure from the western model. In other, significant, parts of the east German economy, whether in agriculture, electricity supply or social housing, distinctive structures or regimes remain in place, which reflect an incomplete transformation to the federal German system. Lastly, the scale of industrial subsidies, and in cases their misapplication, represents also a major departure from federal German practice and a continuing source of tension with Brussels. In each of these areas, developments and policy remain different from those in the west, and one may pose the question whether they display an incomplete transformation towards the western social market model, or whether they represent a more 'eastern' model, which may persist. Furthermore, given the stresses at European level of integration, both among states in the eurozone, and consequent upon the accession of central European states, one may seek to draw some general conclusions for EU integration from the policy experience in east Germany itself.

Adaptation or Erosion of the Collective Wage Bargaining System in the East?

The *Stufentarifverträge* (wage harmonisation contracts) which were negotiated by west German unions such as IG Metall and IG Druck in autumn and winter 1990 for their industrial sectors in east Germany imposed a staged adaptation of the eastern wage levels to the western by mid-1994.[33] The western collective bargaining system had been extended to the east by the State Treaty and so the negotiated, rapid wage increases became almost programmed in the new *Länder*. They were mandatory for all employers who were members of their trade association, and they spread generally throughout the economy, because of the pilot nature of the early wage settlements and because of the broad coverage of the collective wage agreements. Of course, the Treuhand managers who helped negotiate these harmonisation agreements had little personal stake in the survival of their large 'combine' monopolistic enterprises, soon to be broken up: it was argued that wage equality was needed to ensure equality of living conditions in east and west, and to prevent large-scale migration of labour to the west. It might also be added that social benefits were closely linked to earnings and therefore rising collective wage rates would guarantee higher social benefits for those displaced from their jobs. Equally, the western unions feared above all else the undercutting of their wage levels by a cheap labour region on their doorsteps.[34] After a serious strike in the metal industry in 1993 over employer attempts to break the harmonisation commitment, harmonisation was delayed until mid-1996. Among analysts, there are marked differences of view in their assessment of the impact of this application of west German collective bargaining practices to the east. Industrial relations analysts tend to stress the adaptability of the system, with flexibility and innovation being displayed in the east. Among economists, as here in this study, the stress is placed on the damaging impact of wage harmonisation on the competitiveness of eastern firms: it generated unit wage costs, taking account of the low productivity levels, which in 1993 were 70 per cent above the west German rate, and therefore possibly the highest in the world. Even at the end of 1998, eastern unit costs lay on average about 25 per cent above those of the west. The fact that social benefits were index-linked to wages offered the assurance of a safety net, but drove the financial cost of welfare spending to previously unimagined levels, and imposed ever-higher social insurance rates on employers and employees.

In principle, tariff wage rates, as set out by the collective wage agreements, became aligned on western levels in mid-1996. This was the case for employees in the public sector, and in sectors such as metalworking, mechanical and electrical engineering and chemicals. However, even where the tariff weekly wage equates to the western, there are large differences in the hourly wage, the effective wage paid and total wage costs. Thus, since the east German working week stands at 38 hours (35 hours in the west), hourly rates paid differ, west Germans receive better holiday pay, a thirteenth month payment, higher shift bonuses and, generally, their employers pay at rates above the tariff wage. Hence, the effective pay rate in the east can be significantly lower; non-wage labour costs borne by the employer are also far less for similar reasons.[35] Thus, the average gross (monthly) wage in the east in June 1998 amounted to DM3,130 or 79 per cent of the western level. In eastern manufacturing, the proportion was 69 per cent. Small firms often paid significantly lower rates, such that in firms of fewer than four employees the average wage was of DM2,460, compared with DM3,900 in firms of more than 500 employees.³⁶ Overall, the narrowing of pay levels with the west has come largely to a halt in the last two years.

It was clear from early in the transition that newly established small firms, particularly those in the service sector, were paying at rates below the collective wage. For established firms to do so legally, they had to leave their employers' association and establish a firm-level wage agreement negotiated in the works council, or to issue individual pay contracts to each staff member annually. Employer–union tensions in the metalworking and engineering sector in the east had been running especially high because of the high 1995 IG Metall pay settlement and because of IG Metall's insistence that the working week in the east be reduced to 35 hours. An upstart rival union, the Christliche Metallgewerkschaft, had begun to sign house agreements with engineering firms at much lower rates, and the VDMA, the Saxony and Thüringian engineering employers' association, threatened to negotiate with this rival to the seemingly all-powerful IG Metall. In 1996, the IG Metall proposed an 'Alliance for Jobs in the East', which would allow, by joint agreement, special measures to be taken by firms in chronic financial difficulties to offer lower opening pay rates and less than tariff rates, on the basis of an agreed 'hardship' clause. Although such clauses had been negotiated earlier by the chemical industry and its union, nevertheless, these innovations by IG Metall represented a breach, however, small, in the general application of the collectively agreed tariff wage. More recently, in September 1998, IG Metall agreed with the eastern representatives of Gesamtmetall, the engineering employers, that, at the price of a delay until after the year 2000 in the reduction of the working week, the eastern employers would accept the nationally agreed collective wage increases for the sector, after an interval of one month. In this way, IG Metall secured a standard wage increase for the country as a whole, so eliminating the prospect of separate eastern negotiations and pay rates. However, with the very high wage settlement effectively imposed by IG Metall in March 1999, many more employers threatened to leave the negotiating machinery and either negotiate a house agreement with the Christliche Metallgewerkschaft (such as Carl Zeiss Jena has done in the optical industry) or negotiate directly with their employees.³⁷

In 1998, 66 per cent of eastern firms with 38 per cent of employees lay outside the collective bargaining machinery (compared with 47 per cent of firms in the west). Within this group, 26 per cent had agreed a branch-level pay rate and 8 per cent had a house agreement. Among east German-owned firms, the coverage of the collective agreements is even lower.³⁸ Some analysts perceive in this the decay of the formal collective bargaining system in the east, while others stress that the locus of bargaining has simply shifted to the level of plant agreements. However, there has been a huge shrinkage in the coverage of the metal-working collective agreement, for example, which points to an erosion. In 1990, there were 1,192 firms in the east with 500,000 employees which were members of the Gesamtmetall engineering employers' association. By 1997, principally as a result of the slump, but also because of *Tarifflucht*, there were 564 firms with only 108,000 employees covered.[39] East Germany threatens to become a 'tariff wage-free zone', which poses the question whether this is a signal for the future for west Germany, or whether reforms can be introduced there to make the collective wage agreement system much more adaptable, before a similar erosion gathers speed.

Incomplete Transformation in the Agricultural, Electrical Power and Housing Sectors

Traditionally, sectors such as these have been regulated in mixed economies for reasons of income support, social justice or natural monopoly, and regulatory regimes continue in place to a greater or lesser extent, although they acknowledge market mechanisms more than in the past. In east Germany, however, transitional regimes remain in being so as to moderate the profound adjustments needed to transform inherited structures more closely to the western pattern.

The agricultural sector

The East German agricultural sector under the GDR regime comprised huge state and cooperative farms, the result of the Soviet imposed land reform from 1945–49, and of forced collectivisation in stages through to a final amalgamation in 1960. In the early 1970s, the 'industrialisation of farming' created huge enterprises, specialised into livestock and dairying or arable, often of 4,000 ha–7,000 ha in size.[40] Compared with the highly fragmented west German farms, often managed by part-time farmers, this structure represented an extreme in concentration. From 1990, legislation favoured the break-up of the state and collective farms, together with the restitution of land to previous owners, except in the key case of expropriations undertaken during the land reform period of 1945–49, which was excluded explicitly by the Unification Treaty. The legislation allowed those in cooperative farms to take back the land and assets they had contributed under the voluntary, later forced, phases of collectivisation: they could then set up as self-employed farmers, establish cooperatives under federal law, or they could create companies of the GbR (Gesellschaft bürgerlichen Rechts) form, which leased extra land or bought re-privatised land. In practice, and to the disappointment of the

Kohl government, many cooperative farmers also chose to adopt this status under federal law.

Unification brought a catastrophic drop in employment in farming, with a fall from the original 880,000 employees to just 180,000, with the impact felt primarily in the first two years, such was the competitive pressure of the change to CAP pricing! Most livestock cooperatives switched to the more extensive cereal growing. The result of these changes has been that the farm structure in the east remains the polar opposite of that in the west, and in the EU as a whole.[41] On average, farms are of 1,160 ha in size, compared with 29 ha in the west, and there are 140 ha per full-time farmer, compared with 40 ha in the west. In the sugar-beet and wheat-growing areas of the fertile *Börde*, together with the morains of Mecklenburg-Vorpommern, these huge farms could become profitable at close to world prices. The Treuhand successor company, the BVVA, responsible for the restitution and privatisation of the 500,000 ha of forest and 1,087,000 ha of farmland still under its control,[42] sold land, until December 1998, at less than one-half the market value to those expropriated under the Soviet land reform, to cooperatives, or to new settlers in farming. This policy was ruled by the EU Competition Directorate to contravene competition rules in respect of the aid shown to new farmers, and so all sales have been suspended.[43] More critically for the farm sector as a whole in the east, the 'Agenda 2000' proposals for the reform of the CAP, to make it capable of extension to central European countries when they gain EU admission early in the next decade, would have had a significant impact on the revenues of these huge farms. The proposals included the key provision that compensation for price cuts would only be paid to farms of less than a specified size, in what would have hit the east German farms badly; 70 per cent of all the cuts in farm aid to Germany under these proposals would have been borne by the east. Clearly, the federal government rejected any such settlement, and the final, heavily diluted reforms agreed in late March 1999 bore no upper limit to compensation.[44]

Electricity supply

On electricity supply, the main regional generating company, VEAG (Vereinigte Energiewerke AG) was granted a quasi-monopoly until 2002, so as to protect and assist the rationalisation of the two main brown coalfields, the Lausitzer Braunkohle AG and the Mitteldeutsche Braunkohle AG. VEAG's main shareholders comprise the largest west German generators, Preussenelektra, Bayernwerk and RWE. In order to promote an orderly restructuring of these lignite fields, a higher electricity price was permitted in the east, which adds to the cost burden of regional

economic activity. Thus the substantial electricity price falls of
approximately 10 per cent for households and up to 25 per cent for
companies, which have occurred following liberalisation in the west, have
not benefited eastern companies. Nevertheless, rapid changes in the
predominantly municipally owned local power distribution networks are
happening in response to the fundamental pressures being exerted by
liberalisation of power supply, and cities such as Berlin and Leipzig have
been in the forefront of privatisation programmes for the municipal
utilities.[45]

The housing market
The housing market in the east exhibits very distinctive features, even nine
years after unification.[46] As would be expected, the inheritance from the
command economy includes a low level of owner occupation (at 31.1 per
cent in early 1999, compared with 41 per cent in the west), and high levels
of social housing, particularly of the workers' apartments in the inner cities
(*Mietskasernen*) and the grey, corroding, tower block estates on the urban
periphery, built on prefabricated lines (*Plattenbau*).[47] A high proportion of
the social housing is owned by housing associations linked to the
municipalities which inherited this decayed stock after unification. The
inevitably large rent rises, from the absurdly low levels prevailing under
central planning, have been less than the rise in average incomes, as
specified by the Unification Treaty. Further, a combination of rent
controls and housing allowances through the 1990s have moderated the
impact of rent rises. Controls remain in place limiting the extent to which
modernisation costs can be passed on to the tenant. However, in the
present context, a key difference with the west remains the overwhelming
dominance of social housing, in spite of the manifest policy aim of the
Kohl government to privatise a part of the stock, partly for ideological
reasons, but perhaps more out of the need to reduce housing debt levels as
well as to raise capital for improvements to the remainder of the public
rented stock.
    Privatisation targets were set in 1993 for public housing associations in
exchange for a write-down of part of their inherited debt from the GDR
regime. However, given the manifest disinterest among the east German
public in purchasing a social housing apartment (though not, it should be
said, in house ownership as such), housing associations have had to resort
to the *Zwischenerwerber* (interim-owner) model. This transfers ownership
of a fraction of the stock to an independent association, created by the
public housing association. The result is the illusion of more market-
related provision, when in practice the social housing character of much
housing provision in the east remains unchanged.[48]

Subsidies and Conflicts with Brussels over Competition Policy

Given the scale of German transfers to the east, it will be of no surprise that the Federal Republic accounted on average for 45 per cent of the total state aid given by the EU 12 member states in 1993–95 and 37 per cent for the same EU12 in the years 1995–97.[49] In practice, in terms of assistance per employee, German aid lies below the Italian level, and if measured in terms of value-added in industry, then German assistance occupies only a middle ranking among the EU's subsidisers. Compared with the UK, however, German aid per employed person was almost seven times the British level in the years 1995 and 1996.[50] These large transfers, which tend to benefit east Germany (if one leaves aside the very sizeable assistance to the coal industry) have naturally attracted the attention of the EU Competition Directorate. In a number of celebrated cases, the EU Commission has insisted on aid repayment, or has at least investigated the detailed level of assistance. Primarily, the cases concern the misapplication by recipient firms of liquidity credits and investment assistance accorded by the Treuhandanstalt to assist restructuring and privatisation; but there have also been disputes with the federal and some *Land* governments over regional aid. Such cases include regional aid to Volkswagen in Saxony (where the company did not abide by capacity limiting agreements with the EU Commission), the mistransfer of funds among the successor companies to the SKET machine tools firm in Magdeburg, the misappropriation of financial assistance by the Bremer Vulkan shipyard group paid to its eastern shipyards, and fraudulent dealings by the Werkstoff Union petrochemical works. Given the scale of assistance by the Treuhand and its successors in the case of the old industrial core, it is scarcely surprising that Brussels competition authorities have paid close attention, particularly as in such industries there can be capacity limiting agreements at European level.[51]

Although the Treuhandanstalt closed its doors at the end of 1994, in 1998 its main successor institution, the BvS, still held significant shares in perhaps the most troublesome of the old industrial core companies. These included a 40 per cent share in the EkoStahl GmbH, which had received several billions of Deutschmarks in Treuhand assistance, a 33 per cent share in the Leuna refinery, a 20 per cent share in the Buna Olefin chemical project, in which DM9bn of public money had already been injected, and holdings in Kali und Salz, the main eastern potash producer. The BvS is still seeking to resolve difficulties over the two successor companies to the SKET machine tools company.[52] When one considers that almost DM30bn of public funds had been paid for the restructuring and clean-up of the chemicals triangle of Buna-Leuna-Bitterfeld (which retains a

workforce in these activities of just 2,800) and that the cost of protecting
the remaining workforce in the shipyards had totalled DM1 million per
job, then scrutiny by the competition authorities may be thought to have
been justified.

THE SCALE OF LABOUR MARKET AND WELFARE SUPPORT THREATENS TO UNDERMINE THE FINANCIAL STABILITY OF THE SOCIAL INSURANCE FUNDS

The fact that three-quarters of public transfers to the east have comprised
income support payments, and that one-half of all transfers were met by
public borrowing rather than by tax or social insurance contribution
increases, shows the extent to which serious public finance problems were
building up as a result of unification. Quite simply, mass unemployment
combined with the application very largely unmodified, of the western
welfare system and its relatively generous income guarantee levels, led to
the build-up of liabilities. Interest charges on public debt rose from 11 per
cent of tax revenues in 1990 to 15 per cent in 1997.[53] Within the DM888bn
of net public transfers from 1991–97, there were DM199bn paid by the
Federal Labour Office and DM80bn paid by the pension insurance
funds.[54] The east German health insurance funds remained separate until
recently, but again required heavy subvention. Of course, the key causes of
these costs are not difficult to perceive. The almost 2 million workers in
1992 who received short-time working or unemployment pay, the 21 per
cent of the eastern workforce unemployed in January 1998 and the 750,000
workers who were early retired in the period 1990–95, all point to the costs
of alleviating mass unemployment. The fact that such individuals had a
claim to income-related benefits points to the social justice in the German
system; it does, however, generate large-scale financial liabilities. In recent
years, there has been endless debate of the crisis in the German welfare
system, with continuing attempts through the 1990s under the Kohl
government to reform the pensions, health and social benefits systems.[55] It
is the case that longer-term secular pressures will force changes in these
welfare arrangements because of their unaffordability, but through the
1990s the so-called crisis of the welfare state has been caused largely by the
burdens of unification, since the western pension and unemployment
benefit funds have themselves shown surpluses over this period.[56]

ARE THERE LESSONS FROM THE EAST GERMAN EXPERIENCE FOR EMU AND EASTERN ENLARGEMENT?

In important ways, the east German experience is *sui generis*. Also, the debates over the design and conduct of the Treuhand's privatisation programme have less bearing on central European countries, since privatisation there is well advanced and the main steps in their transition to a market economy are in place.[57] However, the east German experience does help reinforce a number of principles which remain valid for EMU and eastern EU enlargement. EMU has brought together under a common currency regime countries with quite marked differences in levels of development, in economic structure and productivity. The loss of the exchange rate bodes badly for a country which loses competitiveness. This points to the requirement particularly for wage flexibility, and counsels against any strategy for wage harmonisation. Given the costs to the federal social security budgets outlined above, one should also advise against any harmonisation of social welfare systems which include fiscal transfers between countries, since the risk of large-scale support for a long-term backward region could not be countenanced. Regional assistance measures might also be most effective in developing skills and industries of the future, rather than in propping up at great cost older industries which will in any perceived future shrink in importance. These points also apply in broad terms to central European states acceding to the EU. Above all, the siren voices calling for their membership of EMU should be shunned; they should adopt an appropriate, adjustable peg exchange rate regime (such as ERM membership) and should seek faster growth to converge on EU levels by productivity improvements and by keeping a keen eye on their competitiveness. In this way they may restructure and re-equip over a longer time period without the destruction and employment losses endured by east Germany.

NOTES

1. EC Commission, *General Report on the Activities of the Community* (Brussels: EU Commission, 1991).
2. E. Owen Smith, *The German Economy* (London: Routledge, 1994).
3. For discussion see 'Sachverständigenrat zur Begutachtung der gesamtwirtschaftlichen Entwicklung', *Jahresgutachten, 1995/6, 1997/8* (Stuttgart: Metzler-Poeschel, 1995, 1997).
4. K. Dyson, 'The Economic Order – Still Modell Deutschland?', in G. Smith *et al.* (eds), *Developments in German Politics*, 2 (London: Macmillan, 1996), pp. 194–210; E. Owen Smith, 'The German Model and European Integration', in K. Larres (ed.), *Germany since Unification* (Basingstoke: Macmillan, 1998), pp. 151–73.
5. D. Swann, *The Economics of the Common Market*, 8th edn (London: Penguin, 1995).
6. See Swann, *The Economics*; K. Armstrong and S. Bulmer, *The Governance of the Single European*

Market (Manchester: MUP, 1998).

7. C. H. Flockton, 'The German Economy and the Single Market', *Politics and Society in Germany, Austria and Switzerland*, Vol. 2/3 (1990), pp. 54–71.
8. C. H. Flockton, 'The Federal German Economy in the early 1990s', *German Politics*, Vol.2/No.2 (1993), pp. 312–27.
9. J-M. Lohse, *Die grosse Blockade* (Frankfurt am Main: Campus Verlag, 1997); 'Sachverständigenrat zur Begutachtung der Gesamtwirtschaftlichen Entwicklung', *Jahresgutachten 1997/98* (Stuttgart: Metzler-Poeschel, 1997); J. Story and I. Walter, *Political Economy of Financial Integration in Europe* (Manchester: MUP, 1997).
10. *Financial Times*, 22 April 1999; *Handelsblatt*, various.
11. C. H. Flockton, 'The Federal German Economy'; E. Owen Smith, *The German Economy*; G. Sinn and H-W. Sinn, *Jumpstart* (Cambridge, MA: MIT, 1992); A. Ghanie Ghaussy and W. Schäfer, *The Economics of German Unification* (London: Routledge, 1993).
12. G. A. Akerlof *et al.*, 'East Germany in from the Cold: The Economic Aftermath of Currency Union', *Brookings Papers on Economic Activity*, Vol. 1, 1991, pp. 1–105; A. J. Hughes Hallett and Y. Ma, 'East Germany, West Germany, and their Mezzogiorno Problem: A Parable for European Economic Integration', *Economic Journal*, Vol. 103 (1993), pp. 416–28.
13. C. H. Flockton, 'The Federal German Economy'.
14. H. Nick, 'An Unparallelled Destruction and Squandering of Economic Assets', in A. Behrendt, *German Unification: The Destruction of an Economy* (London: Pluto, 1993).
15. Arbeitsgruppe Alternative Wirtschaftspolitik, *Memorandum '92* (Köln: PRV, 1992).
16. Report by BvS, *Handelsblatt*, 6 March 1999.
17. Bundesministerium für Finanzen, *16ter Subventionsbericht*, Bonn, 28 August 1997; Bundesministeriumfür Wirtschaft, *ERP-Wirtschaftsförderung für den Mittelstand*, Bonn, April 1997.
18. Bundesministerium für Finanzen, *16ter Subventionsbericht…* ; EU Commission, *6th Survey on State Aid*, Brussels, 1997.
19. EU Commission, *7th Survey on State Aid*, Brussels, April 1999.
20. C. H. Flockton, 'The German Economy since 1989/90: Problems and Prospects', in K. Larres, *Germany since Unification* (Basingstoke: Macmillan, 1998).
21. C. H. Flockton, 'The German Economy'.
22. Deutsche Bundesbank, 'Zur Wirtschaftslage in Ostdeutschland', *Monthly Report*, April 1998; 'Zur Wirtschaftslage in den neuen Ländern und Berlin-Ost', in *Wirtschaft und Statistik*, March 1998, pp. 183–212.
23. *Wirtschaft und Statistik*, various.
24. *Handelsblatt*, 6 March 1999.
25. 'Gesamtwirtschaftliche und unternehmerische Anpassungsfortschritte in Ostdeutschland, 18ter Bericht', *DIW Wochenbericht*, 33 (1998), pp. 571–609.
26. E. Kolinsky, 'In Search of a Future: Leipzig since the Wende', *German Society and Politics*, Vol. 16, No. 4 (1998), pp. 103–21.
27. 'Gesamtwirtschaftliche'.
28. 'Betriebspanel Ostdeutschland', IAB Report, *Handelsblatt*, 27 March 1999.
29. 'Betriebspanel', 'Gesamtwirtschaftliche'.
30. 'Gesamtwirtschaftliche'.
31. 'Betriebspanel'.
32. *Handelsblatt*, 29 March 1999, p. 7.
33. K. Koch, 'The Impact of German Unification on the German Industrial Relations System', *German Politics*, Vol. 4, No. 3 (1995), pp. 145–55.
34. L. Turner, *Negotiating the New Germany* (Ithaca: IRL, 1997).
35. 'Einkommensanpassung in den neuen Ländern verliert an Tempo', *DIW Wochenbericht*, 37 (1998), pp. 707–15.
36. 'Betriebspanel'.
37. *Handelsblatt*, various.
38. 'Betriebspanel'.
39. *Handelsblatt*, 2 February 1999.
40. Deutsches Institut für Wirtschaftsforschung (ed.), *Handbuch DDR-Wirtschaft* (Reinbek: Rowohlt, 1985).
41. Statistisches Bundesamt, *Statistisches Jahrbuch 1998* (Stuttgart: Metzler-Poeschel, 1998).
42. *Handelsblatt*, 13 January 1998.

43. *Handelsblatt*, 27 March 1999.
44. *Handelsblatt*, 24 March 1999.
45. *Handelsblatt*, various.
46. C. H. Flockton, 'Housing Situation and Housing Policy in East Germany', *German Politics*, Vol.7, No. 3 (1998), pp. 70–82.
47. 'Haus- und Grundbesitz sowie Wohnverhältnisse privater Haushalte in Deutschland', *Wirtschaft und Statistik*, 3 (1999), pp. 210–20.
48. C. H. Flockton, 'Housing Situation'.
49. EU Commission, *7th Survey on State Aid* (Brussels: EU Commission, April 1999), p. 30.
50. EU Commission, *7th Survey*, p. 30.
51. *Handelsblatt*, various.
52. *Handelsblatt*, 1 January 1999.
53. Deutsche Bundestag, *Jahresbericht zum Stande der deutschen Einheit*, Drucksache 13/8450 (1997).
54. U. Heilemann and H. Ruppen, 'Sieben Jahre deutsche Einheit: Rückblick und Perspektiven aus fiskalischer Sicht', *Aus Politik und Zeitgeschichte*, B40–1 (1997), pp. 38–46.
55. C. H. Flockton, 'Germany's Long-Running Fiscal Strains: Unification Costs or Unsustainability of Welfare State Arrangements?', *Debatte*, Vol. 6, No. 1 (1998), pp. 79–93; *OECD Economic Survey*, Germany (Paris: OECD, 1997), p. 66ff.; (1998), pp. 65–6.
56. 'Vereinigungskosten belasten Sozialversicherung', *DIW Wochenbericht*, 40 (1997), pp. 725–9.
57. EBRD, *Transformation Report*, 1996, 1998 (London: EBRD).

Part II

Ten Years On: The New Germany since Unification

5

Perceptions of GDR Society and its Transformation: East German Identity Ten Years after Unity

Mike Dennis

AMBIVALENT ATTITUDES CONTINUE TO DIVIDE

Drawing on an extensive corpus of empirical research, both before and after 1990, and a variety of theoretical insights, this chapter seeks to explore the contours of the identity of east Germans – *Ostidentität* – and to explain why a psychological unity and a common social identity have not been achieved a decade after political unification. Despite an apparent reaffirmation of ethnic solidarity and the establishment of a 'normal' nation-state with a clearly defined territory, it soon became clear that the issue of German national identity had lost none of its capacity to generate controversy and taxonomic confusion. Towards the end of 1992, the weekly magazine *Der Spiegel* homed in on opinion poll results which testified to a *'Mauer im Kopf'* (Wall in the head), with a clear majority of east and west Germans concurring with the statement that: 'The Wall has gone but the wall in people's heads grows'.[1]

This east–west mental divide is perhaps hardly surprising in the light of the fact that the turbulent unification process of the 1990s had been preceded by the asymmetrical socio-economic, cultural and political development of the two German republics for more than four decades. Furthermore, despite GDR citizens' vicarious experience of a 'cultural community' through west German television and radio programmes, the construction of a national identity had been impeded by the former east and west German states' ambivalent attitudes and divergent approaches to the national question. The heated objections to Helmut Kohl's decision in the early 1990s to utilise Schinkel's *Neue Wache* (New Guardhouse) on Unter den Linden as a national memorial to the 'victims of tyranny and war', on the grounds that the chancellor's project implied an equality between German oppressors and their victims, aptly demonstrates the intractable problems inherent in constructing a national identity out of a fractured past and and a fractious present.

Although *Ostidentität* is not a monolithic construct and needs to be differentiated according to criteria such as age, social position, political affiliation and gender, the wide gap between easterners (*Ossis*) and westerners (*Wessis*) as regards perceptions of unification, interpretations of the past and mutual stereotyping justify the use of the term in the singular. Indeed, *Ostidentität* is so distinctive that it transcends the traditional regional disparities which have long persisted between the north and south of the old Federal Republic. Eastern identity comprises a series of shared values, common traditions and shared experiences of the GDR past as well as a feeling of segregation – even estrangement – from the dominant culture of west Germany. However, while the east–west divide is undoubtedly substantial, two qualifications need to be made. The territorial integrity of the new nation-state, unlike that of many communist successor states, is not under challenge as few east Germans call for a restoration of the GDR. And, second, inner disunity must not be overstated as value convergence manifests itself in the widespread support in both east and west Germany for political pluralism, the principle of consensus in policymaking and consumerism.

Like German national identity, *Ostidentität* is not an 'essentialist, Herderian quality'[2] but a set of changing attitudes and values. The severe disruption since 1990 to so many lives has produced changes not only to the value hierarchy but also to the content of certain values inherited from the GDR era. Thus, for example, of the values central to *Ostidentität* – work, social security and personal safety – the latter has gained in importance as a result of a higher incidence of crime and violence. In contrast, while partnership, having children and good health retain a high position, they no longer enjoy their former pre-eminence.[3] Perceptions of work have changed dramatically as employment has become far more crucial as a determinant of social status and financial security. This shift can be seen in the above-average rating of 97 per cent attached to the importance of work as a facet of their lives by people in labour creation schemes as against the 73 per cent rating attracted by 'partnership'. Other attributes deemed to constitute *Ostidentität* are: a feeling of inferiority shared by many towards west Germans; a keen awareness of the benefits and losses of unification; and a multiplicity of identifications with the locality, the *Land* and the national community, albeit with a stronger bias than in the west towards the (eastern German) region.

While *Ostidentität* is certainly not coterminous with GDR identity,[4] it draws on experiences, norms and behavioural traits manifest in the GDR as can be seen in the high expectations of the state as a social provider. In addition, eastern approval of socialism as an idea runs at a much higher level than among *Wessis*. In the east, support fluctuates between 58 and 72 per cent and in the west from 30 to 35 per cent.[5] Nowadays, many east Germans associate socialism with positive features such as the right to a job, social justice, fixed rents and the right to pre-school childcare.[6] This perception of socialism resonates with the *soziale Geborgenheit*, that is, the social protection and security extended by the SED regime to its subjects in the form of guaranteed jobs, low prices for basic foodstuffs, cheap rents, free health care and so forth. While the paternalistic social welfare system may be regarded as the 'friendlier' face of the GDR, in contrast to the many coercive aspects, its drawbacks must not be overlooked. For example, the strategy of social pacification and the reduction of risk, belittled by some observers as reducing east Germans to 'babes-in-arms',[7] left many *Ossis* ill-equipped to adjust to the acute stresses of economic and social transformation and is a major reason for the development of the 'wall in people's heads'. Although this chapter will focus on this aspect of the 'socialist legacy', it would, of course, be misleading to treat it as the sole determinant of the east–west mental divide; consequently, alternative and/or complementary explanations of 'inner disunity' and popular dissatisfaction will be examined in later sections, notably the current socio-economic context and east Germans' response to, and perception of, their treatment by *Wessis*.

TRANSFORMATION BY UNIFICATION

The introduction of the Deutschmark and the rapid transformation of the GDR by incorporation into the Federal Republic were legitimised by the *Volkskammer* election in March 1990. Unification was the outcome, above all, of east Germans' wish to share in the prosperity and freedom of west Germany, but it was also facilitated by a sense of a common German ethnic identity. The unification process was initially accompanied by a wave of optimism which bordered on euphoria. Between February and October 1990, public opinion polls conducted in the GDR indicated that between 62 per cent and 72 per cent were 'optimistic' or 'optimistic rather than pessimistic' about their personal future. Belief in an economic miracle was widespread: 13 per cent confidently expected one, 51 per cent believed it probable.[8] And unification has indeed brought many benefits: the incorporation of the GDR into proven west German institutions, laws, and regulations; access to a wider range of consumables; freedom to travel; political pluralism; and the constitutional commitment to ensure the equality of living conditions in the Federal Republic. Financial transfers from west to east, amounting to DM1.37 trillion gross between 1991 and 1998, provide east Germans with a far higher level of social security and consumer power than in any other post-communist state. Net wages and incomes have risen so rapidly that they stand at about 86 per cent of west German levels in 1998 as against 54.7 per cent in 1991.[9] Pensions, which take full account of years of working in the GDR, are even closer to western levels, making pensioners major beneficiaries of unification. The improvement in living standards finds expression not only in income increases but also in the virtual parity between eastern and western households in the possession of TVs, video recorders, mobile phones, refrigerators, washing machines, new cars and video cameras. Such benefits have not gone unnoticed. Many easterners appreciate that they are better off than in 1990 and only a small minority favour a renewed socialism or the communist economic system over the market variant.[10]

GROWING APART TOGETHER?

Yet, growing together has proved far more difficult and painful than anticipated. Disenchantment mounted in the course of 1991 when unemployment and short-time working rocketed in the wake of price liberalisation, the sudden exposure to global markets and the privatisation of state assets. The vale of tears predicted by Ralf Dahrendorf, rather than Helmut Kohl's blossoming eastern landscape, appeared to be the lot of the new *Bundesbürger*. In an investigation carried out in June 1991 among 4,200 east Germans by the Socio-Economic Panel of the German Institute for Economic Research, the proportion of those expressing confidence in the future had dropped by 10 per cent over the preceding 12 months, with the fall being more pronounced among the unemployed and short-time workers.[11] After a rise in optimism during the election year of 1994, fed by promises of improvements in income and employment, 1995 marked another low in popular perceptions of the unification process. Fears were quickened by the slowing down in income convergence, by changes to the health system and by the introduction of legislation allowing for the removal of rent controls. By 1997, only 22 per cent of east Germans were 'mainly optimistic' as against 27 per cent who were 'primarily worried' about developments in the near future; 48 per cent were both hopeful and fearful.[12] In the later 1990s, the major worries and fears concerned unemployment (80 per cent), violence and crime (80 per cent), cuts in social services (68 per cent) and the economic situation (65 per cent).[13] A cleavage is apparent, on the one hand, between pensioners and those with a job and, on the other, persons in labour market schemes and the unemployed. In comparison to the beginning of the decade, the latter two groups exhibit greater concern about the future and a lower level of satisfaction with their living conditions.

The more realistic and sober assessment of the general situation was influenced by the emergence of a conscious eastern identity as well as by what some observers decried as a misguided hammer-and-sickle nostalgia for life in the GDR.[14] Many east Germans believe that the losses of unification outweigh the benefits and hold numerous areas of life in the GDR in higher regard than in today's Germany. In 1995, a majority of easterners rated the GDR as considerably superior to the FRG in seven out of nine areas, notably in social security, equality of opportunity for women and personal safety; five years earlier, it had only been in the latter three areas. However, recognition of the clear superiority of the FRG in living standards and science and technology did not waver.[15]

Life in the GDR, in retrospect, no longer seems so bleak. According to *Der Spiegel*, as many as 75 per cent of east Germans insisted 'I can be proud of my life in the GDR'.[16] The data from 1997 reproduced in Table 5.1 provide high approval ratings for central aspects of the old regime, notably full employment, social security, employment of women, cheap foodstuffs, a sense of well-being in the collective and the country's anti-fascist credentials. The picture is by no means unblemished as the GDR is closely associated with restrictions on travel, shortage of supplies and, though not quite so negatively, being held under tutelage, doping, spying on colleagues and the squandering of achievements. Although a small minority of east Germans express a desire for the return of the GDR,[17] this wish is more pronounced among the unemployed and those in labour market schemes. Not only does such a finding suggest that an

TABLE 5.1

EAST GERMANS' PERCEPTIONS OF LIFE IN THE GDR, 1997 (%)

Life in the GDR was associated with:

Full employment	89	Disguised unemployment	13
Social security	85	Squandering of achievements	7
Employment of women	84	Neglect of children	2
Cheap foodstuffs	77	Shortage of supplies	42
State holiday provision	76	Restrictions on travel	62
Sense of well-being in		Spying on colleagues	5
the collective	65	SED dictatorship	38
Anti-fascism	54	Doping	3
Mass sport	52	Tutelage	18
Co-determination	12		

Source: Winkler, *Sozialreport 1997*, p. 49. The data are from a survey conducted in 1997 among about 1,500 east Germans.

improvement in the economic situation would help reduce support for a resurrection of the GDR, but it also refutes Marc Howard's controversial claim that *Ostidentität* resides in a separate east German ethnicity.[18]

The successor party to the SED, the orthodox 'anti-capitalist' PDS, has managed to tap into the disaffection with the course of unification and the antipathy towards the key political institutions of the Federal Republic. Although there is a broad acceptance of fundamental democratic values, many east Germans are highly sceptical about the effectiveness of political participation and exhibit a disturbingly low level of trust in the federal government, the *Länder* governments, the police and the courts of law.[19] These circumstances partly explain why, to the surprise of most political commentators, the PDS has managed to survive the debacle of communism's collapse. Not only did it clear the 5 per cent barrier for entry into the Bundestag in 1998 but it also increased its seats from 30 to 36. It owes its success primarily to its eastern stronghold where it obtained 21.6 per cent of the popular vote as against a mere 0.9 per cent in the old *Länder*. This reflects different perceptions of the party: only 27 per cent of westerners regard the PDS as a normal democratic party in contrast to 70 per cent of easterners.[20]

MULTIPLE IDENTIFICATIONS IN THE EAST

With so many east Germans looking favourably on life in the GDR, to what extent is this obstructing the development of an all-German identity and a pride in the new Germany? Since unification the issue of an all-German identity has acquired greater salience as one component of a multiplicity of identifications ranging from Europe to the local community. Research data compiled by the Konrad-Adenauer-Foundation in the early to mid-1990s[21] reveal that westerners and easterners profess an all-German identity in roughly equal measure (57 per cent to 53 per cent in 1993 and 66 per cent to 57 per cent in 1995). However, despite the appreciable support for the national community, the sense of an eastern regional identity is far more pronounced than a *Westidentität* (65 per cent to 40 per cent in 1993 and 71 per cent to 46 per cent two years later). The differences are even sharper according to age and political affiliation, with the more highly educated and younger east Germans and those aged 60 and older identifying themselves far more closely with east Germany than is the case with regional affiliation in the west. This finding indicates that an east German identification is neither confined to one social group nor is it associated solely with proximity to the old regime. On the other hand, as expected, the highest level of self-identification with east Germany and the lowest with Germany (75 per cent and 35 per cent respectively in 1993) occurs among the supporters of the PDS, the party most closely linked to the GDR past. At the other end of the political spectrum, the supporters of the CDU, the party which engineered the unification project and, until the 1998 Bundestag election, the most popular party in the new *Länder*, identify themselves more strongly as Germans (74 per cent) than do any other political group. One additional finding underlines the distinctiveness of *Ostidentität*: while both east and west Germans exhibit a complex mix of identities – Germany, east/west Germany, the *Bundesland* and the local community – an exclusive identification with 'east German only' is much more frequent than with 'west German only' (25 per cent to 4 per cent in 1995).

Further light on collective identity is shed by an examination of the level and nature of east German pride in the nation. Not surprisingly, pride in being German was especially high in 1989–90 (74 per cent) but fell by 16 per cent in 1995 under the impact of economic realities and the reconfiguration of Germany's international role.[22] The sources of national pride identified by easterners in a 1996 ALLBUS survey are predominantly Germany's achievements in the economic sphere, science, art and literature, and sport (41 per cent, 57 per cent, 53 per cent and 54 per cent), followed, at a distance, by the political system and social welfare (24 per cent and 23 per cent).[23]

Turning to stereotypes, *Ossis* and *Wessis* project not only markedly different but also mutually negative images and misperceptions which are, as is in the nature of stereotypes, difficult to eradicate. Asked to address each other in a 1992 poll, the westerners insisted: 'Don't complain so much, most people are better off than before'; 'More modesty and thankfulness'; and 'Shut your mouths and work more'. Among the equally sharp responses of easterners were: 'Don't always think about money'; 'They won't take advice, they think they know better'; and 'Why are we being treated like minors?'.[24] East Germans regard themselves as more friendly towards children, more modest and less greedy than the self-confident and arrogant westerners. Not only do easterners tend to criticise west Germans as neo-colonialists and for failing to share their wealth, but they are far more likely than westerners to fault the federal government for tardiness in closing the gap in living standards between the old and new *Länder* (see Table 5.2). Eastern sensibilities are also offended by some of the current debates on the history of the GDR and by the struggle for control over historical memory. The reapplication of the totalitarian label to the GDR, the unjustified equation of the GDR with the Third Reich and attempts to depict the country as little more than a coercive system with the Stasi at the epicentre offend many east Germans. Indeed most

TABLE 5.2
APPROVAL OF WEST–EAST STEREOTYPES BY WEST GERMANS AND EAST GERMANS 1992–94
(%; all respondents)

Item	West		East	
	1992	1994	1992	1994
'Anti-West' Item				
1. The west Germans have conquered the former GDR in a colonial style	30	33	64	63
2. In spite of all their wealth the west Germans have not learned to share	44	47	71	67
3. In the west, there are people who would prefer to live as if unification had not taken place	66	63	78	72
'Anti-East' Item				
1. Many east Germans tend to feel sorry for themselves	62	60	26	26
2. Many workers and employees in east Germany simply cannot stand the pressures in the west	72	64	23	25
All Respondents	2,037	1,060	1,013	1,046

Source: P. Bauer-Kaase and M. Kaase, 'Five Years of Unification: The Germans on the Path to Inner Unity?', *German Politics*, Vol. 5, No. 1 (1996), p. 6.

assert that only those who have lived in the GDR can fully appreciate the complex nature of society and truly know anything about life in their country. Without desiring a restoration of communist-type rule, many easterners cling on to certain memories and symbols of the past. Some of these symbols are so highly politicised – like the showpiece Palace of the Republic and the Ernst Thälmann memorial in east Berlin – that the question of their preservation divides opinion in the east and, like similar controversies among *Ossis* over the treatment of Stasi agents and members of the SED Politbüro, exemplifies the differentiated nature of *Ostidentität* as well as the difficulties inherent in forging a collective German identity.

It is not surprising that the vast majority of east Germans (87 per cent at the end of 1990, 69 per cent in 1995 and 80 per cent in May 1997) regard themselves as second class citizens, a perception which, according to Emnid data, is less pronounced among pensioners and the more highly qualified.[25] Among the main reasons given for the feelings of resentment and inferiority are: east Germans do not enjoy equal pay for the same type of work as in the west but have to cope with equally high living costs (88 per cent); 40 years of separation cannot be overcome quickly; unemployment is disproportionately high in the east; the ruinous legacy of the SED regime; the east German economy has been laid so low that it is uncompetitive; the devaluation of the achievements of the GDR; and western colonisation of the new *Länder*. The extent of mutual grievances and negative images is underlined by the furore in the summer of 1999 when easterners accused west Germans of seeking to enforce segregation on the beaches of the Baltic Coast between nudists and 'textiles' who prefer to wear bikinis or trunks, thereby overriding the traditional east German preference for mixed beaches. Writing in the *Guardian* on 21 July 1999, Ian Traynor drew the conclusion that: 'East and west Germans can barely stand the sight of each other, particularly with no clothes on'.

GENERAL EXPLANATIONS OF INNER DISUNITY

Although it might be argued that these grievances are evidence of easterners trying to have their cake and eat it, there is undoubtedly good reason for dissatisfaction and anxiety as Dr Kohl's neo-liberal prescription for the ills of the GDR seriously underestimated the problems of the grand experiment of a 'transformation by unification'. While there is a general consensus among researchers and opinion pollsters on the variables which determine political dissatisfaction and inner disunity – notably, the 'socialist legacy', the economic disadvantages of unification, the frustration of expectations and easterners' response to treatment by west Germans – disagreement exists as to how much weight should be attached to them. Whereas many analysts would concur with Dieter Walz and Wolfram Brunner that 'it's the economy stupid' and that inner unity depends primarily on the equalisation of living standards,[26] others prefer an explanation which focuses on 'treatment and response'. In his analysis of political dissatisfaction throughout east-central Europe, Helmut Wiesenthal finds strong evidence for the latter thesis among those *Ossis* over 45 years of age who, unlike the younger groups, have experienced a significant decline in their political influence since 1990.[27] This view can be supported by a wealth of evidence relating to western elites' domination of the transformation of the GDR and a thoughtless suppression of eastern interests. The Treuhand, in particular, became a symbol for an alleged west

German neo-colonisation and destruction of vast swathes of GDR industry. The pertinence of the 'treatment-response' approach is reflected in the experiences of east Germans who though fully committed to integrating themselves into the new system are rejected by westerners. They develop what has been termed a '*Trotzidentität*' (a deliberate contrariness).[28] That there can, however, be no mono-causal explanation of the east–west divide, a point made by Wiesenthal, is apparent from the Konrad-Adenauer-Foundation's multi-factor assessment of the reasons for easterners' self-identification.[29] The main categories comprise an 'anti-west identity' (18.5 per cent), 'differences in living conditions' (17.5 per cent) and a 'common east German heritage' (17.4 per cent). These were followed by an emotional attachment to one's home area (15.2 per cent), positive auto-stereotypes such as the alleged higher trustworthiness of east Germans (11.8 per cent) and differences in the mentalities or the psyches of easterners and westerners (5 per cent).

THE SOCIO-ECONOMIC CONTEXT

Although wages and pensions have been converging rapidly with those in the west, this has been against a backdrop of rapid economic collapse, massive de-industrialisation, the disappearance of entire categories of qualifications and jobs and abrupt social dislocation. The following data and observations underpin the salience for inner disunity of the unprecedented social and economic turbulence.[30] The implementation of the west German labour market model has destroyed the old GDR employment society and wiped out almost 90 per cent of workplaces in branches such as textiles and clothing. The number of gainfully employed persons has fallen from the exceptionally high figure of 9.7 million in 1989 to 6.1 million in May 1997. In the early 1990s, unemployment, both official and disguised, hovered around 30 per cent, with the official rate held artificially low by the exclusion from unemployment statistics of persons in labour market measures. A high job turnover and unemployment are constants of everyday life in the new *Länder*. In 1997, only 69 per cent of employees performed the same activity as two years earlier; among those in labour market schemes the percentage was as low as 27. Since 1990, 57 per cent of persons aged 18 to 59 have been unemployed on at least one occasion and 29 per cent of men and 11 per cent of women under 25 years of age have been out of work for up to 12 months. Behind the bare statistics lies a sense of shame, demoralisation, isolation and marginalisation, especially among the long-term unemployed, and a greater risk of familial conflict.[31]

Expectations of job loss in the future are far higher in the east than in the west.[32] The proportion of households in which both male and female partners were employed fell by more than 50 per cent between 1990 and 1996.[33] And not only have east Germans lost their old job security but, with the destruction of the enterprise structure, they have also been deprived of the contacts in the work collectives and the social environment associated with the state planned economy. While all sectors of the economy have been affected by the collapse of the GDR, the impact has been greatest in manufacturing industry and agriculture. By 1994, employment had fallen by over a half in the former, and 80 per cent of workplaces had disappeared in agriculture – from about 800,000 to 157,000 – with serious repercussions for the age structure of the villages and employment opportunities in the rural areas of Mecklenburg-Vorpommern.

Women have been the main losers of the social transformation, with a consistently higher unemployment rate than among men (21 per cent to 10.9 per cent in 1994); even so, the proportion of households with an employed woman is still higher than in west Germany, with the exception of households where members are over 50 years of age, and east German women remain highly committed to work as a central value of life.[34] Despite a general rise in personal income, east Germans enjoy a lower share of net incomes above the DM2,000 rung, with only 26 per cent as against 50 per cent of west Germans occupying the DM2,000 to DM3,999 band.[35] Income poverty has almost trebled, from 2.8 per cent in 1990 to 7.9 per cent in 1995, and affects, above all, single parents and the unemployed. This finding is based on the proportion of households whose net household income is less than one-half the average household income in the new *Länder*. If the benchmark is the old *Länder*, then it would read 17.2 per cent.[36] A final crisis indicator, although the list could be extended considerably, is the fall in the resident population from 16.7 million in 1988 to 15.4 million in 1997, a consequence of the mass emigration to the west and of a plummeting birth rate in 1994 to only 49.2 per cent of its 1989 level. One expert is persuaded that east Germans have 'come as close to a temporary suspension of childbearing as any large population in the human experience'.[37] The sensitivity of east Germans to the new social and economic uncertainties can also been seen in two other social statistics: in 1991 the marriage and divorce rates were only 41.2 per cent and 17.1 per cent of their 1989 levels.[38]

THE SOCIALIST LEGACY

The role of the 'socialist legacy' in the formation of *'Ostidentität'* is much contested. A retrospective positive assessment of life in the GDR is interpreted by some critics primarily as a defensive measure against what is perceived to be western cultural imperialism; other commentators see it as an outcome of east Germans' internalisation of several core 'socialist' norms and values. However, while many historians and cultural scientists acknowledge the existence of a GDR identity on the basis of experiences and life in the GDR, they refute the notion of a widespread identification with the goals and values of the old regime.[39] If this latter line of argument is adopted, then indicators of support today for socialist values may be interpreted both as a misplaced nostalgia for a world which never existed and as an assertion of east German self-esteem in the new Germany. In other words, this represents the late birth of a 'quasi-socialism' which most east Germans did not endorse before 1989! On the other hand, if certain norms and values from the socialist era were embedded in the GDR population, then this may also help to explain the persistence of a mental wall after the demolition of the physical wall.

Although it is methodologically difficult to separate the former GDR identity from post-unification 'virtual reality socialism', it is argued here that 'real existing socialism' – to use the terminology of the old regime – did indeed leave a strong attitudinal and behavioural imprint on east Germans. This entailed not only the internalisation of certain expectations and official norms – social justice, full employment and social security – but also the development of practices and values which were not congruent with the regime's goals, for example, the development of a work environment and a work identity which, contrary to SED pronouncements on economic modernisation and the more effective utilisation of labour, gave priority to the harmony of the work collective over disruptive performance norms.[40] Consequently, the enterprise tended to be regarded as a 'substitute family' or a 'second home', a role which was reinforced by its involvement in the allocation of jobs and further training places and by its provision of shopping, childcare, sports and health facilities. The Confederation of Free German Trade Unions (FDGB) functioned primarily as the social welfare arm of party and state in the factory, not as the autonomous representative of labour. While recognising the political and bureaucratic constraints on the labour force and the disciplinary measures implemented against 'asocials' who sought to opt out of regular employment, the notion of the workplace as a sphere not under the firm control of the party has considerable merit, especially in the Honecker period, in that friendships were formed there, workers enjoyed considerable legal protection against violations of their employment contract by the enterprise, and much work time was lost through absenteeism and shopping. If one also takes into account a chronic shortage of parts, as well as the technical and organisational disruptions to the work process, then it comes as no surprise to learn that in many areas of the economy no work was performed in about one-third of nominal work time. Before the *Wende*, GDR sociologists drew attention to the role of social relations at work as a barrier to the acceptance of the new technologies and labour intensification programmes which the SED aspired to introduce. Even R&D collectives were not committed to 'management values' such as personal success and the absolute priority of work over leisure, hobbies and the family. However, the argument should not be stretched so far as to overlook a commitment to the 'achievement' value both in official pronouncements and among the work force. Yet, although work in the GDR was certainly not devoid of mental and physical stress and job turnover was quite high, it should be recalled that work was less intensive than in west Germany and eastern employees enjoyed a much higher level of security. It is this kind of time and work pattern which would disappear after unification.

The legacy of 'real existing socialism' extended to a series of other expectations and practices: cheap basic foodstuffs, inexpensive public transport, low rents, free education and free health provision; a standard of living not directly dependent on work performance; and greater equality for women predicated on their employment outside the home. The exceptionally high proportion of women in actual employment (81.7 per cent in 1990 as against 55.9 per cent in west Germany in 1989) was made possible by a comprehensive system of pre-school childcare in crèches and kindergartens. A pattern emerged whereby eastern women bore children earlier than their western counterparts and returned to work, within a short period, usually as a full-time employee. They enjoyed an appreciable degree of economic independence and strove to make work and family compatible. These features of social policy were hailed by Honecker as the social achievements of socialism and, given the SED's perennial problems over the national question and its unwillingness to abandon its power monopoly, were integral to the pursuit of regime legitimation via a social welfare paternalism. The *Versorgungsstaat* (all-encompassing state provision) offered east Germans social security in the sense that life planning enjoyed a high level of predictability and many basic needs were guaranteed on condition that citizens did not challenge the SED political power monopoly. This has shaped *Ossi* perceptions of the role of the state in the area of social welfare. In 1994, 75 per cent of east Germans, as against 47 per cent of west Germans, believed that the state should be responsible for provision in areas such as illness, deprivation, unemployment and old age.[41] It has also meant serious problems since unification in adapting to a rapidly changing work environment, particularly for older workers whose age reduces their opportunities for retraining.

How much support did the GDR's social system enjoy among the population before 1990? This is difficult to answer with any precision but, given the lack of any realistic alternative to SED rule until the end of the 1980s, there is reason to believe that aspects of the regime's social policy enjoyed popular approval – with the important proviso that the Federal Republic was most probably the majority's preferred option.[42] Indicators of popular opinion can be found in the confidential internal surveys which were compiled by the SED Central Committee's Institute for Public Opinion Research and by the Central Institute for Youth Research. Although the findings cannot claim to be GDR representative and obviously contain elements of political bias and self-censorship, the surveys were based on guarantees of anonymity to the respondents. The kind of material from an investigation undertaken by the Institute for Public Opinion Research reproduced in Table 5.3 points to widespread support for the GDR's family policy, education, equality of opportunity for women and job security – in other words to the social security and the paternalistic *Soziale Geborgenheit* (all-embracing state provision) which was terminated by unification and which is germane to today's *Ostidentität*.[43] While it may be objected that the percentages are misleadingly high, it can be countered that some of these areas also

TABLE 5.3
EVALUATION OF THE DEVELOPMENT OF SOCIALIST CONSTRUCTION IN THE GDR IN SPECIFIC AREAS, 1970 (%)

	Good	Satisfactory	Unsatisfactory	No answer
Social security	65.8	25.5	3.5	5.2
Education system	77.2	11.2	1.0	10.6
Economic development	33.5	38.4	10.6	17.5
Science and technics	51.0	30.1	7.4	11.5
Socialist democracy	34.0	31.8	14.1	19.2
Cultural development	45.3	32.7	9.0	13.0
Free development of personality	34.4	29.3	19.9	16.4

Source: Heinz Niemann, *Meinungsforschung in der DDR. Die geheimen Berichte des Instituts für Meinungsforschung an das Politbüro der SED* (Cologne: Bund-Verlag, 1993), p. 43. The data are based on the responses (by questionnaire) of over 4,000 persons in craft and agricultural cooperatives, private enterprises, nationalised enterprises and extended secondary schools. The survey was conducted in 1970.

received high levels of approbation in 1988–90, at a time when the GDR was unravelling. For example, the Institute for Sociology at the Central Committee's Academy for Social Sciences found that most respondents were satisfied with the attention paid by the state to social security, the equality of women and childcare. They were, however, highly critical of living standards and the limited opportunities for political participation.[44]

SOCIAL POLICY PROBLEMS

Despite the positive features of the GDR's social welfare network, care must be taken not to create unfounded myths around the SED's social policy. The first and most obvious problem is that the public purse could not support the escalating costs of the system. The combined subsidies of basic foodstuffs, rents and public transport, the most heavily supported items, rocketed from 16.9 billion GDR Marks in 1980 to 49.8 billion in 1988. Planning and finance officials frequently pressed the political leadership to cut back on the subsidies for social consumption, a nettle which Honecker was not prepared to grasp. Second, although the GDR provided social security for its citizens, many were becoming increasingly dissatisfied with the supply of consumer goods and foodstuffs, the privileged position of east Berlin *vis-à-vis* the regions, the pollution of the environment and, in the Gorbachev era, the lack of political freedoms. This is the impression one gets from Stasi materials on popular opinion as well as from sociological investigations conducted in the late 1980s by the Institute for Sociology which provide social scientists with an understanding of the background to the revolutionary events of 1989.[45] Even though the social achievements such as 'women's equality' and 'social security' received high ratings, mention should be made of the many drawbacks. The egalitarian principle was undermined by special categories of pensions and privileges. When the privileged existence of the members of the Politbüro in the Wandlitz compound was revealed during the *Wende*, it provoked great anger among a population in which social and material egalitarianism was engrained. The pension scheme was not without its disadvantages for women for, although the basic pension was intended to guarantee a minimum level of existence, their average pension of 417.73 Marks in 1989 was about 100 Marks less than that of men.[46] Nor was sexual equality attained at the workplace, where a gender-specific segregation prevailed according to occupation and economic sector and, as in the case of the unequal household division of labour, generated tensions between men and women. Moreover, despite the high value attached to marriage by the SED, as well as by the east German population, there was a high incidence of divorce and lone-parent families. As for the central plank of social policy – the housing construction programme – official targets were not met, many new housing estates were soulless, older buildings continued to decay and apartments were considerably smaller than in the west. Finally, the price of luxury items such as cars, washing machines and television sets bore no relation to average income and the purchase of western goods for hard currency in the Intershops opened up a cleavage in society between those citizens in possession of Deutschmarks and those without access to them.

THE DISTINCTIVENESS OF THE EAST GERMANS MUST BE ACCEPTED

The negative features of social welfare provision, together with the coercive apparatus of the Stasi and the constraints on political pluralism, are necessary antidotes to any romanticised picture of the 'good old days' and underscore the argument that today's *Ostidentität* is, in part, a defensive shield against the social and personal losses connected with unification. Yet, as has been argued elsewhere in this chapter, *Ostidentität* also has its roots in a positive assessment of the guarantees for job and social security and the overall *soziale Geborgenheit* which engendered conformity to – if not the legitimation of – the communist system. Furthermore, as an unfavourable assessment by most easterners of the social welfare provision in the new Germany, in comparison to that of the GDR, has been found to correlate with a disproportionately high negative evaluation of democracy in the Federal Republic, this constitutes a serious impediment to the consolidation of the democratic system in the five new *Länder*.[47] While it is reasonable to assume that an improvement in economic performance and social welfare provision would lower such barriers, several problems must be borne in mind. East German expectations are high and are deeply embedded in the socialist inheritance; the east German economy is unlikely to achieve self-sustaining growth in the near future; and federal budgetary constraints will eat into social welfare provision.[48] Indeed, an elimination of the east–west divide cannot be expected in the near future given the strong sense of injustice prevailing among many east Germans concerning inequities in income, employment and housing, the existence of a strong post-communist party and nostalgia for the socialist past. In these circumstances, it is important that the distinctiveness of east German identity be accepted and then, as has been argued elsewehere,[49] a recognition of this distinctiveness will perhaps facilitate the process of integration in the long term.

NOTES

1. 'Erst vereint, nun entzweit', *Der Spiegel*, 8 January 1993, p. 170.
2. H. Krisch, 'The Changing Politics of German National Unity', in P. Merkl (ed.), *The Federal Republic at Fifty: The End of a Century of Turmoil* (Basingstoke and London: Macmillan, 1999), p. 34.
3. For details see G. Winkler (ed.), *Sozialreport 199: Daten und Fakten zur sozialen Lage in den neuen Bundesländern* (Berlin: Verlag am Turm, 1997), pp. 40–3. The data are based on surveys conducted between 1990 and 1997 by the Berlin-Brandenburg Social Science Research Centre.
4. GDR identity was not so uniform as is sometimes presumed. For example, considerable dissonance existed between popular and official values as regards the socialist nation concept. Value divergence between the generations is also observable, with a growing trend towards self-individuation among younger cohorts, despite the Honecker regime's efforts to rein in autonomous tendencies. See A. Göschel, 'Kulturelle und politische Generationen in Ost und West. Zum Gegensatz von wesenhafter und distinktiver Identität', *Berliner Debatte INITIAL*, Vol. 10, No. 2 (1999), pp. 29–40.
5. D. Pollack and G. Pickel, 'Die ostdeutsche Identität – Erbe des DDR-Sozialismus oder Produkt der Wiedervereinigung? Die Einstellung der Ostdeutschen zu soziale Ungleichheit und Demokratie', *Aus Politik und Zeitgeschichte*, No. 41–2 (1998), p. 20.
6. See 'Sozialpolitik und Demokratie', *WZB Mitteilungen*, No. 85 (1999), p. 28.
7. B. Bohley and E. Neubert, *Wir mischen uns ein. Ideen für eine gemeinsame Zukunft* (Freiburg, Basle and Vienna, 1998), p. 49.
8. 'Das Profil der Deutschen. Was sie vereint, was sie trennt', *Der Spiegel-Spezial*, No. 1 (Hamburg: Spiegel-Verlag), p. 80.
9. See 'Gesamtwirtschaftliche und unternehmerische Anpassungsfortschritte in Ostdeutschland. Neunzehnter Bericht', *DIW Wochenbericht*, Vol. 66, No. 23 (1999), pp. 422–3 and K. Bedau, 'Völlige Angleichung der Ost-West Arbeiternehmereinkommen nicht in Sicht', *DIW Wochenbericht*, Vol. 66, No. 15–16 (1999), p. 277.
10. For the evaluation of the two economic systems, see the details from a 1993 survey in R. Rose and E. C. Page, 'German Responses to Regime Change: Culture, Class, Economy or Context?', *West European Politics*, Vol. 19, No. 1 (1996), pp. 10–11.
11. Arbeitsgruppe Sozialberichterstattung, 'Stimmungseinbruch in Ostdeutschland', *WZB Mitteilungen*, No. 56 (1992), p. 71.
12. Winkler, *Sozialreport 1997*, pp. 13, 15–16.
13. Ibid., pp. 17, 22. The results are from a 1996 survey.
14. H-J. Misselwitz, *Nicht länger mit dem Gesicht nach Westen. Das neue Selbstbewußsein der Ostdeutschen* (Bonn: J. H. W. Dietz Nachfolger, 1996), pp. 26–8.
15. 'Stolz aufs eigene Leben', *Der Spiegel*, 3 July 1995, p. 43.
16. Ibid., p. 52.
17. Thirteen per cent according to a 1997 Emnid survey; see D. Walz and W. Brunner, 'Das Sein bestimmt das Bewußtsein. Oder: Warum sich die Ostdeutschen als Bürger 2. Klasse fühlen', *Aus Politik und Zeitgeschichte*, No. 51 (1997), p. 19.
18. M. Howard, 'An East German Ethnicity? Understanding the New Division of United Germany', *German Politics and Society*, Vol. 13, No. 4 (1995), pp. 49–70.
19. For further details see E. Priller, 'Demokratieentwicklung und gesellschaftliche Mitwirkung', in Winkler, *Sozialreport 1997*, pp. 293–5, 307–9.
20. A. L. Phillips, 'The Third Victor: The PDS after the Elections', American Institute for Contemporary German Studies, http://www.aicgs.org/After-the-1998-Election/phillips.htm, pp. 2–3; K. Arzheimer and J. W. Falter, '"Annäherung durch Wandel"? Das Wahlverhalten bei der Bundestagwahl 1998 in Ost-West Perspektive', *Aus Politik und Zeitgeschichte*, No. 52 (1998), p. 34.
21. The 1993 survey data appear in H. J. Veen and C. Zelle, 'National Identity and Political Priorities in Eastern and Western Germany', *German Politics*, Vol. 4, No. 1 (1995), p. 12, and those for spring 1995 in C. Zelle, *Ostalgie? National and Regional Identifications in Germany after Unification*, Institute for German Studies, University of Birmingham, IGS Discussion Papers Series, No. 97/10 (1997), pp. 11–24.
22. Ibid., p. 39.

23. B. Westle, *Kollektive Identität im vereinten Deutschland* (Opladen: Leske & Budrich, 1999), p. 190. The categories in the ALLBUS survey are not identical to those used by Zelle.
24. 'Stolz aufs eigene Leben', pp. 58–9.
25. This section is based on data in Walz and Brunner, 'Das Sein', pp. 13, 16.
26. Ibid., pp. 16–19.
27. H. Wiesenthal, 'Post-Unification Dissatisfaction, or Why Are So Many East Germans Unhappy with the New Political System?' *German Politics*, Vol. 7, No. 2 (1998), pp. 22–3.
28. T. Koch, 'The Renaissance of East German Group Awareness since Unification', in M. Gerber and R. Woods (eds), *Studies in East German Culture and Society 14/15* (Lanham, New York and London: University Press of America, 1996), pp. 199–200.
29. Zelle, *Ostalgie?*, pp. 31–5; 1,100 east Germans were included in the survey.
30. See in particular Winkler, *Sozialreport 1997*, pp. 20–2, 100–3, 130–1, 142–6; R. Geißler, *Die Sozialstruktur Deutschlands. Zur gesellschaftlichen Entwicklung mit einer Zwischenbilanz zur Vereinigung* (Opladen: Westdeutscher Verlag, 1996), pp. 106–7; B. Vogel, *Ohne Arbeit in den Kapitalismus. Der Verlust der Erwerbsarbeit im Umbruch der ostdeutschen Gesellschaft* (Hamburg: VSA-Verlag, 1999), pp. 42, 206–10.
31. S. Foster, H. Liljeberg and G. Winkler, *Arbeitslosenreport 1996* (Berlin: Verlag am Turm, 1996), pp. 96–100.
32. In 1994, among a sample aged 25 to 50 in the year of unification, 20 per cent of easterners but only 7 per cent of westerners expected to lose their job. Details of the investigation in M. Diewald, 'Aufbruch oder Entmutigung? Kompetenzentfaltung, Kompetenzentwertung und subjektive Kontrolle in den neuen Bundesländern', in M. Schmitt and L. Montada (eds.), *Gerechtigkeitserleben im wiedervereinigten Deutschland* (Opladen: Leske & Budrich), 1999), p. 101.
33. 'Private Haushalte in Ost und West', *WZB Mitteilungen*, No. 84 (1999), p. 30.
34. Ibid.
35. J. H. P. Hoffmeter-Zlonik, 'Zur soziodemographischen Entwicklung in Ostdeutschland: Ein Vergleich 1990 mit 1996', in M. Häder and S. Häder (eds), *Sozialer Wandel in Ostdeutschland. Theoretische und methodische Beiträge zur Analyse der Situation seit 1990* (Opladen: Leske & Budrich, 1999), p. 180.
36. Winkler, *Sozialreport 1997*, pp. 143–4.
37. N. Eberstadt, 'Demographic Shocks in Eastern Germany, 1989–93', *Europe–Asia Studies*, Vol. 46, No. 3 (1994), p. 521.
38. J. Dobritz, 'Der Wandel in den generativen Entscheidungen in Ostdeutschland – ein generationenspezifischer Prozeß', in Häder and Häder, *Sozialer Wandel*, pp. 125–6.
39. K. Schroeder, 'Die blockierte Vereinigung. Gemeinsamkeiten und Unterschiede der Deutschen in Ost und West', *Gegenwartskunde*, Vol. 41, No. 3 (1992), pp. 304–5.
40. See R. Hachtmann, 'Arbeitsverfassung', in H. G. Hockerts (ed.), *Drei Wege deutscher Sozialstaatlichkeit. NS-Diktatur, Bundesrepublik und DDR im Vergleich* (Munich: R. Oldenburg Verlag, 1998), pp. 40–2; J. Roesler, 'Probleme des Brigadealltags. Arbeitsverhältnisse und Arbeitsklima in volkseigenen Betrieben 1950–1989', *Aus Politik und Zeitgeschichte*, No. 38 (1997), pp. 12–17; Vogel, *Ohne Arbeit*, pp. 22–33.
41. D. Fuchs, E. Roller and B. Weßels, 'Die Akzeptanz der Demokratie des vereinigten Deutschland. Oder: Wann ist ein Unterschied ein Unterschied?', *Aus Politik und Zeitgeschichte*, No. 51 (1997), p. 7.
42. L. Fritze, *Die Gegenwart des Vergangenen. Über das Weiterleben der DDR nach ihrem Ende* (Cologne and Weimar: Böhlau Verlag, 1997), pp. 96–105.
43. See also the Central Institute for Youth Research material in P. Förster, 'Die deutsche Frage im Bewußtsein der Bevölkerung in beiden Teilen Deutschlands', in Deutscher Bundestag (ed.), *Materialien der Enquete-Kommission "Aufarbeitung von Geschichte und Folgen der SED-Diktatur in Deutschland"*, Vol. V/2 (Baden-Baden: Nomos Verlag, 1995), pp. 1273, 1239.
44. Thomas Gensicke, 'Mentalitätswandel und Revolution. Wie sich die DDR-Bürger von ihrem System abwandten', *Deutschland Archiv*, Vol. 25, No. 12 (1992), pp. 1276–8. The survey involved 1,376 respondents. The average age was 36.7 years, 96.5 per cent were in full employment and 4.5 per cent in part-time work.
45. Ibid., pp. 1281–3.
46. G. Scholz, 'Soziale Sicherung von Frauen und Familien', in Hockerts, *Drei Wege*, p. 132.

47. 'Sozialpolitik und Demokratie', p. 29.
48. The persistent economic problems of the new *Länder* can be illustrated by several key indicators for 1998: gross domestic product was only about half the west German level, unit labour costs were 24 per cent higher and labour productivity 40 per cent lower. See 'Gesamtwirtschaftliche und unternehmerische Anpassungsfortschritte', p. 422, and 'Die Lage der Weltwirtschaft und der deutschen Wirtschaft im Frühjahr 1999', *DIW Wochenbericht*, Vol. 66, No. 17 (1999), p. 311.
49. H. A. Welsh, A. Pickel and D. Rosenberg, 'East and West German Identities: United and Divided?', in K. Jarausch (ed.), *After Unity: Reconfiguring German Identities* (Providence and Oxford: Berghahn, 1997), p. 136.

6

Employment, Gender and the Dual Transformation in Germany

Hildegard Maria Nickel

TWO INTERWOVEN PROCESSES OF TRANSFORMATION

The Federal Republic of Germany is undergoing a dual social transformation. On the one hand, there are the economic, social and cultural processes associated with political unification, which have primarily been taking place in the east, in the new federal states. On the other hand – and this is often forgotten – this transformation of eastern Germany is set within a process of social transformation in the west, the old federal states, which began long before German unification. This more general process relates to the constellation of post-war growth,[1] and is evidently undergoing a crisis. At least, the process is no longer smooth, and has not yet entered a new phase of prosperity leading to a noticeable decrease in high basic unemployment.

From the outset, west Germany's post-war prosperity went hand-in-hand with reforms achieved after tough conflicts over the distribution of wealth. The results were high levels of employment, prolonged economic growth, cushions for social inequality, a broad expansion and individualisation of educational and career opportunity, a diversification of freely chosen forms of cohabitation, and broad democratisation. The basic social consensus of the post-war period was founded on a social contract that was not legally enshrined but was nonetheless observed in practice, which aimed to achieve compromise on the distribution question and which was inspired by the idea that all members of society were 'social partners' with a more or less equal right to benefit from economic growth. During those years, federal government policy did not merely trail along in linear fashion behind the (upward) development in GNP. Social spending actually grew faster than GNP, as in all western European countries; it also played a pro-active part in shaping the social structure by compensating and regulating, and to some degree the emancipatory interests of the individual made gains from this. The rights implied by this intention were actually assertable. This was the narrow material basis for a whole series of emancipatory steps forwards for women in the Federal Republic of Germany from the mid- or late 1960s onwards.[2]

Following the structural crisis in the mid-1970s this overall social construct grew unstable; mass unemployment nibbled insidiously at the financial foundations of social state mechanisms for secondary distribution. From 1982 a policy in effect began gradually modifying established relations of distribution in the name of deregulation, labour market flexibility and the 'restructuring' of the social state, its aim evidently being to discard the social compromise, and in this it was not entirely unsuccessful. The nature and intensity of this project to resize the social state, however, are such that the control potential of capital accumulation is at risk. The fulfilment of individual social and cultural needs is flung back to the level of primary income distribution, ignoring the fact that societies today are stratified in terms of status, power and access to resources along lines of class, gender, age and ethnic origin.[3] In the long term, there is a danger that civil consensus will be undermined.

The process of transformation does not affect all the men and women in Germany at the same time and in the same way. The differentiations between the sexes, and also between women, are huge. Struggles over the distribution of resources, above all employment, are exacerbated. In the same breath, the old bourgeois order of gender, which had long since been abolished in the GDR anyway, has finally vanished in the Federal Republic, or to put it another way, the contract between the sexes associated with the industrial era of capitalism is becoming obsolete, with both parties, women and men, challenging it increasingly. The old gender order centred on the 'normal family' and the ideal of a 'family income'[4] and was founded on the division and bipolar gender allocation of gainful employment and domestic labour.

> This world was characterised by the idea that people should be organized in a heterosexual nuclear family with a male as its head, living primarily off the man's earned income. The male head of household received a 'family income' which was enough to feed children and a wife-and-mother who performed the housework unpaid.[5]

Even if this breadwinner marriage has been eroding in Germany since the late 1960s at the latest, and in spite of the fact that many families did not fit that industrial model before, it is ultimately the foundation on which the German social state, modifications apart, is built. It is certainly one reason why there are structural limits to integrating women into the world of paid employment. East German women are feeling this particularly at present, but they may be the ones who bring to a head the conflict over who gets the jobs, which is the very core of the equal rights issue, and who show up the need for renewal in employment policy and the social state. At least, they illustrate problems which affect women generally in Germany.

EAST GERMAN WOMEN: THE DOUBLE SOMERSAULT

Ursula Schröter maintains (and she is not alone in this) that east German women can be divided into two distinct groups,[6] and in May 1993, according to her representative random sample, 35 per cent of all east German women belonged to the group of losers.[7] I have my doubts as to whether this blanket approach is correct. What is the yardstick? Is it the social situation of women in the GDR? Is it a comparison with east German men? Or with west German women, or foreigners living in Germany? Or does it simply mean that many east German women are worse off than others? Dichotomy hinders our insight into the multiple facets of reality. Besides, clinging to the thesis of losers and winners assumes that women are the lucky or unlucky victims of a structural process over which they have no influence. The opposite is true. Women, like men, were active protagonists in the changes which led to the end of the GDR. Women, like men, voted in the majority at the GDR's first free elections in March 1990 for rapid economic and currency union. Now, however, what many did not wish to recognise at the time is becoming very clear. The crisis of transformation in the west, with a still incomplete transition to a post-Fordist stage, is hitting (eastern) women harder than (eastern) men.[8] It is a waste of time celebrating the 'winners' among women who, in spite of massive job losses in industry and agriculture, in spite of the erosion of once reliable social measures, such as childcare, and all the manifestations of political exclusion, have managed nonetheless to stay on keel, just as it is a waste of time to lament the 'losers', who are still not able, or else are less able than ever, to extract themselves and their children from the nightmare of fears and uncertainties. It is rather more useful to address the transformation crisis in the Federal Republic of Germany and ask how it is affecting women at various levels, and also to recall and demand those mechanisms which society can employ to regulate such matters.

True enough, there is a variety of factual evidence – from rising long-term unemployment in eastern Germany to the feminisation of poverty – that women are worse off. That is absolutely not at issue, but the over-simplistic picture needs to be placed in perspective:

1. The employment rate for east German women remains higher than for west German women; 66 per cent of women in eastern Germany have

jobs which require them to make social insurance contributions, whereas in western Germany the figure is 45 per cent. In other words, western women are in a less satisfactory situation than eastern women when it comes to having their own welfare entitlements.[9]

2. The transformation process in eastern Germany has turned many women into the principal family 'breadwinner', and in the average eastern household almost 50 per cent of the income is earned by women, compared with a third in the west. This has consequences for the gender relationship and could, in the medium term, encourage a pact between the sexes which is based on complementary functions with a low 'depth of hierarchy'. Moreover, the participation of women with young children in the labour market is considerably higher in the new states than on original federal territory. This is presumably a major reason why the proportion of married couples with children described as being in an 'economically difficult position' (children being a poverty risk!) is lower across the board than in the east than in the west.[10]

3. The difficulties of transformation have not so far triggered the expected return to a traditional gender model in eastern Germany. Rather, the 'data suggests the people in the new federal states acquired useful experience in the past with women's dual role', so that in 1995 attitudes to women working was summarised as 'growing approval in the east, stagnation (or else decline) in the west'.[11] And the 1997 Data Report observes astonishing differences between east and west: according to every second west German, women should stay at home to look after the children and the housework (47 per cent women/53 per cent men). In eastern Germany, this opinion is held by 'only' a quarter.[12]

4. The overall picture confirms that women enjoyed a certain 'home advantage' in the transition to a market economy due to a pronounced gender segregation in structures of employment in the GDR and the fact that in 1989 women were heavily over-represented in the service sector. On the one hand, this also meant that women did less well in the GDR's employment system than men, in that the large number of women in this sector was inversely proportional to income distribution and social prestige in the service industry. On the other hand, it also means that a large percentage of women with jobs were not directly affected to begin with by the mass redundancies which accompanied de-industrialisation in eastern Germany, and their experience of labour market restructuring took place against a lower-key gender competition.

If we look back at the dramatic changes of 1989/90, we can see – in spite of all the myths to the contrary which now seek to impose a different interpretation – that when the men and women of the GDR took recourse to 'Exit and Voice' (leaving the GDR or demanding the right of expression)[13] and acceded to the Federal Republic, they were relinquishing their claims on a system which included a 'head start on equality'[14] for east German women. Job security, full employment for women and mothers taken for granted, gainful employment compatible with motherhood, government measures to assist women and families, abortion available in the first 12 weeks with the costs (if the option was taken up) borne by social insurance, and a countrywide network of childcare facilities: these were the as yet unparalleled trademarks of the GDR's 'head start on equality' which, quite possibly, caused more women than men to ponder a while back in 1990 before beginning their democratically elected free fall into a different social configuration, their 'crash landing in the modern age'.[15] Ultimately, however, these familiar manifestations of a social state in paternalistic form were unable to withstand the tide of history. The men and women of the GDR had broken out of a society which took decisions for them and provided for their wants, in order to participate in a modern world which drew its legitimation from other mechanisms – mass consumption, parliamentary democracy and the welfare state – and which, in times of economic prosperity, had provided universal access to its highly developed mass culture. Social polarisations seemed to have been erased, and the social state seemed to present a reliable framework. But once the men and women of the GDR had arrived in the modern Federal Republic, it turned out that this other kind of society was already 'evaporating'.[16]

The stable development which men and women of the GDR had perceived from the outside as the dominant feature of the Federal Republic was founded, not on the elimination of social inequality, but on its regulation by means of high wages, full employment (extending increasingly to women) and a redistribution, or 'transfer' of resources, by the social state to cushion the 'weaker strata' and overcome crasser differences in the standard of living. The cracks which began to permeate this prosperous society in the mid-1970s were less visible on the outside or else appeared to be temporary and, if everyone knuckled down to the task, capable of repair. So the men and women of the GDR were not simply set down upon unification in a different society ridden with modern imponderables and replete with alien challenges which they had chosen of their own will to confront. Instead, the social fabric which they expected to encounter in Federal Germany was already being eroded by the time of unification, or had at least stumbled against own limits. Nevertheless, the *Wende* of 1989, set in motion an irreversible, dynamic social process, and the head start on equality was plunged into the ambivalent maelstrom of modernisation which had already held the west in its grip for some time. It is also buffeting the gender relationship, which is being redefined, while the gender contract hitherto taken for granted and practised by east Germans is losing its structural basis. Suddenly, jobs for women require legitimation, and are the centre of bitter rivalry over this 'strategic resource'.[17]

By now, however, it is becoming clear that, for all the self-assertion and resistivity mustered by east German women in defending their employment, the battle to nudge them out of the market has long since been raging. Moreover, huge social differentiations have been making their mark on female employment generally, and having a job no longer ensures independence, because earnings may not be enough to make ends meet.

By way of concluding this section, I should like to ask a few questions. If at the moment we can observe a tenacity about the east German gender arrangement and a resistivity by women in eastern Germany to being elbowed out of the job market, is that merely a 'temporary aberrance' which will vanish for once and for all as the next generation takes over? Or will the 'eastern model' shape the future for western men and women? Have structural changes perhaps been leading to a feminisation of male employment (with low incomes, precarious jobs, pseudo-self-employment, and so on), to an equalisation downwards, democratising the gender pact only in the sense that a man's working life is now more like a woman's? Is this equalisation downwards a foretaste of the future which awaits the united Germany? Or – and this brings me to the last question – is the gender relationship going to continue unscathed because, to turn Beck's image for the 1970s and 1980s on its head, the 'elevator effect' has become a nose-dive in the 1990s, dragging all social groups down together?

WHAT HOPE FROM THE SERVICES? THE SHADOWS AND COLOUR SPECTRUM OF THE JOBS FOR WOMEN

I shall confine my attention in what I have to say next to large-scale structures in the private service sector in eastern Germany, where the majority of women are still employed. Basically, we can describe the situation as follows:[18]

1. In the wake of German unification and the accompanying boom of 1990–92, a dynamic evolution of the service sector was predicted and occurred, not least in the new federal states. Commercial and savings banks, insurance companies, wholesalers and retailers profited from

and played a leading role in the 'construction effort'. There was a definite expansion of employment in this field. After this impressive increase during the 'build-up phase', the number of jobs passed the zenith in late 1993/early 1994, and in terms of employment the sector has found itself since then in a 'consolidation' phase. In figures, compared with an ongoing decline in the number employed in the primary sector (from about 900,000 to 200,000) and secondary sector (from about 4 million to 2.3 million), the tertiary sector has witnessed an increase in jobs from 3.6 million to 4 million.

2. Unlike the situation in industry from 1990, the big structures in the private service sector took over entire companies and departments almost completely in many fields, including their staff. There is no uniform pattern as to how the organisational and employment structures of these 'western models' were adopted in the new federal states. Modifications occurred, depending on variegated corporate strategies, and active support from east and west German managers gave rise to some specifically eastern features which can still be discerned.

3. In GDR days, service sector employment was almost exclusively female (90 per cent). Even in 1995/96 it still reflected a relatively high segregation (70 per cent). However, as the internal labour markets are restructured, the women still employed by these companies are increasingly being subjected to a subtle displacement ('the new genderisation'), which is achieved not only through the staff recruitment mechanisms, but also by means of company policy on working hours, mobility requirements and – especially at managerial level – long hours and greater pressure.

4. Our latest study,[19] begun in 1996, already indicates that the federal German labour market crisis has now also taken complete hold of the service sector in the new states. The services, therefore, are not the new hope for employment, at least not at present. Deutsche Bahn, the German rail company, is an example. Privatisation is casting its shadow ahead, so that staff have to cope with constant breaks in continuity, change is the 'norm', and there is nothing secure to rely on. To sum up, the effect of corporate integration is long-term discontinuity.

As work in the service sector is extremely heterogeneous, I shall attempt now to avoid generalisations by skirting along some specific segments where empirical research has been conducted, as it has for the financial services[20] and to some extent for the retail trade.[21] Care services[22] have been subjected to comparatively little gender analysis, although this is still a women's domain in the new federal states. We also have some studies under way, although not yet completed, with regard to women affected by the corporate transformations in the transport sector, that is, the German railways.[23]

THE RETAIL SECTOR: FEWER FRUITS FOR LABOUR?

The process of corporate transformation affecting the retail trade has been accompanied by gender-specific restructuring in internal labour markets. Although the retail trade could still be classed as a women's sector in 1994, with a workforce which was 64.2 per cent female (and evidently women will retain their majority here), the percentage nonetheless dropped dramatically between 1991 and 1994.[24] Those employees of former east German institutions who lost their jobs – despite the overall increase in employment until 1994 – were primarily (older) women. By contrast, new contracts during the corporate build-up were given more frequently to (young) men from outside the sector than to women. While the personnel was being restructured, only limited value was attached to managerial training and experience gained specifically in the retail trade. In 1988, 62 per cent of these managerial positions in the GDR's retail and supply sector had been held by women. Instead, the existing corporate hierarchies were 'slimmed down', and west Germans, mostly men, were appointed to managerial posts. In this way, an excessive proportion of women lost higher-grade jobs, and in very few cases were they able to acquire middle-management positions after obtaining qualifications which were formally acknowledged.

Gender restructuring in the retail sector in eastern Germany is also reflected in more precarious employment patterns and in monthly income: in 1994 the net monthly income of women employed in the retail sector averaged 1,354 Deutschmarks, compared with 1,893 Deutschmarks for men.

THE FINANCIAL SERVICES: WOMEN ON THE WAY UP?

Because of the gender-specific segregation which had characterised employment in the GDR, east German women in banks and insurance had a healthy chance of continuing in employment during the build-up phase. Not only were they usually not fired, they actually benefited in 1990/91 from a hiring boom for staff with commercial training.

This was followed by a corporate 'training offensive' which enabled most of these women to acquire basic qualifications which met the latest western standards in the sector. This not only meant an opportunity to stay in work, but created a bridge during that first period for young women to obtain more skills which would grant them access to a supervisory function in middle management or else enable them to specialise in financial products. Today, the percentage of women in third-grade and particularly fourth-grade management (that is, branch managers and team heads) is still higher in the east than in the west in most of the companies studied.

During the consolidation phase – that is, from about 1993/94 onwards – the 51,000 employees, notably women, have gone increasingly on to the defensive. There are several reasons for this: the financial sector has now acquired a greater economic and social significance in eastern Germany, which is reflected in more training applications from men; personnel policy has led to the practice of granting preference to male applicants during the selection procedure, even if their school record is poorer; and streamlining-out all manual activities, especially in the central offices of insurance undertakings and the back office of commercial and savings banks, has primarily hit low-skilled women. The older ones in particular have poor chances of keeping their jobs even by obtaining more qualifications. The financial services seem to be copying a few methods from lean banking, by outsourcing operational functions (such as IT) and shifting previously centralised responsibilities (such as personnel) down to the branches. Lower and middle area/divisional management is being thinned out. As these are the posts where women are well represented, this could turn out to be one of those 'modernisation traps' for women with career ambitions.[25]

The financial service companies reveal the same phenomena which we find right across the tertiary economy: women are disadvantaged by gender-related models of working hours – although there is a general trend for eastern women to cling to full-time jobs – and by the widening wage gap. Nevertheless, it is not yet clear whether, in this particular sector, the restructuring of employment towards jobs for men will continue smoothly as a *linear* process. Since late 1993/early 1994 these internal labour markets have been more or less closed, with a majority of up to 68 per cent consisting of women with newly acquired basic training and also up-to-date specialist and managerial qualifications. In the light of this, it might be assumed, on the one hand, that women will be able to assert their position in the medium term, and even increase their share of management posts. On the other hand, owing to the drastic staffing cutbacks forecast for the sector from the late 1990s, women's current 'home advantage' is more than shaky. It is not yet clear to what extent women will be able to respond to these structural changes steadfastly and actively, especially given intensified requirements of flexible commitment in terms of time and place, and structures of employment that seek increasingly to make 'holistic', total use of skilled human labour. This development, however, will also encourage demands for the *extra-functional virtues*, such as an ability to work in teams, a responsible attitude and a friendly manner with clients. This, in turn, could open the door to female skills and provide a slight boost for women as their position in the field generally deteriorates.

NEW TRACKS TO 'RESET THE POINTS' IN GENDER
RELATIONS? IMPRESSIONS FROM DEUTSCHE BAHN

A team of researchers at the Humboldt University is currently contributing to a project on 'Women in the corporate transformation process in the new federal states: Female options in the financial and transport sectors', which is supported by the Deutsche Forschungs-gemeinschaft. My own part in this concerns the national railway operator Deutsche Bahn AG (DB AG), a service company with a personnel structure highly dominated by men. The former east German rail operator Deutsche Reichsbahn (DR) employed 32 per cent women, and could thus be classified as a mixed company in terms of gender distribution, whereas its western counterpart at the time, the male dominated Deutsche Bundesbahn (DB), employed only 7 per cent women. The all-German DB AG is a privatised company born from the fusion of these two predecessors on 1 January 1994. Although slightly over 15 per cent of the payroll is female, there are significant differences between the new and old states and also between the company's fields of business. The strong presence of women in the new states is particularly concentrated in the customer-oriented service departments, with their specific profile of qualifications and activities.

Unification of the two German states in 1990 created a new situation on the railways: two nationalised companies, DR and DB, now served a single German (transport) market. The merger triggered major corporate restructuring. It is not surprising, given the state of the east German economy, that DR were first on the operating table.

DR's restructuring began with huge cutbacks in staff. Between 1990 and 1993 the payroll was reduced from 236,121 to 148,161, a decrease of 37.2 per cent. Among those who lost their jobs, women were over-represented. The female proportion of DR's workforce fell from 31.6 per cent to 26.4 per cent.

Dismissals were restricted to specific personal terms under an agreement between the management and employees, so that the reductions were achieved by means of socially cushioned measures such as compensation, partial retirement, premature retirement, and so forth. We have evidence that women made more use of these provisions than did men to leave the company. At the same time, DB was facing a staff shortage in certain departments (such as train stewards and in the technical sector). DB responded to the situation by freezing all new recruitment. Positions were to be filled from the DR surplus, which means that DR employees had to meet above-average demands on their geographical mobility. In spite of the staff reductions and transfers, DR still had a surplus of personnel, which was 'carried along' for an initial period.

The corporate labour market policy of DB AG, i.e. since the merger on 1 January 1994, is under three-corner pressure from subsidies (which have to be phased out), the development of company personnel to handle the new market orientation of the various business areas, and social cushions for restructuring.

Although the company structures of the two corporate milieus we have been investigating – financial services and transport – are very different, and with them the processes of corporate restructuring, two inter-referential paths of development can nevertheless be observed. The aim of the transformation process in both corporate environments is to reconstitute these companies as *modern service providers* offering a highly specialised, flexible spectrum of services addressed to specific target groups. This is reflected, first, in a philosophy of 'maximum' customer orientation on the outside and the development of the services required on the inside. Second, the specialisations and redefined business areas associated with this catalyse internal processes aimed at a more efficient added value chain. Changes in the activity structure of individual employees and the occupational demands made of them are coupled with, on the one hand, staff reductions (notably in administration due to slimmer hierarchies and IT rationalisation) and, on the other, a (controlled) expansion in employment in customer-related services.

Our provisional findings at Deutsche Bahn AG differ from those derived in our earlier research in the financial sector, if only – to start with – because the fusion of the two railway operators east and west came relatively late. The previous period, in which DR had adjusted to DB structures by massively reducing staff, quite unlike the financial sector, was overlaid by the operator's conversion from a public authority into a private company, with far-reaching political and structural implications for the organisation as a whole. Furthermore, the way in which eastern staff were integrated was quite different. It did not so much entail a broad training offensive, which in the financial services also performed the function of a collective transition phase, as call upon individual members of staff to fullfil a variety of mobility demands (in terms of *place*, by working elsewhere, sometimes in the west of the country; in terms of *time*, by adapting to new patterns of working hours; and in terms of *content*, by switching to different departments). Individual response was a key factor in staying with the company.

Our studies at Deutsche Bahn AG, like the studies we have already concluded in the financial services, demonstrate that gender is a feature that without any doubt still exercises a crucial 'usherette' function, allocating people places in the increasingly bitter battle over the distribution of labour, and more especially the battle over income and positions (of leadership). At the same time, however, these studies indicate hugely expanding differentiation and hierarchies among women themselves. Transformation and 'market-oriented' company restructuring at Deutsche Bahn AG have brought new requirements of individual life-style, with changes in the nature of work and the way life inside and outside the company is combined. Partcular points include: more compressed tasking, willingness to be mobile and flexible, cooperation and competition, self-employment and servicing, social competence and optimal enhancement of individual resources.

Servicing – often described as a dead end or a bad job – is not a peripheral activity in the company, associated with low wages and prestige, but a central reference for modernisation. Much of this work takes place either around direct customer advice or around inter-company, market-oriented exchange relations. It is ascribed and allocated to women rather than men. This raises opportunities for an enduring source of qualified female employment, but also the risk of new gender demarcations.

At first glance, differentiation among women is a function of motherhood. Provisional analysis suggest that requirements in terms of working hours have become heavier, more flexible and more individualised. The 'normal working week' – especially at Deutsche Bahn, but also in other service companies – is highly differentiated. To keep their job, or improve it, the (female) employees accept limitations on the time they have available for life outside the company, but this flexibility is especially overstretched when they have children of an age requiring care, leading to the 'release' of these women from the workforce. For the most part, the women interviewed – at DB AG most of them work shifts – display a remarkably casual routine in constructing their outside-time requirements around a highly individualized work timetable, rather than the other way round.

This obliges them to synchronise and coordinate on an individual basis, talents which are not evenly spread. We call this skill 'change management'. It applies to a specific ability to coordinate which indicates the active accomplishment of combining various activities and spheres of life into a coherent and consistent whole, thereby achieving 'synergetic effects'. It is regarded, then, as an 'individual resource'. Whether east German women in general have more of this resource to draw on, as a result of their habitualised experience of combining work inside and outside a company, remains to be seen. However, our findings to date confirm that east German women do still make use of specific know-how in tackling new demands on their time, and these routines provide a resource in coping with the pressure to adapt.

Overall, we also find confirmation of something which other analyses have already illustrated.[26] It is not the fact that women have children that underlies their growing exclusion from gainful employment; quite the reverse: 'children' are used to justify exclusion in retrospect. Exclusion and inclusion are determined primarily by qualifications. Along this axis, (east German) women are being elbowed out of the labour market in a process which has not been addressed or researched at all adequately.

SUBTLE DIFFERENTIATIONS OR SOCIAL POLARISATION

The studies show that the gender label still plays a key role in 'assigning people to their place' as the battle for employment heats up, and especially in the tussle for income and rank. At the same time, these studies indicate new and rapidly increasing differentiations and hierarchies among women in the samples. We realised that there was one group of women – at least in the financial services and above all in the insurance field, where few women are to be found in western Germany – actually have excellent chances of promotion and know how to use them. These are middle-aged women (aged 30 to 40 when unification came) who had already been highly motivated to train, achieve and climb in GDR days, who have managerial experience and had finished raising their families when the changes began, or else whose children were now independent beings. These women showed in the GDR that they could be and were persistent and determined about pursuing their careers. Many of them acquired their formal training, usually a university degree, by means of distance study while working and having children. This means that they had to learn to use their time efficiently under GDR conditions, practising 'change management' techniques and learning how to coordinate a variety of demand complexes. These skills, combined with a 'pressure of circumstance' which evidently ignited tremendous potential in these women, now seem to offer an excellent basis for making the grade under new conditions. These women are now well-anchored in the management of east–west mergers in the new federal states, having taken additional or continuous training. In these positions they are profiting from the store of knowledge and experience they acquired in east German institutions and from the fact that they speak a 'common language' with the staff inherited from the past, often functioning as buffers and mediators between western managers and eastern employees (and clients).

THE 'PATH DEPENDENCY' OF GENDER RELATIONS

Our research has illustrated the value of treating societal transformation in Germany as a dual, interwoven process. This two-way interplay with its dovetailed dynamics is of particular relevance to gender relations. The bi-focus is as follows:

- On the one hand, those processes which concern the societal transformation and structural change that were set in motion in former west Germany long before unification and which, since the mid-1970s, have been building into a structural crisis which encroaches upon all fields of social life.
- On the other hand, those economic, social and cultural processes which were triggered in eastern Germany from 1990 onwards by incorporating the former GDR into the old Federal Republic. From the outset, this societal restructuring of eastern Germany has been embedded within the structural changes affecting the old Federal Republic and is also deeply moulded by the character of this western model with its unresolved, crisis-ridden constellation of problems.

Economic reconstruction in eastern Germany has not (yet) created a mirror image of west German structures in (gendered) employment relations. Although institutional structures have been largely appropriated, the social relations inlaid within them are not identical. Furthermore, this transformation (in eastern Germany) has not yet reached its conclusion. It would be accurate to say that it is entering a new, protracted, complex second phase. The points of departure are, first, a drastically shrunken industrial base with the risk of 'tertiary crisis' and, second, the contradictory economic, political and socio-cultural 'knock-on effects' of the first phase. This period of development could be condensed into the hypothesis that the first phase presented an image of 'rupture', dealt with at structural level by rigid institutional transfer and at the level of individual response by the mobilisation of familiar resources which people have proved unwilling to give up, even though they may have adjusted to new requirements. The second phase, by contrast, is characterised by 'enduring discontinuity' in the economic, corporate context and in the personal (occupational) context, linked at the structural level of sector and company with an orientation towards 'new production concepts' and which, at the level of individual action within an interplay of workplace and non-workplace demands, unleashes the 'exploration', 'coordination' and 'fine-tuning' of contradictory and often contrary orientations.

The power and internal dynamics of cultural (habitual and symbolic) influences – and that includes either gender – are inherent in this briefly outlined process of dual transformation. Whereas in the old federal states of Germany the model of the male family breadwinner and the female family carer is institutionally dominant, although undergoing erosion at the level of life scenarios and concrete arrangements, in the new states of eastern Germany we observe an eroding model of combined activity, in which gainful employment for women is the norm, but where domestic labour is unambiguously women's responsibility. Given present income patterns, east German women are expected as individuals to reconcile work inside and outside the home. Gender relations remain very different in concrete practice, both in the private world and in the corporate world. There are, however, also empirical indications that the (re)structuring of gender relations is 'path dependent'. The effect of this is that structural asymmetries in the federal employment system and the division of activity into public and private spheres tend to be 'self-regulating', so that even if east German women cling individually to the combination model and are proving resistant to the mechanisms which exclude them from company labour markets, these asymmetries will tend to be replicated in the new states even against their will.

The process of company change, inlaid within the process of societal transformation, moves along a time axis and, as far as gender relations are concerned, it is still to some degree open; path dependency does not rule out the influence of agents. That is something which (transformation) research by social scientists would need to describe more accurately. We know from studies carried out in core sectors of industry that increasing flexibility in production, being geared to performance criteria, generates new types of segmentation and that these are disadvantageous to women. New patterns of rationalisation in industry clearly indicate trends towards reorganising gender relations, stabilising rather than countering gender hierarchy in the division of labour.[27]

By contrast, studies on new organisational strategies and patterns of labour in certain service segments may well indicate 'that opportunities arise here for redefining the gender division of labour, with some equalisation of career prospects for women and men ... besides, it is becoming harder to draw a boundary between male and female domains, which has hitherto been the decisive segregation mechanism in implementing integrated strategies'.[28] The unification process – as we know from our own empirical analyses – began, for example, by opening up unprecedented scope for action, especially for western male managers, which was utilised very differently as a function of different corporate philosophies, but rarely in conscious pursuit of equality, the promotion of women and/or a democratisation of company gender relations. If we compare companies, we discover major differences in the specific constitution of company gender relations which negate hypotheses seeking to generalise either a negative or a positive scenario. The concrete structure of opportunity for women can sometimes vary substantially even within the same service segment. The empirical research also makes it very obvious that the (corporate) process of reorganisation has 'time windows' which (can) open to varying degrees and for varying periods of time in the sense of opportunity structures for exerting an active influence. More academic reflection is needed to understand this link between the time axis and the design of employment options for women.

NOTES

1. The main features: creation and expansion of a social security system (secondary distribution), public regulation of income distribution (fiscal policy), creation and social regulation of a network of industrial relations ('tripartism'), and creation of a system of intermediate institutions to defend particular interests and to perform public, non-governmental functions (associations, societies, etc.).

2. An analysis that breaks down federal German women's policy into stages shows, for example, that the concept of 'free choice' (career or family) gained ground between 1966 and the early 1980s, although by the late 1970s discussion about 'new motherhood' was gradually beginning, reminding women more insistently again of their alleged 'nature'. Cf. *Frauen im mittleren Alter, Lebenslagen der Geburtskohorten von 1935 bis 1950 in den alten und neuen Bundesländern*, Schriftenreihe des Bundesministeriums für Frauen und Jugend, Vol. 13 (Stuttgart, Berlin, Cologne: Kohlhammer, 1993).

3. N. Fraser, *Widerspenstige Praktiken. Macht, Diskurs, Geschlecht* (Frankfurt am Main: Suhrkamp, 1994), p. 255.

4. N. Fraser, 'Die Gleichheit der Geschlechter und das Wohlfahrtssystem: Ein postindustrielles Gedankenexperiment', in A. Honneth (ed.), *Pathologien des Sozialen. Die Aufgabe der Sozialphilosophie* (Frankfurt am Main: Suhrkamp, 1994), p. 360.

5. N. Fraser, 'Die Gleichheit der Geschlechter', p. 351.

6. U. Schröter, 'Ostdeutsche Frauen im Transformationsprozess', *Aus Politik und Zeitgeschichte*, B20 (1995), p. 40.

7. U. Schröter, 'Ostdeutsche Frauen', p. 41.

8. See also 'Aspekte der Arbeitsmarktentwicklung in Ostdeutschland', *DIW Wochenbericht*, No. 23 (1995), pp. 461–9.

9. E. Holst and J. Schupp, 'Erwerbstätigkeit von Frauen in Ost- und Westdeutschland', *DIW Wochenbericht*, No. 28 (1996), pp. 461–9.

10. B. Eggen, 'Einkommenslagen und wirtschaftlich schwierige Situationen', *Sozialer Fortschritt*, No. 3 (1997), p. 97.

11. *Informationsdienst soziale Indikatoren*, No. 13 (January 1995), 'Einstellung zur Berufstätigkeit der Frauen', pp. 6–9.

12. Statistisches Bundesamt (ed.), *Datenreport* (Bonn: Bundeszentrale für politische Bildung, 1997).

13. W. Zapf, 'Der Untergang der DDR Und die soziologische Theorie der Moderne', in Bernd Giesen/Claus Leggewie, *Experiment Vereinigung. Ein soziologischer Großversuch* (Berlin, 1991), pp. 38–51.

14. R. Geissler, *Die Sozialstruktur Deutschlands* (Opladen: Westdeutscher Verlag, 1992).

15. H. Wiesenthal, 'Institutionelle Dynamik und soziale Defensive. Eine vergleichende Betrachtung der Akteurskonstellation im Transformationsprozeß der neuen Bundesländer', *BISS-public 11*, p. 523.

16. U. Beck and E. Beck-Gernsheim, 'Individualisierung in modernen Gesellschaften. Perspektiven und Kontroversen einer subjektorientierten Soziologie', in U. Beck and E. Beck-Gernsheim, *Riskante Freiheiten* (Frankfurt am Main: Suhrkamp, 1994), p. 35.

17. R. Kreckel, *Politische Soziologie der sozialen Ungleichheit* (Frankfurt and New York: Campus, 1992).

18. H. Hüning and H-M. Nickel, 'Grossbetriebliche Dienstleistungen. Rascher Aufbau und harte Konsolidierung', in Lutz, H-M. Nickel, Schmidt, Sorge (eds), *Arbeit, Arbeitsmarkt und Betriebe* (Opladen: Leske Budrich, 1996).

19. H-M. Nickel and H. Hüning *et al.*, 'Frauen im betrieblichen Transformationsprozess am Beispiel Deutsche Bahn', DFG Projekt 1996–98. The project team consists of Hasko Hüning (Free University of Berlin), Michael Frey, Irina Kohlmetz, Iris Peinl, Susanne Völker and two students, Alexandra Manske and Ulrike Stodt, all of whom are at the Humboldt University in Berlin.

20. H-M. Nickel and H. Hüning (eds), *Finanzmetropole Berlin. Strategien betrieblicher Transformation* (Opladen: Leske & Budrich, 1998).

21. H. Hilf and H. Jacobsen, *Einzelhandel in den neuen Bundesländern*, final report by SfS Dortmund 1995; O. Struck-Möbbeck, 'Transformation und Modernisierung im ostdeutschen Einzelhandel', in H. Hüning and H-M. Nickel (eds), *Grossbetrieblicher Dienstleistungssektor in den neuen Bundesländern* (Opladen: Leske & Budrich, 1997).

22. M. Skogvall, 'Das weibliche Handlungsfeld "Pflege"', in H. Hüning and H-M. Nickel (eds), *Grossbetrieblicher Dienstleistungssektor*.

23. Hüning and Nickel, *Finanzmetropole Berlin*.

24. The reference figure for the retail trade in the new federal states in the late 1990s is a workforce of 490,000, 73 per cent of them women. The Federal Statistics Office reports the following development from 1991 to 1994: in 1991 there were about 591,000 jobs in the sector, 71.9 per cent held by women; until 1994, the workforce continued to grow, with 632,000 jobs that year. Yet in percentage terms, the women's share fell to 64.2 per cent (406,000 women and 226,000 men).

25. In the project seminar on 'Women in the corporate transformation process' at the Humboldt University in Berlin, we have taken up the question we asked in 1993 about what happened to the women who used to manage branches of the east German savings bank in East Berlin. To begin with, it looked as though they would be offered promotion paths once they had completed the right training. Now, however, it seems that not one of the 73 women has obtained promotion. In fact, most of them have not even been able to hold their rung on the ladder. See H. Hüning and H-M. Nickel *et al.*, 'Transformation – betriebliche Reorganisation – Geschlechterverhältnisse', special issue of *Zeitschrift für Frauenforschung* (Hannover: Institut Frau und Gesellschaft), Vol. 16, Nos 1 and 2 (1998).

26. Friedrich Ebert-Stiftung, *Wirtschaftliche Leistungsfähigkeit, sozialer Zusammenhalt, ökologische Nachhaltigkeit* (Bonn: Dietz, 1998).

27. B. Aulenbacher, 'Technologieentwicklung und Geschlechterverhältnis', in B. Aulenbacher and M. Goldmann (eds), *Transformation im Geschlechterverhältnis* (Frankfurt and New York: Campus, 1995).

28. M. Goldmann, 'Globalisierungsprozesse und die Arbeit von Frauen', in E. Altvater, E. Haug and O. Negt (eds), *Turbo-Kapitalismus* (Hamburg: VSA, 1997), p. 157.

7

Pre-school Education and Childcare in East Germany: Transformation and New Challenges

Rosalind Pritchard

Provision in the GDR

The German Democratic Republic (GDR) was well-equipped with daycare facilities (*Krippen*) for babies and toddlers, kindergarten education for pre-schoolers, and after-school organisations (*Horte*) for pupils whose parents were out at work. The extent of these provisions was among the highest in all the eastern bloc countries. The fate of these childcare institutions is worth studying because they were an important agent of political socialisation and personality structuration. They were intended to help mothers combine work and child-rearing and, in so doing, to contribute to equality of the sexes. They also constituted a form of social protection for families at risk (though 'risk' would hardly have been explicitly admitted). Most east Germans would have had contact with state childcare provision. This chapter discusses what became of these all-pervasive institutions after the *Wende*, and explores the implications of system transformation in this field.

The *Krippen* (and their weekly equivalents) took children from 10 weeks to 3 years of age and, as a rule, were open from 6 a.m. to 6 or 7 p.m. By the 1980s, the *Krippe* care-givers had become the second largest group of health care professionals after nurses and by 1989 numbered 75,000 in a sector which had the capacity to accept 353,203 children.[1] By the middle of that decade, about three-quarters of all GDR children under 3 years attended these institutions, whereas this was the case for only 2 per cent of the age range in the Federal Republic of Germany (FRG).[2] The children were tended in groups of about 18, homogeneous by age; there were supposed to be three care-givers per group, but in practice there were usually just two, so in real terms the ratio of care-givers to children was about 1:9 – the same as in the Old *Bundesländer* (OBL).[3] Single parents were treated so favourably that many people deliberately chose not to get married. If their children were not able to attend the *Krippe* through illness, or had no *Krippe* place available, the GDR state paid between 250 and 350 Marks monthly (depending on the number of children in the family) to cover the cost of care in the home.[4]

The kindergartens took children from age 3 until they started school at 6 or slightly older. The availability of places in proportion to the age group rose from 20.5 per cent in 1950 to an almost saturation coverage of 94 per cent in 1988; this contrasted with provision in the FRG where there were places for about 80 per cent of the age group, but with large regional differences.[5] In the mid-1980s, *Krippen* and kindergartens were often combined in the same building to facilitate parents who had children spanning the age range of 0–3 and 3–6.[6] By 1989, there were 13,113 kindergartens in the GDR of which 1,477 were run by business concerns (*Betriebe*), 383 by churches, and the rest by state authorities; the number of children in the childcare system was 785,905.[7] The kindergartens provided free childcare with food at very low cost (0.35 Marks per day).[8] A substantial staff was required to run them; in 1989, the relative proportions of staff categories within the system were: full kindergarten teachers 61,823 (68.1 per cent); assistants 8,732 (9.6 per cent) and helpers 20,221 (22.3 per cent).[9] Teachers underwent a three-year period of training, assistants did one-and-a-half years, and helpers were untrained.

In the *Hort*, staff looked after children from the end of school until their working parents were able to come and collect them. From 1982 onwards, the *Hort* formed an integral part of schools' educational provision, and by 1989 85 per cent of GDR children in years 1–4 attended one of these institutions, sometimes spending as many as 8–10 hours a day in school premises. Understandably, utilisation tended to become less intensive as the children gradually became more self-sufficient: thus, in schoolgrade 1, 93 per cent of children used the *Hort*, whereas in grade 4, the figure fell to 40 per cent.[10] *Hort* care-givers (38,000 in 1989) trained for four years, studied two subjects and had the same status as teachers; consequently, they could be asked to give classes at school and could be used interchangeably with the teaching staff.[11] The director of a *Hort* had the status of deputy head.

After the birth of a child, there was a period of 20 weeks' leave during which parents could claim an allowance at the level of the last net wage. When this time had elapsed, men or women could claim a 'baby year',[12] during which they received payment at 90 per cent of their earlier net wage for the first 20 weeks, thereafter 70 per cent. If a second child was born, they were also allocated 90 per cent of their wage during the first 20 weeks, and from the twentieth week onwards, 75 per cent.[13] The state gave women flexibility in hours of work and even provided a couple of paid 'housekeeping days' every year to allow them to attend to domestic matters. Working mothers with more than two children had their weekly hours cut from 43¾ hours to 40 hours per week; children's clothes were state-subsidised, and families with several children were accorded preferential treatment in the allocation of living accommodation.[14]

IDEOLOGICAL UNDERPINNINGS OF GDR
CHILDCARE STRUCTURES

In the GDR, childcare was collectivist and intended to help integrate children into group life. At first it was meant to be emancipatory for females but later it assumed the central function of enabling women to combine family life with gainful employment; this was very necessary since it was almost impossible for a family to live on one wage. Childcare was meant to contribute to equality between men and women; to provide social education for the children; to bind them into a political system and to help establish loyalty to the GDR. The state for its part squarely accepted responsibility for providing pre-school childcare.[15] More than 90 per cent of women aged between 15 and 60 worked, and the state made it as easy as possible for them to do so. Working was both their duty and their right; thus the 1950 Act governing childcare was revealingly entitled 'Law for the Protection of Mothers and Children and for the *Rights* of Women'.

This contrasts with the pre-*Wende* situation in the Federal Republic where the need for an increased labour force was met to some extent by importing foreign workers; this made it less necessary to increase the number of women in the workforce. Hence, the *Krippen* and kindergartens were not as developed as in the GDR, and demands for an improvement in provision were rejected with the argument that this would undermine the family.[16] Some people also were critical of the type of childcare they provided. Manfred Schmidt[17] points out that demand for female labour is influenced by policy, politics and cultural tradition, and that the (western) German-speaking nations have high levels of inequality in female–male ratios of labour force participation. He argues that Catholicism (and the lower level of secularisation associated with it) is the central variable accounting for the small improvement in these ratios in German-speaking countries. He also takes heed of the fact that the small and medium-sized enterprises (SMEs) which predominate in German-speaking countries are more likely to resist recruitment of female labour. Religious parties of

Christian Democrat complexion have incorporated the conservative stance of Catholicism into family policy, and institutionalised its attitudes towards matters such as social security, childcare, education and taxation. Public childcare has been promoted more by leftist governments or Protestant countries: 'Protestantism', Schmidt believes, 'is more open to a non-traditional division of labour in the family and in the nation as a whole'.[18]

The GDR socialist state was proud of its childcare provision which it regarded as an admirable achievement (though its flaws will be discussed below). There is recent empirical evidence from a longitudinal study of subjects in Rostock and Mannheim[19] that the *Krippe* and *Hort* helped to protect young GDR people against psychiatric disturbances in later life. Since GDR families were usually small, the authorities recommended institutional care on the grounds that it gave much-needed social experience to children who had no siblings or came from small families. The fact of coming together with other youngsters was intended to make them socially more skilled, and better at forming relationships with others later on in their lives. The *Krippen* provided structure and a sort of elementary education. It is sometimes argued retrospectively that they may have helped to even out disparities in children's social backgrounds and compensate for possible social disadvantage on the part of children from poor families. In the GDR, however, there were supposed to be *no* poor families, and so officially the concept of compensatory education was unnecessary. From the Party's angle, the *Krippen* served as a kind of pre-conditioning for a Collective, and the early institutionalisation of the young provided an opportunity for laying down the rudiments of political socialisation. Children were taught songs about soldiers (such as *Hör' ich die Soldaten singen; Mein Bruder ist Soldat; Lieber Soldat, du trägst ein Gewehr; Des Peters großer Bruder*) which sounded innocent enough but were intended to predispose them favourably towards the military; and of course they all learned that Erich Honecker was a 'good person'. However, the children were carefully looked after, often with a high degree of professionalism especially in respect of medical care. The service offered was widely appreciated, and helped individuals undertake the long-term planning of their lives. Women were not condemned to be 'just housewives' for long periods of their existence, and this 'mediated a special feeling of self-esteem to young women'.[20]

SHORTCOMINGS OF GDR DAYCARE

Case Study: David's Experience of the Krippe

Any criticism of the GDR *Krippen* tended to be taken as an implied criticism of female emancipation (perhaps conceived somewhat differently in the GDR and the FRG). Yet they were not suitable for all children. The subject in the following case study is a young woman teacher, and her account has been included because it embodies concerns experienced by many people, not just by her, and vividly illustrates the themes which were later taken up by paediatricians and politicians.[21]

> Interviewer's Question: How did your son react to the *Krippe*?
> Mother's Answer: My son David was nine months old when I first brought him to the *Krippe*. I had to go back to work because my husband was still a student at the time and I had to earn money. David had been accustomed for nine months to spending his time alone with me and it was extremely difficult for him to leave me in the mornings. At the weekends my husband was at home, and from morning to bedtime we spent the whole day together with our child. We played, laughed and sang with him a lot; we went for walks and met up with other parents and children in the playground. In the family, there are two other children of the same age with whom we were in frequent contact. My husband and I often visited his grandparents or my brothers and sisters or my in-laws so that David did not live solely in the company of grown-ups; in those nine months he also had the company of other children.
> David could not get used to the new rhythm of life at the *Krippe* and to the fact that he was parted from me. We tried to manage it for five months: that morning parting which took place very early – at half past six in the morning because I had to be at school at a quarter past seven. Each time, there was a lot of crying, clinging to me, and I myself had to ... it sounds awful ... more or less push the child away and put him into the arms of the care-giver. It created a lot of problems for him and for me too. Both of us found it very difficult to live with this state of affairs. The time in the *Krippe* was hard. He did not like being there – I think because everything was too organised. There was only one room in which 15–18 children between 6 months and a year old were all accommodated and in this room they played, ate, slept and had their nappies changed. Everything took place in the same room with two care-givers and a

great deal of noise. The children didn't have a single moment to themselves and could not sleep or play in peace or eat and drink when they felt like it. The day was organised from morning to night.

I think David was never longer than 3 or 4 days there before he began to run a temperature usually associated with bronchitis, colds, coughs or some other infection – perhaps sinusitis; he was always suffering from something. I used to go to the doctor and get a medical certificate so that I could stay at home to nurse him. After about a week he was better, then the whole thing began again. I brought him back to the *Krippe*, and there was a lot of crying and resistance. He simply didn't want to be there and I felt his distress. At first I could not devise any alternative because I just had to go to work and there was no relative who could have looked after him. However, one day a mother of one of my pupils – I had a first form at the time – offered to take care of him. She called for him in the morning and he seemed to react well to her. He was by himself in her house and she was there just for him, not like in the *Krippe* where there are a lot of children. She lived near the school and I was able to go there in my free periods to tell him stories and play with him.

When he was not quite two, I had another child and was at home with the two boys. It was a lovely time with both the little ones. My days were full. When David was three, ... his brother Tobias went to the *Krippe*. By that time, however, the conditions had changed and there was more space so that the children no longer had to do everything in one room; there were separate rooms for sleeping and for playing and for eating. The conditions were really different and had improved a lot. To this very day, Tobias is a different sort of person who likes being with other people in groups, and has a lot of friends, whereas David needs time to himself. I knew that when he was small, he must have thought: 'My mother is farming me out and abandoning me'.

In December, David was 3 years old and Tobias was 6 months old, and at the age of 3 children were supposed to go the kindergarten. I was told by a community social worker that it would be much better for him to go the kindergarten, that he would learn much more, that a lot of activities took place there which were much better for the upbringing of a child. This is what they said to my husband and me but even so the two of us decided to keep the child at home.

The young mother in this interview takes some trouble to emphasise that David was not isolated from other children, and that she and his father were in a position to provide a lively social environment. For this family the pain of separation predominated in their experience of professional childcare, and the child reacted by manifesting a whole series of psychosomatic illnesses. The liability of *Krippe* children to acute respiratory illness – especially just after entering it for the first time – is well-documented and was used against these institutions after the *Wende*. As a matter of principle, the east German authorities were unsympathetic to the concept of psychosomatic illness (Freud was regarded as 'bourgeois' and 'decadent'), and they treated respiratory disorders by insisting on extreme rigour in the matter of hygiene within the *Krippe*; this was used as a pretext to exclude outsiders, including parents, on the grounds that they might bring germs and infections into the *Krippe* (though in the mid-1980s, a more liberal regime was established and parental exclusion was no longer so draconian).[22]

David's negative reaction is bound up with the overcrowded conditions which then prevailed in the *Krippen* (mid 1980s) – conditions that had improved by the time his younger brother came along. The population of the GDR was falling even before the *Wende*, and by the end of the decade there was overcapacity in *Krippe* provision.[23] This particular young teacher's husband later became a doctor and her in-laws were independent small-business people who as a societal category were not popular with the authorities (too 'capitalist'). Money did, however, give David's mother the opportunity to buy herself and her son out of the state system and into a childcare situation which was much better suited to his individual needs. It is significant that the authorities made an effort to persuade these parents to put the child into a public kindergarten on the grounds that it would be 'much better for him'.

Criticism of GDR Pre-school Education

The *Krippe*-kindergarten childcare system was so all-pervasive that it marked whole generations of GDR people. The Max-Planck-Institut authors[24] report on speculations about whether the high divorce rate characteristic of the GDR was related to disorders in primary socialisation arising from too much exposure to state daycare. It is of course impossible to prove such an assertion, but it is clear that up to the point of unification east and west Germans were socialised very differently. It was alleged that the GDR institutions were not good in the promotion of giftedness; that they encouraged conformism rather than individualism; that the children developed communicative malfunctions like apathy or forms of autism in which they withdrew emotionally from others; and that they were over-protected and over-organised. By assuming so much responsibility, they had a tendency to marginalise parents in the upbringing of their own sons and daughters; and sometimes they used the authority of the health professionals to confront parents with a *fait accompli*, or nudge them towards a decision which they might not otherwise have made but was 'good for them'.

Although the *Krippe* had been viewed in the GDR as much less ideological than the kindergarten, it was still castigated by western pediatricians after the *Wende*. Indeed, pre-school education as a whole emerged as one of the east German institutions subject to the most intense criticism. The Enquête-Kommission of the Bundestag[25] called the GDR kindergarten 'a preparation for the indoctrination methods of the school', and in the west German press it was sometimes positively demonised and used as a pretext for denigrating ex-GDR citizens.[26] Johannes Pechstein, a Mainz university professor, went so far as to call for the reduction of east German *Krippe* provision to the 2 per cent level which then prevailed in the West.[27] J. Niermann in a report to the Bundestag characterised the GDR school as a 'penitentiary', 'a place of denunciation' and a 'factory for producing socialist cadres'; for him the *Krippen* were 'contemptible' and 'unworthy', the GDR parents 'ignorant' and 'psychologically deformed', and the dictatorship of the working class in the GDR comparable to the dictatorship of National Socialism.[28] Of course, this is an extreme view but it illustrates western hostility towards east German state childcare. Eastern professionals in that sector, after undergoing a period of initial self-doubt and insecurity, reacted to it with bitterness.[29]

In the 1980s the GDR had set out to reform its own pre-school institutions. This movement towards pre-*Wende* reform within the GDR actually permeated the whole education System across a wide range of different sectors; it is important to remember that such self-criticism did exist, otherwise a false impression arises of an inert monolithic GDR system devoid of self-insight, frozen in outmoded practice and waiting to be 'rescued' by the west. Although political authority weighed heavily upon the pre-school sector, it was not a monolith: strong disagreements eventually emerged between various factions in relation to reform of pre-school education.

In the 1965 Law on the Unified Socialist Education System, the *Krippe* was designated as the lowest level in the education system, but it was governed by the Ministry of Health, whereas the kindergarten and the *Horte* were responsible to the Ministry of Education and were much more integrated into the mainstream of schooling. Teaching there was carried out according to unified principles and had binding curricula. For the *Krippen*, from 1968–84 the guidelines *Pädagogische Aufgaben und Arbeitsweise der Krippen*, edited by Eva Schmidt-Kolmer, were officially sanctioned and universally accepted by the care-givers. They relied on Russian rather than on indigenous research, and were based on the best practice of the time. They were also hugely prescriptive. The Ninth Youth Report[30] narrates how the head of a *Krippe* was discovered literally testing the temperature of the children's food with a thermometer, and how a trainee care-giver worried about whether it was preferable to apply soap to a face-cloth or the face-cloth to the soap. Christine Weber[31] tells us that the diameter of toys was specified (at least 2 cm) so as to discourage swallowing by young children; pets such as hamsters, fish and birds were discouraged to minimise the danger of allergies. It must have been difficult for the care-givers to promote freedom in their young charges when they were themselves so tightly restricted in their operations.

Eva Schmidt-Kolmer, who was leader of the *Institut für Hygiene des Kindes und Jugendalters* (IHKJ) until its dissolution in 1990, exercised enormous personal influence on pre-school education. She energetically refuted theories like those of Bowlby[32] on maternal deprivation, and attributed problems to deficits in daily organisation or lack of assiduousness on the part of the care-givers.[33] Certainly, she regarded the *Krippe* as the first step in developing the socialist personality, and the care-giver as the mediator of social and cultural values. Games were exercises with objectives to be accomplished and formally entered in developmental records – an approach which somewhat negated their significance as an individual form of experience and as *fun*. Pedagogical leadership and control were over-emphasised, as were the 'leading role of the care-giver' (linked, of course, to the leading role of the SED Party and the working class); any dissent from the dominant orthodoxy was suppressed.[34] A poor relationship often existed between advisers and care-givers who experienced their interventions as heavy-handed and oppressive, and who after 1990 rejected them – sometimes with vehement hate. The accumulated negativity surrounding the whole relationship between the care-givers and 'authority' figures made implementation of western reform after the *Wende* more difficult than it might otherwise have been.[35]

But a reforming tendency did exist, and by the end of the 1970s, a rift had already opened between Eva Schmidt-Kolmer and more modern thinkers. In 1985, the *Pädagogische Aufgaben* were superseded by the more research-based *Programm für die Erziehungsarbeit*. Disagreements between childcare professionals were hushed up, and the fiction was maintained that the *Programm* was just a working over of the 1968 *Aufgaben*. It was the doyenne of GDR pre-school education – Schmidt-Kolmer herself – who in 1983 successfully presented the revised *Programm* to the Council of Medical Sciences for its approval. The new model showed more respect for the child's individuality and for human diversity, and interpreted 'learning' as a process which took place throughout the day, with or without the help of the care-giver. The role of the adult was not just to plan activities for an end-result, but to facilitate and promote them, paying greater attention to spontaneity and creativity.[36] In the settling-in phase for tiny children at the *Krippe*, it was deemed acceptable for a member of the family to be present; this would have helped to mitigate the separation anxiety so graphically described by David's mother in the case study above.

The *Programm* was approved in 1983 but did not come into force until 1985, and thereafter was implemented gradually until it became fully mandatory in 1987. The reason for this delay was political. Despite its successful defence in front of the medical authorities, it involved a restructuring of basic principles and was vetoed by Margot Honecker personally! She objected to the section on the environment, to finger painting, and to the fact that not enough was being done to promote socialist ways of thinking and behaving. The leading role of the care-giver was at variance with increased freedom for the children, and had apparently been down-graded: this had to change. Greater clarity in the formulation of objectives was demanded, and the *Programm* was referred for revision to the pre-school department of the *Akademie der Pädagogischen Wissenschaften*. Here the 'correct' political terminology was inserted (the 'leading role of the care-giver' was reinstated), concessions were made and a certain amount of 'fudging' took place – all of which rendered the *Programm* much more vulnerable to denigration after the *Wende.*[37] Prompt publication of a new training textbook for care-givers was desperately needed, and should have been synchronised with the appearance of the 1985 *Programm*, but there was so much political in-fighting about its content that its appearance was delayed until 1990. In the circumstances, it was very difficult for the care-givers to discern the new emphases of the *Programm*, and to base reform on them. They were accustomed to being *required* to carry out certain actions, and in the end they tended just to fall back into their old habits conditioned by the 1968 guidelines. In this way, the liberalisation potential of the *Programm* was largely neutralised and wasted.

CHANGES AFTER THE *WENDE*

During the existence of the GDR, criticism of childcare and pre-school education had been repressed. After the *Wende*, however, a number of organisations within the New *Bundesländer* campaigned for change; *Der Unabhängige Frauenverband* and the *Deutsche Forum Partei* (DFP) wanted to free the kindergarten from bureaucracy, *dirigisme* and formalism in organisation, and from militarism in content. The *Liberal-Demokratische Partei Deutschlands* (LDLP) and *Demokratischer Aufbruch* wanted parents to be able to choose between institutions offered by different providers and characterised by different pedagogical approaches.[38] There were also demands for reduction of the ratio between care-givers and children and for the formation of small groups (not necessarily to be homogeneous in age); for more parental involvement in *Krippen*; for continuity in contact between children and specific individual care-givers; and for children to spend shorter daily periods in pre-school care. The overwhelming consensus was that daycare institutions should be retained but improved in quality.[39]

The legal basis at national level for the reform of childcare was the Child and Youth Support Law (*Kinder- und Jugendhilfegesetz* (KJHG))[40] which came into force in the New *Bundesländer* on 3 October 1990. In the government commentary on the Ninth Youth Report, it is argued that the changes were endorsed and approved by the last GDR government and can in no way be regarded as having been 'imposed' on the New *Bundesländer*.[41] However, the KJHG was in many respects a continuation of existing FRG law; it originated in the west under different social conditions, and although well received, was not always easy to implement. Daycare of children under 3 years was enacted by a series of *Länder* laws between 1991 and 1993. Local providers of public childcare are legally obliged to ensure that it corresponds to 'need' which is differently defined in different *Länder*. Four of them (Saxony, Saxony-Anhalt, Thuringia and Mecklenburg-Vorpommern) do not distinguish between *Krippe* and kindergarten in this respect, but Brandenburg, which is the only *Land* to provide a numerical target, sees the letter of the law being fulfilled if *Krippen* are provided for 40 per cent of the age group, and kindergartens for 90 per cent of 3–6 year olds; moreover, it accords to parents a legal right to a *Krippe* place for their child.[42] The Brandenburg Ministry[43] sees state financial commitment to childcare not just as a form of 'consumption' but as an investment in the future, and a precondition for a possible increase in the birthrate and in parental employment. Mecklenburg-Vorpommern does not give a legal right to a *Krippe* place, but in 1992, 40.2 per cent of its 0–3 year olds were accommodated – a figure which can be broadly regarded as corresponding to need. Saxony and Saxony-Anhalt give a legal right to childcare without distinguishing between children under and over 3 years, but do not define exactly what the numerical provision should be. Some of the New *Bundesländer* (Brandenburg, Mecklenburg-Vorpommern, Saxony-Anhalt and Thuringia) have provisions in their law stating that public childcare must be geographically accessible to parents. Since Mecklenburg-Vorpommern is an especially sparsely populated region, there is under-provision in some rural areas, estimated at 10 per cent.[44] Obviously, in cases where public daycare is under-provided or difficult in terms of access, private daycare *(Tagespflege)* can be an important safety net. Thuringia, which insists that provision must correspond to need, subsidises these at the rate of DM200 per place and month, and Mecklenburg-Vorpommern at DM120 (figures for 1993).[45] Other *Länder* also have provisions for subsidy, but these are usually more restrictive than in Thuringia, and have the effect of favouring public provision. Clearly, the provision and the use of *Krippen* is subject to considerable regional variations in the New *Bundesländer*, but the official figure is that in 1994 they were used by 41 per cent of the age cohort.[46]

The update of the KJHG of July 1992 gave the right to a kindergarten place for all 3–6 year-olds. For Old *Bundesländer* citizens, this represented a significant development because it contributed to a new balance between private and public responsibility for children (though for many Old *Bundesländer* local authorities, scarcity of resources made it difficult to implement the new requirement). For New *Bundesländer* citizens, however, it was no improvement on the situation in the erstwhile GDR; indeed the fact that in most New *Bundesländer* the legal right to a pre-school place was limited to 3–6 year-olds, thereby excluding the *Krippe*, was retrograde and based on a much narrower concept of entitlement than in the GDR.[47] This formal legal right existed in a context of massive reduction of kindergarten places in the New *Bundesländer*.[48]

In the West the *Hort* has played a minor role, often being used most intensively by single parents or parents in distress; its negative image makes it conceptually difficult to develop, and many people feel that, after school, children need a change of scene rather than staying on in the same building. In an attempt to contribute to equality of opportunity, the Old *Bundesländer* have made use of the All-Day School (or variations of it); this is almost unknown in the New *Bundesländer* which feature the *Hort* instead. In an attempt to find a rationale for the *Hort*, the Tenth Youth Report suggests that it should promote socialisation processes and develop independent personalities; also that it could extend traditional concepts of gender roles; its development in all *Bundesländer* and its diversification in the New *Bundesländer* is advocated.

Horte are governed by the same laws as those which relate to *Krippen* and kindergartens. Only in Brandenburg and in Saxony-Anhalt do parents have a legal right to daycare for children over 6 years, the former until they finish primary school, the latter even up to the age of 14. Opening times are supposed to be set in collaboration with parents, and in Thuringia and Saxony-Anhalt have been legally fixed at 6 a.m. to 6 p.m.[49] There is no legal right to subsidy of *Hort* places in any of the New *Bundesländer*, so it is optional and varies from *Land* to *Land*. Parents in the New *Bundesländer* spend less on average on their children than those in the Old

Bundesländer,[50] probably because their incomes are smaller, and their contributions are means-tested; and the fact that *Horte* now have to be paid for whereas they were free in the GDR has led to withdrawals.[51] In 1989, the provision of *Hort* places for schoolgrades 1–4 was 88 per cent with an actual takeup rate of about 80 per cent.[52] At the end of 1990, only 5 per cent of 6–10 year-olds in the Old *Bundesländer* had access to a *Hort* place, whereas in the New *Bundesländer* the figure was about every second child in this age group.[53] By 1992, the actual take-up rate in the New *Bundesländer* was as follows: Brandenburg, 35 per cent; Mecklenburg-Vorpommern, 48 per cent; Saxony, 32 per cent; Saxony-Anhalt, no figures; Thuringia, no figures.[54]

In the New *Bundesländer*, the *Hort* is not difficult to justify because many families are under pressure. Many young people live in increasingly threatening and destabilising conditions. Schools in difficult areas have had to accustom themselves to their pupils sometimes going without proper nourishment and clothes, or even to the fact of them becoming homeless. A survey carried out by Maria Fölling-Albers[55] in Berlin-Mitte showed that childhood is becoming increasingly isolated there. Forty per cent of all children grow up without brothers and sisters; 40 per cent have only one sibling; 30 per cent of all children experience the separation of their parents while still at primary school; and 35 per cent live in one-parent families. These figures are for Berlin which is in a special situation, and does not represent the whole of east Germany, but the day-to-day reality is that many children lack emotional backup, and parents are not always in a position to look after them competently. In the GDR, they were accustomed to the state taking on a lot of responsibility for the organisation of children's free time. Pre-conditioning has given them the expectation of state help in the upbringing of their children. However, now that things have changed, the parents need to assume a much greater role in structuring their offspring's leisure, but not all of them feel equipped to do so.

This increased imperative of parental childcare coincides with a period in which the adults themselves, especially if unemployed, are under great psychological, social and financial pressure. Rather than 're-possessing' their children from the grasp of a socialist state, many parents, particularly the worse-off, seek to divest themselves as far as possible of childcare responsibilities and expect the school to compensate for the home's shortcomings. Even those who are unemployed do not necessarily use their enforced leisure to look after their children. Some lack parenting skills; some lack self-confidence and need counselling or therapy for their own problems. Violence and frustration among children is increasing concomitantly with regional and social inequality, exposure to the mass media, uncertainty about values and economic hardship.[56] The challenge to the education authorities is enormous: if parents are often not in a position to 'bring up' their young successfully, then other compensatory arrangements must be made. The All-Day Schools constitute one such response but they do not come cheap. Changed family circumstances, the increasing isolation of children, the fact that many adults are inexperienced in childcare or are under too much pressure themselves to give it the time it needs – all these factors necessitate a political response on the part of the education authorities, and a great deal of money which is in increasingly short supply.

In the process of its implementation, the KJHG predictably ran up against historically conditioned differences between Old and New *Bundesländer*, each of which had quite different concepts of the relative importance of state and family in the upbringing of children. Whereas in west Germany, the educational role of the state had been clearly subordinated to that of parents and family, the GDR parental role had been supplemented by other agents such as teachers, colleagues and the Collective who had all exercised a legitimate and state-sponsored influence in pursuit of socialist ideology and the 'all-round developed socialist personality'.[57] It is easy to criticise the GDR, but at least it regarded children as important and had a clear concept of its aims for them. By contrast, when east German care-givers went west after the *Wende* to observe their counterparts' work, one of the things they noticed was that the westerners did not have any real, conscious rationale for what they were doing – *'kein Konzept'*.[58] The Tenth Youth Report is implicitly recognising a pre-existing deficit in the Old *Bundesländer* when its authoring Commission notes that in the west, more attention is now being paid to the very young than in preceding years: this is being reflected in the development of policies for children and in giving them a legal right to a kindergarten place.[59]

The KJHG emphasises the right of children to their own individual personal and social development. This contrasts with the collectivistic process of socialisation in the GDR according to which care-givers were supposed to avoid any preference or partiality for individual children, and instead had to give priority to group integration. The concept of childhood was based on a deficiency model, and children were oriented towards adult norms as quickly as possible. The question needs to be posed as to whether new forms of childcare are now producing different sorts of people with different norms and outlooks. Lieselotte Ahnert and colleagues[60] carried out research comparing educational attitudes of parents with small children in Russia and in both parts of Germany. Their conclusion was that the Russian child-rearing style differed substantially from the German style, and that there was a considerable degree of commonality between east and west Germans. They attribute this to a common nineteenth-century heritage, and conclude that there is a basic compatibility in the early socialisation patterns espoused by east and west German mothers. They believe that state socialist doctrines of education for small children were not a very effective agent of socialisation in (east) German families.

The aim of the KJHG is to produce equality of opportunity for children, and to level out structural or individual deficits; it is based on a concept of participation, dialogue and cooperation between families and childcare professionals which should result in children being able to exercise more influence over their life, learning and leisure. Ideally, the power differential between those in need of youth services and professionals proffering those services should be reduced. There is even a concept that the child and youth social services should actively *fight* the cause of children in all domains of politics and public life, and liaise with the *Länder* and local authorities. The youth services are enjoined to work towards a more collaborative integrative model, cooperating, for example with schools and educational administration bodies (KJHG Article 81). It will be interesting to see what becomes of this aspiration: many New *Bundesländer* citizens experienced the new school structure as divisive, pulling apart school and leisure, school and home, school and professional life. They are therefore very receptive to notions of cooperation between school and youth welfare services as enshrined in the KJHG.[61] Under the old regime, they rarely ventured to make criticisms and suggestions, and there was no *Mitbestimmung* (joint decision-making), so they are being confronted with new opportunities. There is already evidence[62] that care-givers are moving from a commitment to creating a positive *group* atmosphere to an increased focus on *individual* children and their needs.

In Article 5 of the KJHG, the principle of mixed public/private provision is espoused, provided this does not lead to 'disproportionate expenditure'. New laws allow New *Bundesländer* churches, welfare associations, parents and commercial organisations to offer pre-school education – as has long been the case in the west.[63] Although the New *Bundesländer* do not have the same tradition of voluntary childcare associations as the Old *Bundesländer*, they now have about the same number of institutions; but these tend to be small in size and are not perceived as equal in weight to their western equivalents.[64] The state assumes a large element of the costs of private institutions, and savings are small even if they are taken over by independent providers.[65] Hence, many east German local politicians do not understand why they should privatise. The official rhetoric is that privatisation is part of a client-centred approach in which diversity of provision is perceived as appropriate for a pluralistic society and is even expected to stimulate new ideas within the system. Pluralism of provision and of values is advocated, but the demographic trend forces mergers and closures of institutions, and is therefore somewhat in tension with pluralism.

Historically speaking, the churches have had quite a long-standing, if quantitatively minor, involvement in east German pre-school education: for example, in 1979 the *Evangelische Kirche* maintained 320 kindergartens with 17,000 children.[66] These church institutions were much less rigid than the state kindergartens, more oriented to western models and more willing to involve parents.[67] In 1989, about 11.3 per cent of childcare institutions were maintained by firms, 86 per cent by local state authorities, and 3 per cent by churches.[68] In the New *Bundesländer* the churches are now much freer than they were in the GDR to provide voluntary childcare institutions, yet their commitment to *Krippe* development remains small and they have been slow to use their rights as *Freie Träger*. In principle, the existence of sound childcare makes it easier for women to continue with unplanned pregnancies; certainly the provision of such care has traditionally been one of the responses of churches to women considering abortion, and it is suggested in the Tenth Youth Report that the churches' dilatoriness in organising this care undermines their claims to provide religious protection for unborn life.[69] In the GDR, there were special institutions for the handicapped. Now, however, the trend is towards the integration of these children into the mainstream and there is convergence between east and west in the extent of such integration. Mainstreaming handicapped youngsters is an important policy trend but has not recast provisions in eastern Germany. In the mid-1990s, some 60 per cent of children with disabilities were still looked after in special institutions, more so in rural areas (72 per cent) than in towns and cities (48 per cent).[70]

QUANTITATIVE PROVISION AND THE IMPACT OF COMPETITION

Despite new laws and promising changes, developments in east German society as a whole are causing significant problems in childcare provision. The birthrate in the New *Bundesländer* halved between 1989 and 1994.[71] In 1992, the proportion of unemployed was twice as high in the New as in the Old *Bundesländer*. It was officially given as 15.6 per cent, but if one counted those in work creation schemes, vocational re-training, premature retirement and so-called *Warteschleifen*, the percentage of 'potentially unemployed' was about 40 per cent.[72] The economic performance of east

Germany is plagued by high interest rates and wage demands, low productivity and public finance deficits.[73] Taken together, these factors all have implications for the development of childcare and pre-school education. Factually, provision of *Krippen*, kindergartens and *Horte* has been as shown in Tables 7.1 and 7.2.

TABLE 7.1

DEVELOPMENT OF CHILDCARE PROVISION IN THE NEW *BUNDESLÄNDER*

(Numbers and Percentage of Places Available in Relation to the Relevant Age Group)

	1989	1990	1994
Krippe places:	353,203	255,280	103,689
for the <3s	56.4%*	54.2%	41.3%
Kindergarten places:	880,420	713,306	552,865
3–6½	112.0%	97.7%	96.2%
Hort places:	818,821	246,860	284,505
6–12	60.6%	32.4%	22.6%

* Counting the mothers who claimed the baby year, the percentage of *Krippen* places available was 82% in 1989.

Source: Tenth Youth Report, p. 200.

TABLE 7.2

DEVELOPMENT OF CHILDCARE PROVISION IN THE OLD *BUNDESLÄNDER*

(Numbers and Percentage of Places Available in Relation to the Relevant Age Group)

	1986	1990	1994
Krippe places:	28,353	38,153	47,064
for the <3s	1.6%	1.8%	2.2%
Kindergarten places:	1,472,819	1,583,622	1,918,832
3–6½	69.3%	69.0%	73.0%
Hort places:	102,874	128,789	145,775
6–12	3.0%	3.4%	3.5%

Source: Tenth Youth Report, p. 200.

The demographic decline works itself out soonest at the level of the youngest children, and by 1995 this had already happened in the New *Bundesländer*: the number of 3–6 year-olds (656,000 in 1989) had by 1995 sunk to 385,000 (less than 60 per cent of the 1989 baseline) and was then expected to rise slightly though not to anything like the 1989 level.[74] In the GDR of 1989, at least 12 per cent of the kindergarten places were unoccupied, and so even at that stage there was a considerable over-provision of facilities. Add to this the fall in the birthrate, and there is no escaping from the fact that many *Krippen* and kindergartens have had to be closed. It is, however, still possible to meet parents' requirements: although by 1992/93 the New *Bundesländer* had only 55 per cent of the 1989 provision, the coverage still corresponded to *need*.[75] The only problem is that if sparsely populated areas lose their childcare facilities, then it may not be practicable for parents to transport their children further afield. Falling rolls make the kindergartens acutely conscious of the threat to their viability, and they are increasingly assuming the functions of the *Hort*, thereby threatening to put the latter out of business. A different strategy used by some local authorities – under legal pressure to provide kindergarten places – is actually to close *Horte* in order to save money while simultaneously developing kindergartens to fulfil their statutory obligations.[76]

In the light of demographic trends the question can legitimately be posed as to whether there is any real need at all for private sector development since independent providers are clearly in competition with state institutions of which there are plenty. There is also a real concern about quality assurance. Giving one's children over into another family for daycare (*Tagespflege* by *Tagesmütter*) was rare in the GDR.[77] In the New *Bundesländer*, *Tagespflege* is seen as a competitor to the mainstream childcare institutions which will contract if daycare continues to increase. From the state point of view, however, it is quite attractive since it does not need investment, and salaries are not linked to *Bundesangestelltentarif* (BAT) rates; but quality is much harder to monitor. In fact large discrepancies exist in quality between different childcare institutions, and quality assurance is weak.[78] In some *Länder*, the requirements for their foundation and functioning have been loosened up; this, however, can potentially lead to larger group sizes, lower building standards and perhaps less qualified staff.[79] In relation to buildings, it should be pointed out that in 1989, only about half of the kindergarten rooms were in good condition;[80] and that from 1 January 1991 to 30 June 1991, the federal government made enormous efforts and spent DM1bn in improving provision and ensuring that the network of kindergartens did not contract too steeply as a result of the falling birthrate.[81]

Pre-school institutions that are well run, conveniently located and have good opening hours are important reflections of political goodwill and commitment to childcare. After all, they now cost real money: parents pay between DM200 and DM300 a month (means-tested) plus about DM50 for food; yet the service is not altogether user-friendly. Most kindergartens are only open for about four hours a day; although this is the norm in the west, the authors of the Tenth Youth Report[82] believe that it should be extended to six hours. Even this is still not enough to enable a parent to do a full day's work; and with six hours' opening time, provision would still be vastly inferior to what existed in the GDR. There is obviously a discrepancy between public provision and parental needs which has not yet been reconciled. Closures have resulted in long journeys for some parents and children; catchment areas have become bigger, and in some locations the earlier organic connections between neighbourhood, place of residence and childcare institutions are being destroyed.[83]

Childcare policies are very vulnerable to economic crisis, of which there is no shortage in the New *Bundesländer*. In 1990, just after the *Wende*, children brought up in one-parent families were at minimal risk of poverty because the state 'safety-netted' them but now, because of the post-*Wende* privatisation of childcare facilities, this has changed: children in numerous families with single parents who are either unemployed or working part-time are at the greatest risk of poverty and chronic dependence on social welfare. The resultant economic deprivation can be expected to have significant adverse effects on their development and life chances. Nauck and Joos[84] point out that before the *Wende*, the GDR and the FRG were already dissimilar in their family profiles and thus did not start from the same baseline after 1989: the GDR birthrate was falling and the illegitimacy rate was rising; children living with unmarried parents, in one-parent families or with step-parents were more frequent in east than in west Germany. Moreover, since marriage was relatively easy to terminate, it carried less weight in east than in west.[85] These social factors were, however, mitigated by the exercise of socialist state power.

The main change in benefit after the *Wende* was that child-funding and financial responsibility were transferred to the family, and so became subject to much greater variability. Despite the widening of income differentials, the poverty risk of east German children living with *married* parents increased only slightly from 3.4 per cent to under 10 per cent.[86] The New *Bundesländer* marriage rate, however, dropped from 7.9 per 1,000 inhabitants in 1989 to 3.1 in 1993,[87] and the percentage of children being brought up by single parents and living below the poverty threshold rose almost threefold from 13 per cent in 1990 to 36.3 per cent in 1993.[88] Mothers as a group were the most vulnerable to becoming unemployed, and children whose mothers were single parents, living alone, and working part-time had the highest risk of poverty: in 1993, 66.4 per cent of them lived under the poverty threshold.[89] An interaction effect exists between poverty and the educational level of parents: the lower the level of parental education, the higher the risk of children being poor. In this correlation, the achievement of the matriculation examination *Abitur* seems to be the watershed: if parents have no school leaving certificate at all or only that from a *Hauptschule*, 22.5 per cent of the children live under the poverty level; if, however, they have *Abitur*, this risk falls to only 4.8 per cent.[90] Moreover, regional factors leading to inequality of life chances among children play a more significant role in east than in west Germany.

Whereas adult benefits such as pensions and unemployment pay are centrally regulated and distributed, child benefit payments are mainly the responsibility of local authorities, most of which are suffering from financial stringency and lack adequate resources to invest in a child infrastructure. Hence, children's welfare is influenced by the relative prosperity of each region; their benefits are easily squeezed and more variable than adult benefits.[91]

THE IMPACT OF CONTRACTION AND OF EDUCATIONAL REFORM ON CARE-GIVERS' ROLE AND STATUS

In the west, the legal right to a kindergarten place has brought about an expansion in childcare professions, whereas in the east they are contracting (due to the fall in the birthrate, and reduction in the provision of childcare institutions).[92] In 1989, there were 75,000 GDR *Krippe* care-givers; since then, the number has about halved.[93] The implications of this loss are many and far-reaching. Obviously, the loss of a job causes great personal pain to the individual. Staff reductions are ubiquitous and have led to loss of motivation, chronic worry about redundancy, short-time working, and competition between childcare institutions.[94] They have a bad effect on the age structure: in the New *Bundesländer*, it is the younger care-givers who have tended to lose their jobs or go west; it is also they who are physically the fittest and in that respect best up to the demands of the job. New *Bundesländer* care-givers are on average much older than in the west (about half are aged between 40 and 60); they tend to suffer from burn-out.[95] There is a move towards part-time staffing, especially among those care-givers who have left the profession temporarily and then return. This part-time pattern, however, makes it more difficult to coordinate staffing plans and timetables, and is not conducive to innovation.

Care-givers' professional qualifications have been seriously devalued as a result of the *Wende*, and if they suffer unemployment, these qualifications are of little transferable value in other vocational areas. Nevertheless, a study carried out by Ursula Rabe-Kleberg[96] for the KSPW (*Kommission für die Erforschung des politischen und sozialen Wandels in den neuen Bundesländern*) reveals that the care-givers in her sample had a strong residual loyalty and commitment to their profession. They had been well satisfied with their jobs before 1990, and the majority of them (69.6 per cent) wanted to continue in the same field, working with children. Only 6.8 per cent were willing to give up work and concentrate on looking after their own families. Faced with threatened or actual unemployment, they had developed their own strategies of 'holding on' and adapting. They were not, however, very keen to move elsewhere in search of a job – a lack of mobility doubtless explained by the fact that most of them were married or in established relationships, and over 90 per cent had children. It is clear from the study that the process of professional socialisation before 1990 had made them identify very strongly with their profession, and this identification helped them to endure loss of status and downward mobility.

The care givers in the New *Bundesländer* were accustomed to a highly prescriptive framework which on the one hand constrained their freedom of action, but on the other conferred a certain degree of security. Now the demise of compulsory programmes makes them feel insecure.[97] After the *Wende*, they found it a major challenge to move from this closed conceptual framework to more differentiated and individualised objectives.[98] The new concept is not 'what children should learn', but rather 'what can we offer them to help them develop their identity'.[99] There is even a notion that older children have their own claims to a self-defined culture, and this would involve adults refraining from interference so that independent, peer-mediated learning can take place.[100] The balance of power between the childcare institutions and parents has changed in favour of the latter who are officially conceded to have primary responsibility (KJHG Article 1(2)); this of course is to the detriment of the care-givers who no longer have the 'leading role' they enjoyed in the GDR, and are suffering from status deficit – in common with their counterparts in the Old *Bundesländer*.[101] As Calder[102] points out: 'Although in absolute terms, they had previously not been paid much, and were getting more now, they had felt a more central part of society in the GDR and had felt they were carrying out a worthwhile job.'

BOTH WEST AND EAST NEED TO CHANGE TO ACHIEVE HARMONISATION

In the west, the family was 'privatised', and the labour force was more strongly gendered than in the east.[103] Until the mid-1960s, west German state-organised care was regarded as a way of helping out those women who could not afford to be with their children full-time, and was considered second-best; childcare was regarded as essentially the concern of the individual.[104] Now, however, that is changing. Even in the west parents no longer see responsibility for the next generation as exclusively a private matter, and family demands for help are increasingly finding public and political support.[105] In the Old *Bundesländer*, women's rights to combine family and gainful employment are being asserted and accepted, and the state is having to adapt childcare institutions to help them. This is a sea change in the Old *Bundesländer*. The east, however, has long had all the relevant structures in place which are now having to be created in the west at great expense.[106] The Brandenburg Ministry of Education, Youth and Sport [107] certainly believes that the Old *Bundesländer* can learn from its projects, pilot studies, initiatives, experiences, competences and search for new ways of doing things. There is an increasing convergence between family policy in the Old and New *Bundesländer*, and the east's role in stimulating change throughout the whole of Germany has been officially recognised. Members of the Ninth Youth Report Commission[108] claim that west German discussions of pre-school pedagogy had been stagnating for years, and have received new impulses from the New *Bundesländer*. In the same volume, the government in its position paper 'shares the view of the Ninth Youth Report Commission that important impulses for the development of institutions complementing the family *should emanate from the New Bundesländer towards the Old*'[109] (my italics). This is a rare phenomenon: a post-unification plaudit from west to east. It indicates that transformation in the new Germany is a dialectical process, and that the west needs to change as well as the east if synthesis or harmonisation is to take place. The west is increasingly accepting this responsibility.

NOTES

I wish to thank Professors Hans Oswald and Lothar Krappmann for helpful comments in the preparation of this chapter.

1. *Neunter Jugendbericht: Bericht über die Situation der Kinder und Jugendlichen und die Entwicklung der Jugendhilfe in den neuen Bundesländern* (Bonn: Bundesministerium für Familie, Senioren, Frauen und Jugend, 1994), p. 482.
2. Max-Planck-Institut, 'Kindergarten, Vorschule und Grundschule (Elementar- und Primarbereich)', in *Das Bildungswesen in der Bundesrepublik* (Reinbek bei Hamburg: Rowohlt, 1994), p. 295. (No editor's name is given in this book.)
3. Ibid., p. 483.
4. Bund-Länder-Kommission (BLK) für Bildungsplanung und Forschungsförderung, *Entwicklungen und vordringliche Maßnahmen in den Tageseinrichtungen für Kinder/Elementarbereich in den neuen Ländern* (Bonn: BLK, 1993), pp. 8–9.
5. 'Kindergarten, Vorschule und Grundschule', p. 295.
6. K. Klemm, W. Böttcher and M. Weegen, *Bildungsplanung in den neuen Bundesländern: Entwicklungstrends, Perspektiven und Vergleiche* (Weinheim and Munich: Juventa, 1992), p. 46.
7. *Neunter Jugendbericht*, p. 507.
8. *Entwicklungen und vordringliche Maßnahmen*, p. 4.
9. Ibid., p. 30.
10. *Zehnter Jugendbericht: Bericht über die Lebenssituation von Kindern und die Leistungen der Kinderhilfe in Deutschland* (Bonn: Bundesministerium für Familie, Senioren, Frauen und Jugend, 1998), p. 201.
11. *Neunter Jugendbericht*, p. 518–19.
12. The baby year was introduced from 1976 for the second child, and from 1986 for the firstborn.
13. *Entwicklungen und vordringliche Maßnahmen*, p. 8.
14. C. Weber, 'Erziehungsbedingungen im frühen Kindesalter in *Kinderkrippen* vor und nach der

Wende', in G. Trommsdorff (ed.), *Sozialisation und Entwicklung von Kindern vor und nach der Vereinigung* (Opladen: Leske und Budrich, 1996), p. 176.

15. *Zehnter Jugendbericht*, p. 192.
16. L. Liegle, 'Vorschulerziehung', in O. Anweiler *et al.* (ed.), *Vergleich von Bildung und Erziehung in der Bundesrepublik Deutschland und in der Deutschen Demokratischen Republik* (Cologne: Verlag Wissenschaft und Politik, 1990), p. 158.
17. M. Schmidt, 'Gendered Labour Force Participation', in F. G. Castles (ed.), *Families of Nations: Patterns of Public Policy in Western Democracies* (Aldershot: Dartmouth, 1993).
18. Ibid., p. 214.
19. W. Ihne, E. Esser, M. H. Schmidt, B. Blanz, O. Reis and B. Meyer-Probst, 'Die prospektive Bedeutung von Risikofaktoren des Kindes- und Jugendalters für psychische Störungen des Erwachsenenalters: Ergebnisse zweier Längsschnittstudien in Rostock und Mannheim', in *Zeitschrift für Soziologie der Erziehung und Sozialisation*, 2 Beiheft (Weinheim: Juventa, 1998), pp. 265–81.
20. 'Erziehungsbedingungen im frühen Kindesalter', p. 176.
21. The interview for this case study was conducted by the present author in Schwerin on 25 March 1995 during research for the book authored by her and entitled *Reconstructing Education: East German Schools and Universities After Unification* (Oxford and New York: Berghahn, 1999).
22. 'Erziehungsbedingungen im frühen Kindesalter', pp. 195–7.
23. *Neunter Jugendbericht*, p. 496.
24. Kindergarten, Vorschule und Grundschule, p. 294.
25. Deutscher Bundestag, *Enquête-Kommission, Aufarbeitung und Geschichte des SED-Diktatur in Deutschland. Rolle und Bedeutung der Ideologie, integrativer Faktoren und disziplinierender Praktiken in Staat und Gesellschaft der DDR*, Band III (Frankfurt am Main: Suhrkamp, 1995), p. 21.
26. H.-D. Schmidt, 'Erziehungsbedingungen in der DDR: Offizielle Programme, individuelle Praxis und die Rolle der Pädagogischen Psychologie und Entwicklungspsychologie', in G. Trommsdorff (ed.), *Sozialisation und Entwicklung von Kindern vor und nach der Vereinigung*, p. 17.
27. *Neunter Jugendbericht*, p. 487.
28. J. Niermann, 'Schriftliche Stellungnahme zum Thema Identitätsfindung von Jugendlichen in den neuen Bundesländern anläßlich der Anhörung durch den Deutschen Bundestag' (Bonn: Ausschuß für Frauen und Jugend am 18. September 1991, manuscript copy).
29. *Neunter Jugendbericht*, p. 496.
30. Ibid., p. 482.
31. 'Erziehungsbedingungen im frühen Kindesalter', p. 188.
32. J. Bowlby, *Child Care and the Growth of Love* (Harmondsworth: Penguin, 1965).
33. 'Erziehungsbedingungen im frühen Kindesalter', p. 206.
34. Ibid., p. 207.
35. *Neunter Jugendbericht*, p. 484.
36. 'Erziehungsbedingungen im frühen Kindesalter', p. 211.
37. Ibid., pp. 213–14.
38. H.-W. Fuchs, *Bildung und Wissenschaft seit der Wende* (Opladen: Leske und Budrich, 1997), pp. 42–4.
39. *Neunter Jugendbericht*, p. 487.
40. 'Kinder- und Jugendhilfegesetz', in *Jugendrecht 22. Auflage* (Munich: Deutscher Taschenbuch Verlag, 1998).
41. *Neunter Jugendbericht*, p. XXI.
42. Ibid., p. 496.
43. Ministerium für Bildung, Jugend und Sport, *Kinder- und Jugendbericht 1994: Der Aufbau der Jugendhilfe im Lande Brandenburg* (Potsdam: MBJS, 1994), p. 103.
44. *Neunter Jugendbericht*, p. 498.
45. Ibid., pp. 498–9.
46. *Zehnter Jugendbericht*, p. 133.
47. Ibid., p. 194.
48. *Neunter Jugendbericht*, p. 526.
49. Ibid., p. 527.
50. *Zehnter Jugendbericht*, p. XII.
51. *Neunter Jugendbericht*, p. 528.
52. Ibid., p. 518.

146   *The New Germany in the East*

53. Ibid., p. 530.
54. Ibid.
55. M. Fölling-Albers, 'Kindheit heute', *Die Grundschule*, No. 5, 1989.
56. I. Skrypietz, 'Militant Right-Wing Extremism in Germany', *German Politics*, Vol. 3, No. 1 (1994), pp.133–140; Neunter Jugendbericht, pp. XI, 189, 192; J. Böhm, J. Brune, H. Flörchinger, A. Helbing and A. Pinther (eds), *Deutschstunden: Was Jugendliche von der Einheit denken* (Berlin: Argon, 1993).
57. *Zehnter Jugendbericht*, p. 177.
58. *Neunter Jugendbericht*, p. 486.
59. *Zehnter Jugendbericht*, pp. 177–8.
60. L. Ahnert, S. Krätzig, T. Meischner, and A. Schmidt, 'Sozialisationskonzepte für Kleinkinder: Wirkungen tradierter Erziehungsvorstellungen und staatssozialistischer Erziehungsdoktrinen im intra- und interkulturellen Ost-West-Vergleich', in G. Trommsdorff (ed.), *Psychologische Aspekte des sozio-politischen Wandels in Ostdeutschland* (Berlin, New York: de Gruyter, 1994), pp. 94–110.
61. *Zehnter Jugendbericht*, p. 216.
62. L. Ahnert, 'Erzieher-Kind-Bindungen im Vergleich. Ein Beitrag zu Veränderungen in der außerfamiliären Tagesbetreuung für Kleinkinder in Ost-Berlin nach der deutschen Vereinigung', in *Zeitschrift für Soziologie der Erziehung und Sozialisation*, 2 Beiheft (Weinheim: Juventa, 1998), pp. 17–33.
63. H.-W. Fuchs, *Bildung und Wissenschaft seit der Wende* (Opladen: Leske und Budrich, 1997), p. 141.
64. *Zehnter Jugendbericht*, p. 182.
65. I am grateful to Lothar Krappmann for providing this information.
66. D. Waterkamp, *Handbuch zum Bildungswesen der DDR* (Berlin: Arno Spitz, 1987), p. 86.
67. *Neunter Jugendbericht*, p. 509.
68. *Bildungsplanung in den neuen Bundesländern*, p. 46.
69. See *Zehnter Jugendbericht*, p. 201.
70. M. Gawlik, E. Krafft and M. Secklinger, *Jugendhilfe und sozialer Wandel* (Munich: Deutsches Jugendinstitut, 1995), p. 58.
71. Grund- und Strukturdaten 1995/96; 1998/98 (Bonn: Bundesministerium für Bildung, Wissenschaft, Forschung und Technologie, 1995).
72. *Neunter Jugendbericht*, p. 35.
73. A. J. Hughes Hallett and Y. Ma, 'East Germany, West Germany, and their Mezzogiorno: A Parable for European Economic Integration', *Economic Journal*, 103 (1993), pp. 416–28.
74. *Bildungsplanung in den neuen Bundesländern*, p. 48.
75. *Bildung und Wissenschaft seit der Wende*, p. 143.
76. *Zehnter Jugendbericht*, p. 201.
77. Ibid., p. 197.
78. Ibid., p. 191.
79. Ibid., p. 196.
80. *Bildungsplanung in den neuen Bundesländern*, p. 50.
81. *Zehnter Jugendbericht*, p. XXV.
82. Ibid., p. 195.
83. *Jugendhilfe und sozialer Wandel*, 1995, p. 75.
84. B. Nauck and M. Joos, 'Wandel der familiären Lebensverhältnisse von Kindern in Ostdeutschland', in G. Trommsdorff (ed.), *Sozialisation und Entwicklung von Kindern vor und nach der Vereinigung*, pp. 243–98; quotation p. 256.
85. Ibid., p. 262.
86. Ibid., p. 267.
87. Ibid., p. 254.
88. Ibid., p. 267.
89. Ibid., p. 268.
90. Ibid.
91. Ibid., pp. 286–7.
92. *Zehnter Jugendbericht*, p. 204.
93. *Neunter Jugendbericht*, p. 495.
94. *Bildung und Wissenschaft seit der Wende*, p. 144.
95. *Zehnter Jugendbericht*, p. 206.
96. U. Rabe-Kleberg, 'Berufsbiographien in der Transformation. Die Berufsgruppe der Erzieherin.

Bericht über die Ergebnisse einer Fragebogenerhebung' (Halle: Martin-Luther-Universität Halle-Wittenberg, 1994).

97. *Bildung und Wissenschaft seit der Wende*, p. 144.
98. *Zehnter Jugendbericht*, p. 191.
99. Ibid., p. 192.
100. Ibid., p. 201.
101. H. Colberg-Schrader and P. Oberhuemer, 'Early Childhood Education and Care in Germany', in T. David (ed.), *Educational Provision for our Youngest Children: European Perspectives* (London: Paul Chapman, 1993).
102. P. Calder, 'Ideologies, Policies and Practices in East Berlin Before and After the Fall of the Wall', *International Journal of Early Years Education*, 4, 3 (1996), pp. 49–60.
103. 'Gendered Labour Force Participation', 1993.
104. *Zehnter Jugendbericht*, p. 192.
105. Ibid., p. 215.
106. *Kinder- und Jugendbericht 1994*, p. 103.
107. Ibid., p. 111.
108. *Neunter Jugendbericht*, p. 496.
109. *Neunter Jugendbericht*, p. XXVI.

8

Unexpected Newcomers: Asylum Seekers and Other Non-Germans in the New *Länder*

Eva Kolinsky

In eastern Germany, unification initiated a transformation of some magnitude. The transfer of the economic and political system from west to east resulted in a 'problematic normalisation' as people tried to cope with a recast social environment and everyday life.[1] A decade after unification, everyday life remains buffeted by unfamiliar challenges and changed circumstances.[2] One such challenge concerns the presence of non-German residents and the continued arrival of asylum seekers. The GDR had kept its borders closed, preventing east Germans from moving to other countries and other nationals from settling there. Migration did not feature in socialist state policy. In 1989, the population of the GDR included just 1.2 per cent foreign nationals, fewer than 200,000 individuals. About half of these were diplomats, students or experts employed by foreign companies, the remainder so called contract labourers, *Vertragsarbeiter*.[3] Occasionally, the state cast itself in the role of benefactor by allowing children from Namibia to attend a school in the GDR or by taking in socialist refugees.[4] Officially, however, GDR sources made no mention of 'foreigners', and academic studies of GDR society, even those published in the west, replicated the silence.

When the new *Länder* replaced the GDR in October 1990, they were nearly completely German in their demographic composition while the old *Länder* had already become home for a sizeable non-German population and the intended home for an increasing number of asylum seekers who entered the country with a view of settling there. This diversification of the west had gone unnoticed in the east. For east Germans, the social environment they demanded instead of socialism had no place for ethnic and cultural minorities but focused instead on national belonging. The 'one people' envisaged by the demonstrators did not include German passport holders of Turkish, Italian or Greek origin, let alone foreign nationals living in Germany or hoping to stay there. The Germany after the peaceful 'revolution' was to be for Germans only. Instead, the treaty that sealed German unity opened the borders and allowed European Union (EU) nationals and other non-Germans to work and live in the five new *Länder* in the same way as they could do in the west and it stipulated that from 3 October 1990 onwards the new Germany in the east should receive non-Germans seeking political asylum in the country. Calculated on the basis of population figures, the quota for the new *Länder* amounted to 20 per cent of Germany's asylum seekers.

THE TREATMENT OF CONTRACT WORKERS BEFORE AND AFTER UNIFICATION.

Before considering how east Germans and their administrations faced up to the unexpected challenge of admitting asylum seekers to their society, we need to review the GDR's record of receiving and accommodating non-Germans prior to unification. Generally speaking, the state pursued an agenda of exclusion by closing the borders and criminalising contacts between Germans and non-Germans. East Germans were expected to celebrate as exotic the cultures of presumably oppressed or endangered minorities, their folk music and outlandish costumes without ever considering them a regular part of east Germans society. In GDR society, ethnic diversity had no place: 'The cultural "other" was like an item in a museum, something at which to wonder. The experience was intellectual, aesthetic or emotional, or all three at the same time but hardly ever real. The "other" did not become part of one's own culture.'[5] Under the guise of *Völkerfreundschaft* – friendship between peoples – Germans were kept apart from non-Germans, even those who had been invited or fêted for their exotic difference by party officials.

Since GDR contract labourers, *Vertragsarbeiter*, worked alongside German colleagues, their treatment constitutes the most accurate indicator of the extent to which an integration of non-Germans had been attempted or achieved in everyday life and civil society.[6] Recruitment commenced in the mid-1950s and was regulated by intergovernmental agreement from 1966. Designed to alleviate labour shortages, it was intensified in the mid-1980s when the Honecker government tried to increase industrial output without new investment by operating a third shift in key industries. The overall number of *Vertragsarbeiter* remained below 100,000 but would have been higher had the GDR survived. In 1989, 60,000 Vietnamese workers were recruited and contracts signed for the recruitment of a further 90,000 workers from Mozambique. Initially, non-German labour had been recruited from neighbouring eastern European countries. As democratic ideas, however, began to spread there, the GDR turned to regimes where the seeds of democracy had not yet been sown and whose nationals could be trusted not to import unwanted notions of liberalism. When the east German state collapsed, its non-German workforce numbered just under 100,000, less than 1 per cent of the total.

Inside the GDR, they were disadvantaged with regard to employment, pay, housing and rights of social participation.[7] Contract workers were not entitled to any kind of social citizenship; were barely tolerated in the employment functions to which they had been allocated; were accommodated in warden-controlled hostels, had limited rights to receive or spend their earnings; and could be expelled without appeal. This treatment as second-class citizens matched the east German government's fear of social or political diversity and it also matched the sending governments' determination to use their workers as pawns in economic and financial relations with the GDR. The east German government remained silent on all aspects of the agreements it concluded with sending countries. The silence about numbers meant that east Germans did not know the picture across the region as a whole and could not form a view as to where contract workers were deployed and why. When numbers began to increase sharply in the late 1980s and moves seemed afoot to replace east Germans departing to the west with contract workers from East Asian or African countries, the silence surrounding the recruitment policy bred hostility. So did the silence surrounding the rights of contract workers that been agreed with the various sending countries. These included a right to language instruction at the place of work but normally confined to ensuring that commands in German could be understood. Contracts also promised skilled employment, a clause largely ignored although many labour recruits, notably those from Vietnam, were highly skilled or even came from professional backgrounds. Stipulated also were wage equality and housing of the quality enjoyed by Germans; both conditions were neither publicly known nor adhered to.[8]

Some special conditions spelt out in the intergovernmental contracts could not be denied as blatantly as those concerning type of employment, levels of pay or quality of housing: agreements included the right to purchase and send home once or twice a year goods up to the value of half the annual wages.[9] Witnessing these shipments east Germans accused contract workers of causing the shortages they had to endure and of buying the country dry.[10] Although contract workers existed on the margins of east German society economically and socially, they were perceived as unwelcome competitors for consumer products and a danger to the economic equilibrium in the GDR.

Not surprisingly, contract workers were the first to feel the brunt when east German state enterprises decided at the beginning of 1990 to prepare for a new economic regime.[11] By the time the Round Table (an advisory body to the GDR government in the interim between the end of SED-control and the first free elections in March 1990, which included all political parties, social organisations that were represented in the *Volkskammer* and the citizens' movement that had spearheaded the system transformation in 1989) addressed the issue in February 1990, at least 60 per cent had been dismissed or faced dismissal while the sudden closure of hostel accommodation or a massive increase in charges left many homeless. In December 1990, just 28,000 contract workers remained; one year later the total had fallen further to 6,670.[12]

Had public sentiment determined policy, the region might have rid itself of its unwanted non-German residents. Neither the Round Table nor the citizens' movements envisaged rights of residency for former contract workers, although at the insistence of the latter, the Round Table addressed what it termed the 'Ausländerproblem' – the fact that thousands of unemployed and homeless former contract workers were roaming the streets – by creating the office of Foreigners' Adviser, *Ausländerbeauftragter,* whose original task it was to implement the removal of these unwanted non-Germans, the former contract workers, from east German civil society. The elections in March 1990, however, produced a government that was to agree and implement the unification process with the Federal Republic and establish democratic principles and practices in the final phase of the GDR. In this context, former contract workers won some protection from social injustice and expulsion. Not all who had been dismissed and evicted from their lodgings wanted to return home. Some lacked the financial means to do so, others refused to accept the one-sided change of terms and insisted on their right to remain in Germany for the duration of their original contract. Workers from Vietnam were particularly outspoken in their refusal to return early, partly because their government would sue them for breach of defaulting on their commitment and partly because they wanted to optimise their chances of improving their material circumstances by working in Germany.

On 13 June 1990 the east German government proposed a *Bleiberecht*, a right to remain on a temporary basis. Modelled on programmes to persuade *Gastarbeiter* (labour migrants originally recruited to western Germany, who had become a settled non-German population) to return to their country of origin, contract workers in the east were offered part of the pay owed to them and the fare for the return journey if they undertook to leave the country. Those who insisted on remaining were permitted to do so up to the original duration of their contract.[13] After unification, former contract workers were barred from applying for political asylum on the grounds that they were already resident in the country. It took until 14 May 1993 for the *Bleiberecht* to be confirmed in unified Germany.[14] To activate this *Bleiberecht*, former contract workers had to provide evidence of adequate housing and income. Employment was restricted to street trading and they were not eligible for any benefits.[15] Despite such lack of generosity, the *Bleiberecht* allowed the most determined of the former contract workers to extend their residency in Germany. Five years after unification, 19,000 remained, most of them (15,000) Vietnamese ex-*Vertragsarbeiter*, who had come to the GDR in 1989. In 1997, a further change in the legislation entitled former contract workers to count their stay in the GDR towards their overall stay in Germany, a concession that improved their chances of remaining.[16] On the other hand, many who stayed on now have a criminal records and face deportation since German police have tended to arrest non-German street traders for alleged offences against customs regulation, notably illegal trade in cigarettes. In addition, former contract workers who accepted financial compensation in the GDR when they lost their employment but then failed to leave Germany forfeited their right of residency. Even those who ventured to become self-employed have to have proof that their business is making a profit before being permitted to extend their stay.[17] On paper, former contract workers seemed to have won the right to rebuild their lives in Germany after unification, but the small print of special regulations seems to threaten most of them with expulsion or force them into illegality. The Vietnamese who have been the most determined to eke out a new living in Germany are now the group most severely affected by the exclusion clauses.

UNINVITED RESIDENTS: ASYLUM SEEKERS IN THE NEW *LÄNDER*

Asylum seekers should have arrived in the new *Länder* as soon as the unification treaty came into effect. The date, however, was put back to December 1990 since the recast administration in the eastern region was unprepared for the task.[18] It took until 1992 for regional quotas to be defined and asylum seekers to be allocated to a specific *Land*.[19] Until then, the numbers actually arriving remained below target, not least since many asylum seekers preferred to be located in the west. Of the new *Länder*, Saxony was the most densely populated and was required to receive the largest number of asylum seekers, 6.5 per cent of the total; at the other end of the spectrum, 2.7 per cent were directed to Mecklenburg-Vorpommern (see Table 8.1).

TABLE 8.1
DISTRIBUTION OF ASYLUM SEEKERS BY REGION

	Asylum Seekers (%)
Old Länder	
Baden-Württemberg	12.2
Bavaria	14.0
Bremen	1.0
Hamburg	2.6
Hesse	7.4
Lower Saxony	9.3
North Rhine-Westfalia	22.4
Rhineland Palatinate	4.7
Saarland	1.4
Schleswig Holstein	2.8
Berlin (West and East)	2.2
New Länder	
Brandenburg	3.5
Mecklenburg-Vorpommern	2.7
Saxony	6.5
Saxony-Anhalt	4.0
Thuringia	3.3

Source: Adapted from *Migration und Integration in Zahlen*, p. 280.

In the absence of published statistics on the actual arrival of individuals, it is impossible to present more than estimates. Based on the overall number arriving as asylum seekers in Germany and the quota allocation mentioned earlier, the total for the new *Länder* for the years 1991 to 1996 amounted to 277,593 persons (Table 8.2). At its peak in 1992, more than 400,000 asylum seekers filed applications in Germany as a whole, of whom 87,615 should have been allocated to the new *Länder*. Since then, the influx of applicants has fallen by nearly three-quarters.

TABLE 8.2
QUOTA ALLOCATION OF ASYLUM SEEKERS IN THE NEW *LÄNDER*, 1991–96

New Länder	*1991*	*1992*	*1993*	*1994*	*1995*	*1996*	*1991–96*
Brandenburg	8,960	15,330	11,287	4,452	4,476	4,070	48,575
Mecklenbg.-Vorpommern	6,914	11,828	8,707	3,424	3,453	3,140	37,466
Saxony	16,646	28,476	20,962	8,268	8,313	7,559	90,224
Saxony-Anhalt	10,244	17,524	12,900	5,088	5,116	4,652	55,524
Thuringia	8,451	14,457	10,642	4,197	4,220	3,837	45,804
Total	51,215	87,615	64,498	25,429	25,578	23,258	277,593

Source: Adapted from *Migration und Integration*, S. 276.

The unprecedented numbers arriving to be accommodated and applying to have their cases processed constituted a formidable challenge for east German authorities, in particular the *Ausländerbeauftragte* charged with administering matters at local level. Before a revised law on political asylum reduced numbers in 1993, a sense of panic prevailed among local authorities who were obligated to house new arrivals and tried to do so in out-of-town sites or former contract worker hostels.[20]

The number of arrivals does not translate easily into the number entitled to stay. At the height of the influx in 1992 and 1993, the success rate of applications stood at 4.3 per cent and 3.2 per cent respectively. By the mid-1990s, it averaged eight per cent.[21] The application procedure has been complex and likely to take several years to complete since it also includes a right of appeal.[22] Official estimates suggest that up to 10 per cent of cases result in a right to stay while at least 65 per cent are turned down since the applicant may be regarded as an economic migrant and does, therefore, not qualify under the terms of the law as a political refugee. Some 25 per cent of cases are resolved by other means – usually by deporting the applicant. After a slow start in 1991 and 1992, deportations in the new *Länder* rose sharply and constituted one in four of all deportations although the region only received one in five applications for political asylum. Yet, administrations in the new *Länder* also complained that most would-be deportees absconded and left the area before the deportation order could be implemented.[23] The authorities in Thuringia complained that asylum seekers who had agreed to be repatriated would resurface a short time afterwards elsewhere in Germany to buy cars.[24]

Official data on benefits paid in accordance with the legislation governing the conditions of stay and support for asylum seekers provide more accurate information on their presence in society while their applications for residency rights are being processed. In 1996, a total of 56,000 asylum seekers in the new *Länder* received benefits to cover basic living expenses; in an additional 21,000 cases, one-off payments or provisions were made to assist in special circumstances such as illness or pregnancy.[25] Benefits were paid to a total of 33,000 households. Two-thirds of recipients were single men, 65 per cent lived in communal reception centres or hostels and most were young. In December 1996, the average age of the asylum seekers was 25 years.[26] In east Berlin, expenditure for asylum seekers' benefits grew by 11 per cent between 1995 and 1996 and by 44 per cent between 1996 and 1997.[27] In Berlin-Friedrichshain, the number of non-German residents increased by 75 per cent between 1995 and 1996 as a new reception facility for asylum seekers began to operate. Generally speaking, there are signs of more non-Germans living in central districts of big cities such as east Berlin and Leipzig than in the region as a whole, a process not dissimilar from urban settlement patterns in western Germany. In Berlin, for instance the number of non-German residents in Mitte and Prenzlauer Berg increased by one-third while other areas saw no change or even a fall in the numbers living there.[28] Leipzig has experienced a similar population shift: as well-to-do Germans leave the city centre to move to the suburbs or outskirts, central areas are accommodating increasing number of non-German newcomers.[29]

Civil society in the east is no longer for Germans only. Although numbers remain small compared with those in the west, the increase since unification is significant. In 1992, less than 1 per cent of new *Länder* inhabitants were non-Germans; by 1998, their share had nearly trebled, reaching almost 250,000, fewer than in any one of the old *Länder* except Bremen, but more than ever during the GDR era, and set to increase.[30] As during the GDR years, Berlin and Leipzig had the largest non-German populations, in the east. In Leipzig, foreign nationals constituted 2 per cent of the inhabitants in 1990 and 5 percent in 1998. In 1990, the city recorded 8,967 non-German residents amidst an overall population of 511,054.[31] By 1998, migration losses had reduced Leipzig's population to 470,523, a decrease of over 9 per cent, while the number of non-Germans had increased by 45 per cent to 19,549.[32] A similar demographic shift is taking place in the region as a whole as the east continues to lose German population, while the number of non-German residents there rises. The arrival and eventual settlement of asylum seekers has been the main reason for an increase in the non-German population in the new *Länder*. The story in the east is one of transformation compared to the situation in the GDR: the development, albeit from a low base, of a multicultural fabric of society. It also differs sharply from the west where multiculturalism had already begun to emerge before asylum-based migration set in on a significant scale. In the east, they are occurring simultaneously in a social environment of unfamiliar risk and dislocating transformation.

MIGRATION AND RISK SOCIETY

In the old *Länder*, the transformation of a labour migrant population to a resident non-German population commenced in the 1970s after the *Anwerbestopp*, the ban on further labour recruitment, forced non-German workers who wanted to remain to settle on a more permanent basis and use their right of family reunion to rebuild their private lives. In the era of labour recruitment, three in four guestworkers were male, and virtually all were aged between 18 and 40. The non-Germans included very few children or old people and relatively few women. Over 90 per cent of those living in Germany were in employment.[33] As the former *Gastarbeiter* turned into a settled non-German population, the demography changed to include children, women and older people. Labour market participation has declined to under 50 per cent as families include non-working members; in addition, employment opportunities for those of working age have fallen since the 1980s, with the unemployment and low incomes resulting from it a major social problem for the former *Gastarbeiter,* their descendants and migrants from other countries who settled in Germany.

In the old *Länder*, today's newcomers arrive after a sizeable non-German population, the former labour migrants, had become resident, defined their identities and cultures and in particular had already established pathways of integration in society. The presence of their children in kindergartens and schools, the participation of adults from cultural and ethnic minorities in the labour force, and the visible involvement of individuals and families from various backgrounds into all aspects of everyday life had already happened in western Germany before asylum seekers began to arrive in larger numbers. Although by the 1990s, a 'multicultural democracy'[34] had begun to emerge and a majority of foreign nationals had lived and worked in Germany for more than a decade, the influx of asylum seekers has posed an unfamiliar challenge: not only do these people arrive without recruitment contracts in their pockets, without a clear destination and often without educational and vocational qualifications that would be useful in their new environment, they also arrive at a time when jobs are scarce and society as a whole has turned from an employment society into a risk society.[35] With unemployment at one million and more in western Germany, employment is out of reach for many resident non-Germans and most newcomers.[36] Those who arrive as asylum seekers feature prominently in this high-risk group of the un-employable.

In eastern Germany, non-German newcomers face additional difficulties. Here, system transformation after unification not only implemented the social market economy, it also recast the labour market in such a way that employment uncertainties became a dominant experience in a population that had previously been used to state-allocated training and employment tracks, and had enjoyed continuous employment biographies between leaving school and retirement.[37] A decade into the new Germany, close to 50 per cent have been phased out of the labour market and of those still in work, nine out of ten had to change jobs at least once. The risk society which had taken several decades to take shape in western Germany has been sprung without transition on the east. It forces east Germans to adapt to its unfamiliar demands and face unemployment, income uncertainty, status loss and a threat of social exclusion.

In this transformed environment, east Germans have been reluctant to accept any newcomer who might compete with them in the labour market. Table 8.3 shows them less inclined than west Germans to accept employment mobility from EU and non-European countries while demands for banning all such mobility have increased since unification. In 1996, 38 per cent of east Germans did not accept the right of EU citizens to employment mobility; for non-EU citizens, non-acceptance was higher in both parts of Germany, reaching nearly 50 per cent in the east. With regard to asylum seekers and ethnic Germans; differences between east and west were less striking as more than two-thirds of both populations called for restrictions. In the west, views were more negative towards asylum seekers than towards ethnic Germans, in the east the reverse was true although there, demands for banning both groups from entering Germany have soared since the early 1990s.

TABLE 8.3
ATTITUDES IN WEST AND EAST TOWARDS ADMISSION TO GERMANY

	West Germany			East Germany		
	1991	*1992*	*1996*	*1991*	*1992*	*1996*
For citizens from EU member states, employment in Germany should be:						
unrestricted	35	35	33	13	13	11
restricted	55	56	55	62	63	51
banned	10	9	12	26	24	38
For citizens from non-EU states, employment in Germany should be:						
unrestricted	11	10	8	6	5	4
restricted	60	62	59	55	59	46
banned	29	29	33	39	36	49
For aslyum seekers:						
unrestricted	13	12	13	15	15	12
restricted	65	64	66	69	67	67
banned	22	24	22	15	18	21
For ethnic Germans from eastern Europe:						
unrestricted	22	19	15	15	15	13
restricted	68	71	74	73	74	69
banned	10	10	12	12	11	18

Source: From *Allbus Surveys*, 1991, 1992 and 1996, quoted in *Datenreport 1997*, p. 458.

The 'problematic normalisation' of sustained labour market uncertainties and a continued sense of individual and collective dislocation inhibited the consolidation of a democratic political culture. Confidence in key institutions of parliamentary government and decision-making remain low and the endorsement of political agendas that had already been agreed prior to unification has not taken place.[38] The European project with its challenge to closed borders and its commitment to social citizenship and employment rights regardless of nationality did not win favour in a social environment where every newcomer, in particular a newcomer with western know-how, was viewed as an unwelcome and unwanted competitor. When east Germans had accepted labour migrants in the past, they dictated the terms and controlled the conditions. In the transformed parameters of a democratic polity and a market economy, control has shifted from the state to the individual who is entitled to rights of social citizenship. The strong preference in the east for preventing labour migrants from entering Germany seems indebted to the authoritarian tradition of imposing restrictions and limiting or curtailing such rights.[39]

The acceptance of asylum seekers in the new *Länder* is also hampered by the GDR's own treatment of refugees. Before unification, the state could grant political asylum to certain fellow socialists who faced persecution or injustice in their country of origin. Hailed as martyrs to the ideological cause, these were not random asylum seekers from various national backgrounds and with diverse personal histories but quasi-official ambassadors of socialist state policy. The asylum seekers who arrived after 1990 had no such approved function or presumed ideological cohesion. This changed scenario may explain that opinion polls around the time of unification seemed to suggest that east Germans were more positively inclined towards asylum seekers than west Germans. As soon as survey questions addressed practical issues such as employment rights and public support for asylum seekers, east Germans were less welcoming and more inclined to refuse entry. In 1995, a civic survey in Leipzig tried to address problems of acceptance by including questions about attitudes of Germans towards non-Germans and contacts between the two populations. Only 3 per cent of German Leipzigers reported positive experiences with non-Germans or asylum seekers, and 66 per cent had no experiences to report. Of the 34 per cent who have had contacts with non-Germans or asylum seekers, two thirds claimed to have had mainly negative experiences.[40] The Leipzig study also found that respondents were less negatively inclined towards non-Germans – *Ausländer* – generally than towards asylum seekers.[41] With the exception of pupils and students, where opinions were evenly divided between good and bad experiences, 60 per cent rated their experiences with asylum seekers as worse than those with Germans while less than 1 per cent thought they were better.[42] Whereas the findings of the Leipzig study indicate that Germans objected in particular to the presence of asylum seekers, a 1997 survey of opinions and preferences revealed that the integration of non-Germans into civil society ranked at the bottom of a 23-item list of policy issues for local government. Sixty per cent of Leipzigers advocated to cut public spending on the integration of non-

Germans; no other issue elicited such strong demands for expenditure cuts and such meagre support for an increase (5 per cent).[43]

The arrival of asylum seekers also differed sharply from previous experiences since they came in need of support from public funds and without employment. As we had seen earlier, the place of contract workers in GDR society was defined mainly in terms of their economic function while other aspects of social integration were deficient or explicitly prohibited. Acceptance of non-Germans without a specific political pedigree outside the employment context of low-level manual labour had not existed before unification and did not develop afterwards in a climate of socio-economic uncertainties and increasing expectations that the state, even in its democratic guise, should prioritise the support and well-being of its native German population in the east.

The policy model, of course, that was transferred from west to east to deal with non-Germans in the state and in society had already been flawed, wavering between integration and exclusion even before being extended to the east. Although *Gastarbeiter* were able to settle and benefit from family reunion, various west German governments offered financial incentives to leave Germany while, at the same time, appealing to the general public to accept their '*ausländische Mitbürger*', their foreign co-citizens. Similar contradictions applied to the treatment of asylum seekers. Until the change of legislation in 1993, all-comers were entitled to apply for political asylum and receive material support from public funds during their stay in Germany. Recognition procedures were highly bureaucratic, drawn out over several years and, in most cases, doomed to fail. This dual system of unrestricted access and sharply restricted admission produced its own pattern of hostility as Germans resented the large number of newcomers and the strain they imposed on public resources while the low number of actual acceptances underpinned suspicions that most applicants were bogus asylum seekers who had no right to enter Germany, let alone remain there. Hostilities towards asylum seekers accelerated as numbers rose after 1990.

Eastern Germany commenced its new era of receiving non-German newcomers who were neither contract labourers nor politically approved quasi martyrs to the socialist cause in a climate of escalating hostility which found fertile ground in a society stunned by socio-economic uncertainties, fears of unemployment and totally unused to ethnic diversity, migration and social pluralism. Since no processes of pluralisation had taken place to develop a democratic civil society, east Germans were not prepared for social integration and unwilling to face this unexpected risk in addition to all the others unleashed by unification and its aftermath.

MIGRATION INTO POVERTY?

Unification opened the borders in the east not only for Germans eager to leave or travel but also for newcomers to enter from other countries. Migration into eastern Germany became possible and has begun to transform the German monostructure of society there. While some non-German migrants arrive as *Werksarbeiter*, temporary labour recruited for a specific project, or are EU citizens with unrestricted employment rights, the majority consist of individuals without a prearranged job to go to. In the unfavourable conditions arising from high unemployment, the *Werksarbeiter* constitute a new and growing problem group. Thus, between 1996 and 1997, applications from non-Germans for a work permit increased by 20 per cent in eastern Germany and by just 2 per cent in the west.[44] In eastern Germany, 58,500 non-Germans held a work permit in 1997, an increase of 9,100 within one year, but this demand for employment is not matched by employment opportunities. Unemployment of non-Germans in the new *Länder* grew by 20 per cent within 12 months to at least 40 per cent of the non-German labour force in 1997 and has continued to rise.[45] That 'foreigners' of working age should live in the country without actually working was (with the exception of a handful of diplomats' spouses) unheard of in the days of contract workers; today, it has become an everyday reality. In Leipzig, for instance, 19,500 non-German residents were registered in the third quarter of 1998, of whom 2,087, less than 11 per cent, were in employment.[46] Nine out of ten were not employed. In Berlin, non-employment was less extensive. At the end of 1997, about 440,000 non-German residents lived in the city, 71,000 or 16 per cent of them in the eastern part. Of these, one in three derived

TABLE 8.4
NON-GERMAN POPULATION IN BERLIN AND MAIN SOURCES OF INCOME, 1997
(in 1,000 and %)

	Overall	Income from employment	Unemployment benfit	Pension	Income via family/partner	Welfare payments or other*
Berlin						
West+East	423	144.9	34.6	13.3	146.7	80.4
West Berlin	84%	83%	88%	90%	90%	72%
East Berlin	16%	17%	12%	10%	10%	28%

* Includes *Bafög*, the government grant for students from low-income homes and payments to asylum seekers.

Source: Statistisches Landesamt Berlin, *Statistisches Jahrbuch 1997*, p. 56.

their income from employment, 28 per cent were family members without an income of their own, while the remaining one-third of the non-German population in east Berlin depended on some kind of public benefit.[47]

Of the non-German population in Berlin, those living in the east of the city were significantly more likely to be out of work and depending on benefit than those living in the west. Not counting asylum seekers whose case is still under review and who receive targeted support from public funds, one in seven non-Germans living in west Berlin in 1997 and one in three in east Berlin were receiving benefit. In both parts of the city, welfare payments to non-German recipients have increased sharply since the early 1990s. Then, the number of non-Germans in the eastern districts was so low that the Statistical Yearbook for Berlin did not record their circumstances. Since 1995, however, data have been published. They show that in the east, benefit dependency among non-Germans increased by 40 per cent from 3,700 in 1995 to 6,000 in 1997.[48] In Germany as a whole, the social integration of migrants has contributed to an increase in households living near or below the poverty line. The rise in poverty can be traced to the problems of employment integration experienced by all groups of migrants: ethnic Germans and Jewish refugees from eastern Europe as well as former asylum seekers. Moreover, low incomes or temporary income poverty also affected a larger number of Germans due to growing income inequalities as well as unemployment risks for many.[49] In the first five years after unification, poverty levels seemed to be higher in western Germany than in the east.

This numerical comparison does not reveal the full picture. On the one hand, income differentiation had only commenced in the east in 1990, incomes remained less disparate although some occupational groups such as managerial staff and civil servants gained much faster than, for instance, blue collar workers.[50] On the other hand, poverty in western Germany hit non-Germans particularly hard, a group which remained too small in the east to impact on statistical overviews. Yet, data for 1996 and 1997 show that the number of high income earners among non-Germans in east Berlin decreased to such an extent as to become statistically invisible (Table 8.5). Leaving aside spouses and children without an income of their own, two-thirds of non-German income earners lived on or below the poverty line (50 per cent or less of average income) which, at the time stood at DM1,000 (monthly). Given the persistent shortage of employment opportunities in eastern Germany and the high level of unemployment among the non-German population – both settled and newly arrived – migration today appears to result in poverty by German standards and existence at the margins of civil society.

TABLE 8.5
INCOME DISTRIBUTION AMONG NON-GERMANS IN EAST BERLIN, 1996 AND 1997 (in %)

	Under DM600	DM600– under DM1,000	DM1,000– under DM1,400	DM1,400– under DM1,800	DM1,800– under DM2,200	No income
1996 N: 69,300	28	12	17	8	9	20
1997 N: 72,900	26	20	22	–	–	24

Source: Author's calculations from Statistisches Landesamt Berlin, *Statistisches Jahrbuch 1998*, p. 60.

OUTLOOK

If the settled non-German population experiences material hardship and a risk of social exclusion, asylum seekers awaiting permission to settle are forced to lead an even more marginal existence without material resources to utilise the promises of the affluent and modern society around them. Within Germany's population generally and also within the country's non-German population, their uncertain residency status and poor material circumstances place them in a precarious position. In an era where opportunities to work and secure earned income contracted significantly for non-Germans generally and virtually disappeared for those without residency rights, non-German newcomers face an uncertain future after migration. In the transformed and harsher climate of the new *Länder*, exclusion from even the 'problematic normalisation' that east Germans encounter seems inevitable for the foreseeable future.

NOTES

1. C. Flockton and E. Kolinsky: 'Recasting East Germany. An Introduction', in C. Flockton and E. Kolinsky (eds), *Recasting East Germany: Social Transformation after the GDR* (London: Cass, 1999), pp. 2–5. E. Kolinsky, 'Everyday Life Transformed', in E. Kolinsky (ed.), *Between Hope and Fear: Everyday Life in Post-Unification East Germany: A Case Study of Leipzig* (Keele University Press, 1995), pp. 17–38. For 'problematic normalisation' see A. Segert and I. Zierke, *Sozialstruktur und Milieuerfahrungen: Aspekte des alltagskulturellen Wandels in Ostdeutschland* (Opladen: Westdeutscher Verlag, 1997), p. 48.
2. H. Welsh, A. Pickel and D. Rosenberg, 'East and West German Identities', in K. H. Jarausch (ed.), *After Unity: Reconfiguring German Identities* (Oxford/New York: Berghahn, 1997), pp. 116–19. Also E. Kolinsky, 'Social Transformation and the Family: Issues and Developments', in E. Kolinsky (ed.), *Social Transformation and the Family in Post-Communist Germany* (Basingstoke: Macmillan, 1998), pp. 1–20.
3. L. Trommler, 'Ausländer in der DDR und in den neuen Bundesländern', in *Beiträge aus dem Forschungsbereich Schule und Unterricht des Max-Planck-Institutes für Bildungsforschung*, July 1992, No. 39, p. 2.

4. A. Stach, 'Ausländer in der DDR. Ein Rückblick', in Der Ausländerbeauftragte des Senats Berlin (ed.), *Ausländer in der DDR: Ein Rückblick* (Berlin: Der Ausländerbeauftragte des Senats, 1994), 4th edition, p. 8.
5. F. Hayek, 'Multiculturality in the GDR', in K. J. Milich and J. M. Peck (eds), *Multiculturalism in Transit: A German–American Exchange* (Oxford/New York: Berghahn, 1998) p. 112.
6. For an informative overview see R. Stoll, 'Ausländerbeschäftigung vor und nach der Wiedervereinigung', in *Institut für Arbeitsmarkt- und Berufsforschung (IAB) Werkstattbericht*, No. 10, 17 November 1994, pp. 1–4.
7. For a comprehensive account see Die Beauftragte der Bundesregierung für Ausländerfragen (ed.), *Die ausländischen Vertragsarbeiter in der ehemaligen DDR: Darstellung und Dokumentation*, Bonn, November 1996. Also Die Beauftragte der Bundesregierung für Ausländerfragen (ed.), *Bericht über die Lage der Ausländer in der Bundesrepublik Deutschland*, Bonn, December 1997, pp. 139ff.
8. *Die ausländischen Vertragsarbeiter*, p. 27ff.
9. Text of the agreement governing contract workers from Vietnam in *Die ausländischen Vertragsarbeiter*, pp. 83–98.
10. *Die ausländischen Vertragsarbeiter*, p. 23.
11. Details in E. Kolinsky, 'Non-Germans and Civil Society in the New Länder', in C. Flockton and E. Kolinsky (eds), *Recasting East Germany*, pp. 196ff.
12. Beauftragte der Bundesregierung für die Belange der Ausländer (ed.), *Daten und Fakten zur Ausländersituation*, Bonn, July 1992, p. 39; also E. Kolinsky, 'Foreigners in the New Germany', in *Keele German Research Papers*, No.1, 1995.
13. R. Stoll, *Ausländerbeschäftigung*, p. 8–9.
14. I. Runge, 'Die Toleranz der Intoleranten. Zur Situation der Ausländer in der ehemaligen DDR', in M. Struck (ed.), *Ausländerrecht und Ausländerpolitik. Entwicklungen und Trends* (Bonn: Friedrich Ebert Foundation, 1990), p. 53ff.
15. E. Kolinsky, 'Non-Germans and Civil Society', p. 199.
16. *Bericht über die Lage der Ausländer*, 1997, p. 140.
17. R. Stoll, *Ausländerbeschäftigung*, p. 9.
18. *Frankfurter Rundschau*, 9 November 1990.
19. Beauftragte der Bundesregierung für Ausländerfragen (ed.), *Migration und Integration in Zahlen. Ein Handbuch*, Berlin, November 1997, pp. 95–9.
20. E. Kolinsky, 'Non-Germans and Civil Society', pp. 201–2.
21. Statistisches Bundesamt (ed.), *Datenreport 1997: Zahlen und Fakten über die Bundesrepublik Deutschland* (Bonn: Bundeszentrale für politische Bildung, 1997), p. 43.
22. *Migration und Integration in Zahlen*, p. 282.
23. Bundesminister des Inneren (ed.), *Bericht über erste Erfahrungen mit den am 1. Juli 1993 in Kraft getretenen Neuregelungen des Asylverfahrensgesetzes. Asyl-Erfahrungsbericht*, Bonn, 25 February 1994, p. 51, 53–4.
24. *Asyl-Erfahrungsbericht*, p. 54.
25. *Wirtschaft und Statistik*, 4, 1998, p. 298.
26. *Wirtschaft und Statistik*, 4, 1998, p. 298; *Wirtschaft und Statistik*, 6, 1998, p. 511, reports an average age of 23.8 for recipients of asylum seekers' benefit.
27. Statistisches Landesamt Berlin (ed.), *Statistisches Jahrbuch 1997* (Berlin: Kulturbuch Verlag), p. 487; Statistisches Landesamt Berlin (ed.), *Statistisches Jahrbuch 1998*, p. 465.
28. Statistisches Landesamt Berlin (ed.), *Statistisches Jahrbuch 1997*, p. 487.
29. Stadt Leipzig, *Statistischer Quartalsbericht*, 4/1998, p. 47.
30. *Datenreport 1997*, p. 39.
31. Stadt Leipzig (ed.), *Statistisches Jahrbuch der Stadt Leipzig 1991* (Leizpig: Amt für Statistik und Wahlen, 1991), p. 45.
32. Stadt Leipzig, *Quartalsbericht*, 2, 1998, p. 38.
33. A good overview in K. J. Bade, *Ausländer, Aussiedler, Asyl: Eine Bestandsaufnahme* (Munich: Beck, 1994; also E. Kolinsky, 'Non-German Minorities in German Society', in D. Horrocks and E. Kolinsky (eds), *Turkish Culture in German Society Today* (Oxford/New York: Berghahn, 1996), pp. 71–111.
34. D. Cohn-Bendit and T. Schmidt, *Heimat Babylon: Das Wagnis der multikulturellen Demokratie* (Hamburg: Hoffmann & Campe, 1992).
35. U. Beck, *Risikogesellschaft: Auf dem Weg in eine andere Moderne* (Frankfurt am Main: Suhrkamp, 1986).

36. W. Hanesch, *Armut in Deutschland* (Reinbek: Rowohlt, 1994), p. 197, shows that in 1994, under-provision with employment and other forms of poverty were particularly grave for non-German residents.
37. For case studies of transformation see H-H. Krüger, M. Kühnel and S. Thomas (eds), *Transformationsprobleme in Ostdeutschland. Arbeit. Bildung. Sozialpolitik* (Opladen: Leske & Budrich, 1995); R. Geißler (ed.), *Sozialer Umbruch in Ostdeutschland* (Opladen: Leske & Budrich, 1993) and the publications arising from the work of an ESRC-funded study group: E. Kolinsky (ed.), *Social Transformation and the Family*, 1998, and C. Flockton and E. Kolinsky (eds), *Recasting East Germany*, 1999.
38. H. A. Welsh *et al.*, 'East and West German Identities', p. 111.
39. E. Kolinsky, 'Non-German Minorities, Women and the Emergence of Civil Society', in E. Kolinsky and W. van der Will (eds), *The Cambridge Companion to Modern German Culture* (Cambridge: Cambridge University Press, 1999), pp. 110ff.
40. Leipziger Statistik und Stadtforschung, *Ausländer und Asylbewerber in Leipzig: Ihre reale Präsenz sowie Erfahrungen und Einstellungen aus der Sicht der Deutschen* (Leipzig: Amt für Statistik und Wahlen, 1996) p. 43.
41. *Ausländer und Asylbewerber in Leipzig*, p. 23.
42. Ibid.
43. Stadt Leipzig, *Kommunale Bürgerumfrage 1997: Ausgewählte Ergebnisse in Kurzberichten* (Leipzig: Amt für Statistik und Wahlen 1997), p. 19.
44. Bundesanstalt für Arbeit, 'Ausländer und Spätaussiedler', in *Arbeitsmarkt 1997*, p. 195.
45. 'Ausländer und Spätaussiedler', in *Arbeitsmarkt 1997*, p. 196.
46. Stadt Leipzig, *Quartalsbericht*, 3, 1998 p. 38.
47. Statistisches Landesamt Berlin, *Statistisches Jahrbuch 1998*, p. 58.
48. Statistisches Landesamt Berlin, *Statistisches Jahrbuch 1998*, p. 462–3.
49. *Datenreport*, p. 518.
50. Details in C. Flockton, 'Economic Transformation and Income Change', in E. Kolinsky (ed.), *Social Transformation and the Family*, pp. 99ff.

9

Legacies of Exclusion:
The Memory of Terror and the
Creation of Civic Values in the New
Bundesländer

Anthony Glees

A decade has passed since the collapse of the German Democratic Republic (GDR), yet there is no end in sight to the debate about the precise nature of the regime and the reasons for its demise.[1] The GDR survived for almost two generations and appeared to have become a permanent feature on the political landscape of contemporary Europe. Thus, Hermann Weber, a leading GDR scholar, wrote in 1988 that 'the GDR has existed for forty years, much longer than the fourteen years of Weimar, or the twelve of the Third Reich. This proves that the GDR, like the Federal Republic, is one of the historically most stable states in recent German history.'[2] Yet in 1989–90 it disintegrated with remarkable and unexpected speed. What brought down the GDR? Were the causes of its downfall external to east German politics or was there an internal dynamic, producing collapse from within, working alongside the wider changes in the communist world after 1985? The answers to these questions do not merely provide an interpretation of the sudden death of the east German communist state, but also offer revealing insights into the establishment of civil society in the new eastern German *Länder* which themselves inevitably impact on the political culture of the new German nation that came to life on 3 October 1990.

It is true that there have been extensive studies of the 'external shocks' to the GDR, as well as a number of studies on the 'causes of the internal implosion'.[3] Yet they usually conclude that internal dissidence was politically insubstantial and had very limited impact. One scholar insists that the 'dissidents failed the test' in the 1980s.[4] The regime, others claim, was certainly not totalitarian in any 1930s sense but able to offer its citizens a 'social contract' in which it bartered consumer and welfare goods for its citizens' willing acceptance at best, or grudging compliance at worst (the German word for both is *Anpassung*).[5] That the GDR fell, it is sometimes said, was merely the outcome of the evaporation of Soviet power.

Such an interpretation, however, is unsatisfactory on several counts. For one thing, by concentrating on *Anpassung*, it ignores the many testimonies to the extent to which communism prevailed for as long as it did by means of the systematic abuse of human rights by the east German secret police, the Stasi (*Staatssicherheitsdienst*). In the 40 years of the GDR some 250,000 individuals suffered serious abuse at the hands of what ultimately became a secret police consisting of 91,000 officers and 173,000 'informal collaborators' or IMs (*Informelle Mitarbeiter*).[6] For another, it plays down the political significance of the internal dissident opposition to the terror of the Stasi state. To do so is both historically inaccurate and politically misleading since it discounts the central role of the east German opposition in the evolution of a civil society in the eastern part of Germany both during and after communism.

Civic values and the acceptance of constitutionalism in the New *Bundesländer* were by no means just the outcome of the transfer on to them of west German political institutions. Rather, they stemmed directly from the contribution made to the east German political culture by enlightened and courageous dissenters such as Ulrike and Gerd Poppe, Bohley, Hirsch and Templin.[7] The examination of witness testimony makes this wholly plain and is, therefore, a valuable resource in constructing a fuller account of the significance of dissidence in the GDR, and of the terror practised with ruthlessness and innovation by the Stasi. But there is an additional dimension, often discounted by researchers, but highlighted in the testimony and documentary evidence. It concerns the support given to dissidents by western governments and institutions who wished to see civil rights and civic values prosper during the lifetime of the GDR.

To ignore these aspects of the collapse of communism in Germany may well have unfortunate political consequences, to leave the scholarly ones aside. If memories of dissidence are ignored or confiscated, the horrors of east Germany's communist past are easily forgotten. This in turn allows those who have abused the human rights of their fellow citizens a real chance of escaping justice. Indeed, the strength of civil values in the new Germany may well depend on the state's readiness to confront this difficult aspect of communism's legacy.[8] However strongly it may be argued that no public good can come from the full legal investigation of the communists' human rights abuses, the fact remains that without it the rule of law is not being seen to be upheld. What this means is that unless memory is properly utilised, the successful transformation of eastern Germany – the New *Bundesländer* – into a stable and consensual *Rechtsstaat* may never take place.[9] Plainly, the *new* Federal Republic can only be a *Rechtsstaat* if eastern Germany's transition into it allows the rule of law to be sustained – and this, in turn, is a problem for the whole of

Germany and not just the new *Länder*. German unity in 1990 has indeed triggered a *dual transformation*: eastern Germany has been transformed, but in the requirement to deal appropriately with the consequences of communist injustice (as with the many other legacies of the GDR), the whole of the Federal Republic has been, and still is, required to transform itself as well. For that process to be completed, due weight must be given to east German dissident testimony.

This chapter, then, aims to examine these matters in closer detail by setting the memory and testimony of some of those whose human rights were abused as dissidents against the official, if top secret, record of that inhumanity kept – carefully – by the Stasi. It seeks to demonstrate the primacy of Stasi terror, rather than *Anpassung*, in securing a long life for the GDR. It, and not any 'social compact', provides the defining dynamic of east Germany. Yet despite the Stasi's best efforts, the dissidents (of whom 2,500 were under surveillance by 1989) won through. Their persistence and courage in promoting civil values was a major cause of political change once the ordinary people of the GDR decided that open support for these values would bring about the collapse of the regime they had come to hate. Without the dissidents, however, there would have been no tradition of human rights to which the wider citizenry could lay claim.

WITNESS TESTIMONY, RESEARCH AND POLICY

Ten years after the collapse of the GDR could be considered the right time to ask whether transformation studies, that is, the study of the process of political, social and economic change in eastern Germany since 1989, have not outlived their usefulness. In 1955, ten years after the collapse of the Third Reich, one might claim, the Bonn Republic had become an important member of Nato, was a core member of the Coal and Steel Community, and was already deeply involved in the creation of the EEC. Many west Germans could have been forgiven for believing the transformation of their country into a democratic republic had been accomplished. By analogy, therefore, it might be thought today that after a decade of political liberalism and economic and social support the transformation of eastern Germany into the new *Länder* of the Federal Republic has been completed. It might be said that its current political condition no longer requires the concept of transformation to comprehend it, still less to fashion it, and that its political culture is now sufficiently secure to allow the communist past to be forgotten.

In fact, of course, in 1955 west Germany's transformation had merited greater attention than it received, particularly in respect of its failure to address properly the impact of the Nazi past on the large numbers of Germans who had been servants of the Third Reich, and also on those Germans and others who had been its victims.[10] With the ending of the first phase of Occupation in 1949 most west Germans seem to have been only too glad to cast a veil of silence over these issues – a silence which in some instances was maintained for the following 50 years. It is therefore hardly surprising that there is much evidence that the transformation of eastern Germany is still ongoing – and in need of monitoring and assessment. The enduring social and economic problematic in the former GDR and, indeed, the very outcome of the federal elections of September 1998 (and the dramatic gains scored by the successor party to the SED – *Sozialistische Einheitspartei* or German Communist Party – the PDS – *Partei des Demokratischen Sozialismus* or Party of Democratic Socialism – in the new *Länder* where it gained an average of 20 per cent of the vote), all serve to confirm that the legacy of communism has, without doubt, not yet been overcome.

Nothing supports this view more eloquently than the appalling record of the exclusion of the SED's political opponents. Over the 40 years of communist rule in eastern Germany, as many as 250,000 Germans suffered serious abuse for political reasons.[11] Although this study is a political and not a psychological one, it would be wrong not to begin it by stressing the grave, and possibly indelible, psychological impact that this abuse has had on the Stasi's victims. Because it is a political one, the political effect of such abuse at the time should also be properly appreciated. After all, it was the purpose of persecution to break the *political* spirit of dissidents by breaking them psychologically.[12] Terror, fear, torture and the recognition of betrayal were merely some of the tools of the Stasi's trade, but all were designed to cause trauma, and all of them, to some extent, did so. For this reason it is also the wish of a large number of the victims of communist human rights violations that their stories should be subject to further research; they have formed associations such as the *Gemeinschaft ehemaliger politischer Häftlinge*, ably chaired by Harald Strunz, to facilitate such investigations.

They seek to counter the view espoused by some politicians, some former supporters of the SED and the Stasi (which itself has set up an active, and dangerous, ex-officers' organisation as well as numerous *Seilschaften*, or secret associations) that the use of terror in the GDR is simply a 'fiction'. Since 1990 those who suffered under German communism have produced a vast archive of eye-witness and documentary testimony. In addition, of course, their activities inside the GDR generated some 180 kilometres of Stasi files – files, it should be added, whose accuracy has to date been consistently reconfirmed (although occasionally evaluations of factual material have been shown to be inaccurate).[13]

If true social peace is defined not as the absence of conflict but as the presence of justice, it must follow that the collective memory of human rights abuse must play its part in the policy process. Whether its input should be confined to support for the idea of financial restitution for damage suffered, or as evidence for use in any legal measures against identifiable perpetrators may be open to debate.[14] Yet it seems hard to believe that, without retribution for wrong-doing, adherence to human rights in civic society can be regarded as wholly secure. And without the record of this memory, the true nature of the SED state will remain hidden.

While no one could support the use of memory to pursue revenge against German communists (which is not an acceptable use of collective memory in any constitutional polity), it is proper to believe that the stories told by victims must be formally heard – and processed – within the framework of the law. It is the duty of a constitutionally defined state to understand such testimony and organise retribution if deemed right, the more so in respect of abuses committed both under communism and Nazism, since under these two regimes the rationale of abuse was that it served the wider interests of the German state.

To move beyond the past requires the past to have been decently evaluated. This is in the interests of victims as well as the state. Two very prominent victims, Wolfgang Templin and Ulrike Poppe, have both recently reiterated their opposition to a policy of official amnesia, or an amnesty for wrong-doers.[15] Poppe states unequivocally that human rights abuses can only be forgiven by those who suffered them, not by the state nor any party or institution claiming to act on their behalf.[16] Yet Johannes Rau, the new President of Germany, is but one of the leading German politicians who have called for a general amnesty for Stasi perpetrators.

One of the strongest supporters of a practical policy of retribution against Stasi perpetrators has been the recently retired Director of the Berlin Police, Manfred Kittlaus. By the time of his departure from office in the late autumn of 1998, Kittlaus and his staff had compiled a list of more than 250 Stasi suspects involved in serious human rights abuses against individuals or serious fraud.[17] The Berlin police are of the view that to date some DM26 to DM30 billion (twice the figure estimated in 1996) have been secretly transferred from German banks by former members of the Stasi (DM3 billion has been recovered). In addition, Kittlaus is inclined to believe that the more than 6,000 cases of savage sentences passed by east German courts for political reasons should be subject to criminal investigation since they may have contravened GDR laws and can thus now be pursued under federal German law (which is the current yardstick in such cases).

It is not only on the testimonies of those who were abused that research is necessary; it is also required to define who was or was not a victim in the first place. While the 'racial' victims of the Third Reich were reasonably easy to identify, its 'non-racial' ones were harder to classify. In the case of purely political persecution, whether from 1933–45 or from 1945–90, the definition is harder still. Those arrested, abused, tortured or even killed for political reasons are plainly victims. But it could plausibly be suggested that those who opposed communism in the GDR – for whatever reason – but chose not to try to leave it and were not subject to imprisonment, or worse, should not be regarded as its victims. Instead, it could be argued, not only were they able to cultivate 'niche' anti-communist values, but were actually left unscathed by regime and secret police while they did so. Indeed, to allege the existence of such niches could be taken to imply that within an overall structure of communism some dissent was possible and those in the niches were not truly victims of the Stasi.

Other observers, however, regard such individuals not only as genuine victims but also as full members of a significant, effective and ultimately successful underground political opposition in the GDR.[18] They were victims, it could be claimed, because, even if they were not imprisoned, they were subject to almost continuous surveillance, and open to the abuses that accompanied it, of which discovery that fellow conspirators, friends and even partners were IMs was but one aspect. They were significant because even they kept alive a faith in civic values for Germany, and effective because an increasing number of east Germans came to support these values as the 1980s progressed. Finally, it might be concluded, they were successful because these east German dissidents were the true political victors of the events of 1989 and 1990 when communism was replaced by constitutionalism in a peaceful revolution sustained by the vast majority of ordinary east Germans who had sensed they were about to become German citizens.

In addition, as Konrad Jarausch has suggested in an internet review, the extent and limit of Stasi power might be revealed most tellingly by an examination of the ultimate success of the dissidents of the 1980s. He notes that 'whilst the Stasi was very effective in combatting traditional anti-Communist and pro-Western enemies of the 1950s, it proved incapable of dealing with a different brand of internal critics of the 1980s, who just wanted Socialism to live up to its own pacifist, feminist and environmentalist claims'.[19] Why, he ponders, was this so. In a broad sense, this present investigation may go some way towards providing an answer.

TESTIMONIES OF DISSIDENCE AND REPRESSION

The 1980s dissidents realised how they could use the internal logic of the regime's stated support for peace and civil rights against itself not least by gaining external publicity for their demands.[20] They were also able to rely on a number of objective external changes which their predecessors did not possess. The old Cold War and *détente* had been and gone. The post-Brezhnev Soviet Union was in rapid decline and new hardline leaders in Britain (Margaret Thatcher) and the United States (Ronald Reagan) had decided to squeeze and possibly even defeat Soviet control over its empire. The British government, supported by the United States, decided to support dissidents everywhere in eastern Europe, and established a new policy for this called 'Maximum Engagement'.[21] We should not forget that by all accounts the most impressive single exhibit in the Reagan Presidential Library in Simi Valley, California, is a 10-foot high, 6,000-pound piece of the Berlin Wall, presented to him by an east German dissident group, in recognition of his efforts to get rid of it.[22]

The argument that where dissidents were not arrested, they were, in effect, permitted to function more or less freely as dissidents is quite untenable when the evidence of the Stasi files is considered. They show that the Stasi permitted such activists to exist only because they were completely confident that they could steer, control and then neutralise them *from within*. The IM 'Karin Lenz', one of a vast army who worked against civil rights and peace activists in the 1980s, said: 'When I have found out where I can hit someone to maximum effect, how I can finish them off – and that is usually with psychological methods – and if that person is my enemy, then that is what I do.'[23] The Stasi term for this was, ironically, 'subversion' (*Zersetzung*). A Stasi directive 'for developing and working upon operational objects' states that it aimed at 'promoting discord amongst hostile-negative forces' by the 'systematic organisation of professional and social failure, the undermining of self-confidence of individuals, and the creation of mistrust and mutual suspicion'.[24] The means to be employed included the use of anonymous letters, phone calls and denunciations to the police and the propagation of specific rumours and acts of indiscretion. Far from existing happily as germs of an alternative political culture, the spying, steering and control of the dissidents demonstrated the extent to which the Stasi believed in the final victory of communist *Gleichschaltung*.[25] As Wolf Biermann famously noted 'we were all like rats in a laboratory'.[26]

It is for this reason that the all-embracing, scientifically constructed and perfectly ruthless work of the Stasi must be deemed the defining dynamic of the political development of the GDR. Timothy Garton Ash is right to argue that, by the early 1980s, the GDR was both totalitarian and a close, real-life example of Orwell's fictional nightmare state.[27] His comments that the corruption practised by the Stasi continues to wreak havoc on both perpetrators and victims, and that it has now unwittingly invested researchers with some of the power over both groups that the Stasi once possessed over its victims are every bit as trenchant as (and well borne out by) this very research.

In the end, of course, the Stasi's calculations proved disastrously wrong. They had overestimated their ability to steer events because they had underestimated the unflinching courage of the dissidents, and because there were some organisations and events outside of the GDR, in the Soviet Union and in the west (especially Britain), over which they had virtually no control. But their failure does not mean that they did not try. Research into their abuse of their victims demonstrates the almost unbelievable lengths to which they were prepared to go in order to win against them. Indeed, careful consideration of the mind-boggling extent and scope of their work allows one to realise that the number of those who must be considered Stasi victims is even greater than one might imagine. This is because an apparently significant number of the 173,000 or so IMs, the all-important foot soldiers in the Stasi's campaigns, were themselves often also Stasi victims in a real sense (although it does not follow that one need have much sympathy for them). They included not just those who were blackmailed into becoming Stasi 'alongsiders', but also ironically those who worked for them out of deep political conviction who include non-Germans as well.

THE STASI, THE DISSIDENTS AND THE UK

The voluminous files of two British IMs 'Armin' and 'Diana', recently uncovered, show that despite possessing great political sympathy for east German communism, these two (one male, one female) were systematically manipulated, deceived and lied to over long periods by the very officers they strained themselves to serve and in whom they had total trust.[28] Examples of the Stasi's readiness to corrupt the lives of ordinary humans included in the case of the two Britons their fabricating a romantic and then sexual relationship between her and a young male journalist (in reality a Stasi agent codenamed 'Schnitter') to secure (or seduce) 'Diana' into becoming an IM. She was seen as likely to gain a post in Nato, the European Community or the Ministry of Defence. They had discovered that she was desperate to have such a relationship, and to tempt her further they produced false publishing contracts. Against 'Armin' (once again, specially selected for the professional promise he showed), no less elaborate and depraved ruses were developed, first to bind him to the GDR, then, once fully signed up, to distance him physically from the GDR (in order to avoid the suspicions of MI5), and finally, when a fillip was needed to spur his treacherous work on behalf of the Stasi, to manufacture a completely fictitious public celebration in the GDR to which he was to be invited. They knew that he would be flattered by what he thought was a genuine invitation to return to the GDR and that once there he could be enticed to commit even worse acts of treachery in the UK. He was also cruelly lied to in order to end his first and happy sexual relationship with an east German girl because it carried security risks for the Stasi, and serious and frightening threats were made to his girlfriend to get her to leave him (which she did). 'Armin' never knew why.

The lives of both these perfectly ordinary British citizens were effectively ruined by the Stasi in ways neither of them could have ever guessed. Even today they will be unaware of the extent to which their work for the Stasi will wreak terrible damage to them in the future, both in terms of their careers (both hold publicly accountable appointments) and privately (within their relationships). It is true that both were committed to 'Socialism' and were knowingly and willingly Stasi spies, and that 'Armin' in particular did serious damage to the groups on which he spied as well as to his colleagues and friends in various British universities. But it is also true that they were manipulated and misled with total viciousness and brazen mendacity by a secret police who served a state which had absolutely no respect for the lawfulness of or the need to protect basic human rights. In this way, then, 'Diana' and 'Armin' and many like them were also victims of the SED state.

VICTIM TESTIMONY: MEASURING POLITICAL REPRESSION AND OPPOSITION IN THE GDR

Victim testimony especially where it can be set beside the Stasi's own documentary evidence is one important measure of the changing methods and purpose of Stasi repression. Yet it also provides accurate and fresh evidence of the growth in the 1980s of a dissident political movement, predicated on support for peace and human rights (values the GDR officially claimed to uphold and promote), and, revealingly, one supported by various western groups, institutions and authorities. In terms of the periodisation of east German political development after 1945 it can be seen that the Stalinist horrors perpetrated as much by German communists as by their Soviet rulers gradually yielded to more modern and usually (the word should be stressed) less brutal but equally effective means of social control. The memories of those interviewed for this present research, as well as those not interviewed but whose files are now available in the archives of the *Bundesbeauftragte für die Unterlagen des Staatssicherheitsdienstes der ehemaligen Deutschen Demokratischen Republik* indicate that there were three main phases of political persecution: the first lasted from 1945 until 1953, the second from 1953 until 1982 and the final phase from 1982 until the collapse of the GDR at the end of that 1989. The main emphasis in this study has been on this final phase.[29]

Political victims of the first Stalinist phase of persecution provide a testimony of almost unbelievable horror which firmly links the behaviour of the two German totalitarian regimes. Margret Bechler, who describes herself as an apolitical German nationalist, though never a Nazi, was married to a senior *Wehrmacht* officer who was a passionate National Socialist.[30] When he was taken prisoner by the Russians at Stalingrad he joined the Free German Movement in Russia and became a communist. A courier was sent to make contact with his young wife (who lived with her two young children in army quarters in Dresden) to tell her this, but out of fear that her children would be taken from her if the courier were discovered, she told the Gestapo about him. He was duly arrested and executed.

After the collapse of the Third Reich she was blamed for the courier's death and arrested by the Russians. Held in various gaols and former concentration camps, including Mühlberg and Buchenwald, she survived quite appalling abuse (while many of those with her did not) before being tried five years after her arrest on 13 June 1950 in an east German court. In the meantime, her husband, by now a leading communist in Brandenburg, had divorced her without her knowledge, gaining custody of their two children. At her first trial her defence (that she had acted to protect her children) was accepted, but she received a life sentence. This was, however, quashed and at a second trial she was sentenced to death for complicity in a war crime. She spent three years on death row at Waldheim before her sentence was commuted to life. She was permitted to go the west in 1956 but was refused permission to have any contact with her husband or her two children and she believed she would never see any of them again.

It is by no means clear that Frau Bechler was guilty of any wrongdoing at all, let alone a war crime. She herself regards her action in 1944 as morally culpable, but is satisfied that her motive, the protection of her children, was honourable and left her with no alternative. Unification in 1990 presented her with a unique but desperately painful opportunity to reassess her past life and relationships. She quickly came to realise that what once had been there – a husband and two children – had been destroyed by German communism and that, even though her family were still all alive, in a deeper sense they had been irretrievably taken from her more than 40 years before. Her suffering has been great but she is also marked today by a complete serenity. She says that, at her present age, compensation or retribution lack any meaning; she is beyond all of that ('*ich bin hindurch*', she says, adding that for her the answer to the reason for her suffering at the hands of German communism is not to be found on this earth).

Other victims of this era have experiences of similar suffering although their 'crimes' were more actively oppositional than Frau Bechler's if equally political (in that they threatened, or seemed to threaten, the supremacy of communism).[31] They included membership of the SPD and opposition to the merger with the KPD; membership of the CDU and opposition to the concept of the National Front; and support for free speech at east German universities.[32] As the years went by, new 'crimes' appeared: in 1961 a chance meeting with American troops visiting east Berlin led a 19-year-old man to ask for help in crossing the recently built Berlin Wall. Arrested, he was tortured for more than seven months, chiefly, he believes, because he refused to become an IM for the Stasi.[33] In the 1970s a young man received a seven-year hard labour sentence for photocopying pages from George Orwell's *Animal Farm*; an 18-year-old in Erfurt was given 12 months for distributing leaflets criticising Solzhenitsyn's expulsion from the USSR;[34] another was given 17 years for a variety of offences sparked off by an attempt to overhear a Rolling Stones concert in west Berlin by putting his ear to the Berlin Wall;[35] another political detainee committed suicide in prison in Jena after being played a tape purporting to be the sound of his pregnant girl-friend being tortured.[36] Ordinary lives were being destroyed with extreme ruthlessness by a secret police who balked at nothing.

THE STASI AND DISSIDENTS IN THE 1980s: THE UK DIMENSION

In the 1980s, however, the GDR's odious but central tradition of political persecution was faced with a new threat: organised dissent based on a demand for peace and civil rights.[37] As Poppe later explained: 'By being incriminated and persecuted, we were pushed into a formal opposition to the regime. This is how we discovered the issue of human rights.'[38]

Victim testimony and Stasi documentary evidence reveal how dissidence developed – and how it was investigated and dealt with. It took roughly three years for the potential magnitude of the threat to be understood by the Stasi, but they were at all times confident they could handle and eradicate it. Their strategy was always clear and consistent: to contain and neutralise the new form of opposition by a mixture of well-tried nostrums, persecution, terror and *Zersetzung* (subversion). It is not possible here to give a comprehensive account of either dissident or Stasi activity in this period.[39] Instead, a specific problematic will be investigated which exposes the Stasi's methods, illustrates their medium-term success but also their final failure. It centres upon the exploitation of peace and human rights issues by those dissident groups *Frauen für den Frieden* ('Women for Peace') and the *Initiative für Frieden und Menschenrechte* ('Initiative for Peace and Human Rights') of whom Ulrike Poppe, Bärbel Bohley, Werner Fischer and Vera Wollenberger were some of the leading figures, upon the Stasi tactic for neutralising them, and on adjunct Stasi activity to this end in Britain.

As far as the Stasi's work in the UK in this regard was concerned (which was by no means, of course, their only sphere of UK activity), they had three main and clearly defined aims. The first was to monitor all UK efforts to support the dissidents; these could – from the SED viewpoint – prove highly dangerous to the GDR. The second was to demonstrate in public in the GDR that there were clear linkages between 'suspect' (anti-communist) parts of the UK peace movement and the dissidents in order to indicate that the dissidents were essentially enemy agents. Thirdly, but no less outrageously, the Stasi actually sought to steer the UK peace movement (the Campaign for Nuclear Disarmament, the CND, and European Nuclear Disarmament, END) away from support for the east German dissidents and into ever closer links with its own SED-run peace movement, the *Friedensrat*, led by an *apparatchik* named Werner Rumpel.

Ulrike Poppe has provided a general account of the Poppe–Bohley circle.[40] Her political story began early in 1980. The decision to re-arm Nato in response to Brezhnev's re-armament of the Warsaw Pact states had led to a considerable, and dangerous, increase in tension between east and west. Nato leaders feared that *détente* might be now be dead; the Soviets appear to have seriously expected a pre-emptive Nato strike and planned accordingly. Poppe and her associates, already worried about militarism, decided to form what was probably the first organised but non-SED run political group in the GDR (*Frauen für den Frieden*).[41]

In the first instance this group opposed the nuclear arms race. By 1982, however, they had constructed an organised opposition movement, which promised annual 'conferences' to attack the planned conscription of women into the east German armed forces. Initially an east Berlin group, it soon had members in all other major east German cities and became a 'group peace engagement' of east German women. At first, their criticism of the SED state was confined to certain aspects of its *militaristic* policies (the conscription of women, as already mentioned, its hostile attitude towards conscientious objectors, and the introduction of toy guns into kindergartens) and the fact that although it claimed to be dedicated to the pursuit of peace, it had merely made a few public declarations and accepted the stationing of Soviet missiles on east German territory. Yet this opposition, however mild at this time and notwithstanding the truth that it was based on support for values that the state *itself* claimed to stand for, was nevertheless opposition to SED control over peace issues.[42] Since it was self-evident that the control of peace activities, like every other political activity in the GDR, was itself a core communist policy, this automatically made the dissidents anti-communist in fact, even if strictly speaking not so in theory. It is generally accepted that the awareness among many dissidents that they were becoming anti-communists, if the definition of communism was what the SED stood for, dawned only very gradually. At the start of their journey into opposition, they regarded themselves as committed 'Socialists' because they genuinely believed in respect of peace what the SED state said about itself. Indeed every primary school textbook in the GDR made its devotion to peace quite explicit.[43]

This had fateful consequences for the dissidents, for their supporters in the west but most seriously of all for the SED and the Stasi themselves. The first of these was that the GDR authorities – the Stasi – moved into higher gear in combating them. They had already been unsettled by the 'Berlin Appeal' of Rainer Eppelmann in 1982. Eppelmann had stated that 'the fear of atomic war amongst the east German people is greater than their fear of participating in the unofficial peace movement' which (rightly) seemed to the Stasi to carry more than a whiff of incitement to dissidence with it.[44] Much more gravely, from the Stasi's viewpoint, an organisation called European Nuclear Disarmament (END), created by the historian and radical thinker E. P. Thompson in 1980, had published the 'Appeal' in the west and gained an impressive set of signatures supporting Eppelmann (two signatories, Robin Cook MP and Michael Meacher MP, were to become leading ministers in the 1997 Labour government).[45] END, led by the enigmatic Thompson himself and, for a period, by the strategic analyst Mary Kaldor, was a most remarkable institution, with a political impact in eastern Europe so great that we are entitled to regard it as one of the main causes of the defeat of communism in central and eastern Europe.[46] Thompson's book *Protest and Survive* reveals much more about his aims in the section entitled 'Appeal for European Disarmament' than in his more widely read opening chapter from which the book takes its title.[47] The Stasi exploited their considerable resources in the UK to investigate END; they were convinced that its leading figures, Thompson, Kaldor and Ken Coates (also head of the Bertrand Russell Peace Foundation), were determined to subvert CND whose unilateralist line suited the GDR very well. The GDR did all it could to assist and comfort CND. And they believed (the word should be stressed) that Thompson and Kaldor were 'close' to the British secret intelligence service and the CIA, and that Coates shared these links but acted chiefly out of a 'Trotskyite' desire to harm the Soviet Union.[48]

What made things considerably worse, in the eyes of the Stasi, was that on 23 November 1981 E. P. Thompson had himself come to 'Westberlin' to give a speech in which he declared that: 'the Havemann initiative is a good example of how eastern and western peace movements should work together ... there is an immediate link between real disarmament and the development of democratic movements in the Socialist states. *Furthermore, the creation of democratic movements in them is a precondition for forcing the Socialist states to disarm.*'[49] Thompson was not simply urging eastern and western peace movements to cooperate, but stating that together they could pressurise the Soviet bloc. To add insult to injury, Thompson had insisted that 'pressure on the Soviet Union must be increased' alongside pressure on the USA: Thompson's line, intriguingly, came increasingly to demand that the Soviets disarm before Nato. Not merely multilateral, rather than unilateral (which was CND's position), it in fact reflected the 'Zero Option' which both Ronald Reagan and Margaret Thatcher came to support.[50]

The east German dissidents took great heart from Thompson's audacious but intellectually irresistible formulation and responded to the Stasi's intimidation of them by coolly adding demands for civil liberty to those for peace. They took the line that both aims were formal state aims of the GDR, and therefore to be sanctioned by the SED, but that the Stasi's attempted suppression of the women dissidents showed that without civil rights, the call for peace could not be properly made.[51] Since the east German constitution guaranteed the right of association and free speech the dissidents' request seemed hard formally to contradict.[52] Poppe recalls: 'Peace to me did not mean simply non–war and rocket-reduction. Peace was indissolubly linked to the human rights issue.'[53] What was particularly significant was that this *junktim* (one thing being conditional on the other) echoed fully the one which had been pressed by the western supporters of the east German dissidents, organised since 1980 END as the 'END–GDR Group' or the 'END–GDR Women's Group' via a letter sent by Thompson to the *Guardian* newspaper.[54] Poppe adds that neither she nor any of her close colleagues believed that any of the Soviet satellites would be able to lead the Soviet bloc but they did feel that a 'staged reform of the system from within' was perfectly thinkable. Dialogue with the SED, they were sure, would deliver it.

The Stasi files show that in the view of the SED dialogue with Poppe and the others was not on the menu. Although the Stasi were fairly certain that Poppe and her circle were not by any manner of means an invention of END, which it had been monitoring via its agents within END as well as outside it, the END link offered an immediate means of dealing with the dissidents, who were already all under constant surveillance (Poppe's flat was also bugged).[55] The Stasi believed that if the opposition leaders could be successfully intimidated, the organisation they led would quickly crumble. They soon began to see that their very work in the UK could provide the necessary means of achieving this. They knew that END and the GDR–END Group within it were offering Poppe support. If they could prove that Poppe was accepting it, and conspiring with END against the Soviet Union and the GDR, she and her colleagues could be charged with high treason and working for foreign intelligence. This, they schemed, would discredit them all as traitors, puppets of the west and enemies of 'Socialism'.

The Stasi found London a relatively easy area for their operations. One Stasi file gives a list of the names of Stasi agents working out of the GDR Embassy in Belgrave Square in London in 1988.[56] Interestingly, it also shows that the *Hauptverwaltung Aufklärung* (HVA) or Stasi Foreign Intelligence Service, led by Markus Wolf, undertook its own security operations against GDR Embassy staff, a fact consistent with our understanding that the internal system for checking and evaluating intelligence within the Stasi was well-developed and thus its information was highly reliable. Agents mentioned by code-name in this file and those dealing with END throughout the 1980s are the IMs 'Hans Reichert', 'Jutta May', 'Tommy', 'Diestel', 'Luis', 'Hammer', 'Michael Linke' and 'Manfred'. A Captain Müller (his real name), based in London, compiled reports for the Ministerium für Staatssicherheit (Secret Service Ministry (MfS)) on these individuals. The Britain–GDR Friendship Society and Berolina Travel in London (which arranged travel to the GDR) were also important sources of information about British issues, especially via academics and journalists who were, allegedly, sometimes offered study visits to the GDR and detailed information in return for reports on events and personalities in the UK.[57] The Society also helped organise the somewhat unfortunately named Intercourse Programme, which brought British German-language teachers to the GDR.

Of these London Stasi agents, 'Hans Reichert' and 'Jutta May' were plainly the most important. Both of them organised the successful penetration of END (and, indeed, CND). However, in their real identities

('Reichert' was, amazingly, the east German Ambassador at the time, Gerhard Lindner, and 'May' a counsellor called Helga Scheibe) they were also supplied with copious sensitive information by individual END (and CND) members who believed it was right for them to do so. According to the investigative journalist Jamie Dettmer, the real names of some of the others were: O. Schneidratus, V. Kempf and Dr H. H. Kasper.[58] In addition, confidential information of use to the Stasi but highly damaging to non-communists in CND was knowingly supplied by those members of END (and CND) who had communist sympathies, including Vic Allen, at that time professor of sociology at Leeds University.

At the same time, the Stasi had a high regard for the British Security Service which was, it must be conceded, demonstrably unwarranted (since none of these agents, and neither of the two British IMs mentioned above were identified before 1995) although their reverence for MI5's technical skills may have been justified. The Stasi commented with awe on their telecommunications brilliance and their ability to tap phones without any audible sign. A Stasi informer inside Chatham House complained that his calls to them were being listened to. He was assured that if he could hear clicks and whirrs, this proved that it could not be MI5 under any circumstances. The Stasi believed that in the 1980s MI5 had stepped up its activities, and were working even more closely with the metropolitan police to catch foreign agents. They even feared that 'neighbourhood watch' schemes in those areas where diplomats lived were run in collaboration with the security service, and warned all their own agents never to be caught drinking and driving, or breaking other minor laws which might prompt further investigation. The Stasi also ordered a stop on '*Treffs*' (covert meetings) or meetings with their British agents at football matches in the London area because they feared, with little substance one imagines, the increased police presence might – inadvertently – lead to discovery.[59]

THE EINHORN TRAP

London also provided the Stasi with an ideal opportunity to scupper Poppe and her circle. On or around 11 October 1983, their London agents discovered that an END–GDR Women's Group contact to the east German dissidents by the name of Barbara Einhorn (a Brighton academic with research and family ties to the GDR) would be travelling to meet them during the period 1–11 December 1983, at which time information would be passed to her about the activities of the dissidents.[60] On 14 November 1983 Markus Wolf began to prepare his junior colleagues in Department XX for action.[61]

To catch Einhorn receiving information from Poppe and Bohley would provide the smoking-gun evidence the Stasi needed to destroy them, and it was agreed on 2 December to make the necessary moves. In addition, Einhorn was due to meet Jutta Seidel and Irene Kuckutz. Since Poppe's flat was under constant surveillance, the Stasi knew exactly when to strike. At 11 p.m. on 10 December Einhorn was arrested as she sought to cross the border back to west Berlin. She was transferred (at midnight) to Hohenschönhausen, a Stasi gaol and interrogation and torture centre in Berlin. At her third interrogation she gave the Stasi the statement they required, and they confiscated the material she had collected from the dissidents and her diary. She was charged with 'crimes against the state, under paragraph 99 of the legal code, carrying a sentence of 2–12 years'. In fact, Einhorn was released after a few days, thanks partly to the fact that she was not the real target and to the efforts of Canon Paul Oestreicher, another remarkably courageous and hugely skilled opponent of German communism. Even so, it is by no means implausible to believe that her incarceration and interrogation was a life event for Dr Einhorn, from whose appalling effects she may still be suffering today, not least because she knows herself to have been betrayed to the Stasi by one of her English END colleagues. What is more, it was assumed by END that the Stasi now knew everything about its organisation and its aim. While this assumption was correct, the knowledge had not come from Einhorn, but from the Stasi's own subversion of END.

As for Poppe and the others, they were arrested at once and also transferred to Hohenschönhausen, where they were incarcerated over the Christmas period (in the knowledge that some, including Poppe, who had young children would be particularly damaged by this). They faced charges of high treason and espionage.[62] Poppe herself states she was not beaten, but was with others who were. They realised that their activities had been betrayed to the Stasi but whether from Britain (and by whom in Britain), or from within their ranks was something they did not know at that time. They did know, however, that some of the group might be Stasi IMs, and they recognised that the tension that this induced was itself part of the Stasi's subversive goal. Today it is certain that they were betrayed both externally and from within. Poppe singles out Ibrahim Böhme as a major Stasi source (and she has refused to absolve him for as long as he continues to attempt to justify his spying). The IM 'Karin Lenz', Poppe has stated, made over 125 secret reports on her group. While there were some matters about which they were in any case quite open, those which Einhorn had merely confirmed to the Stasi, others (for example, the location of their all-important photocopier, which Einhorn did not know) were substantial secrets, to be kept at all costs.

Naturally, the existence of such vital secrets increased the terror felt by those arrested. But they kept silent and were set free in January. In a frighteningly crude and defiant act of victory over Poppe, the Stasi destroyed her *Kinderladen*, the 'children's shop' which had come to symbolise her public presence as a dissident. Very early one morning, a group of secret police (in uniform) turned up in a truck, systematically smashed its windows and walled up the front of the building with bricks, obliterating it entirely from sight. Such state-sponsored vandalism showed, in a single act of violence, that the rule of law, enshrined in the very constitution of east Germany, meant nothing whatsoever either to the SED or its instrument, the Stasi. The physical destruction of Poppe's *Kinderladen*, analogous to the Nazis' burning of books in 1933, was intended to remind opponents of the SED that what could be done to things could also be done to people.

It seems sensible to believe that the Einhorn incident did cause serious damage to the dissident movement in the short and medium term. It is a mark of the courage of Poppe and her circle, however, that their efforts to mobilise east Germans in support of the *junktim* between peace and civil rights increased, rather than declined. END support in the form of practical advice and practical assistance (a photocopier, for example, found its way to east Berlin) was increased. The British Embassy under Tim Everard (believed by the Stasi, not without reason, to be 'close' to MI6, the British Secret Intelligence Service) did all it could to boost the morale of the dissidents and even arranged meetings between various dissidents at the ambassador's private residence.[63] A 'Berlin Citizenship Group' was formed in 1987 in order to plan a major protest at the 1988 Rosa Luxemburg and Karl Liebknecht rally.[64] It included Bohley, the Wollenbergers, Werner Fischer and Ralf Hirsch.

Even though the Stasi knew precisely what the Group planned (Vera Wollenberger's husband, Knud, was, unknown to her, of course, and appallingly, an IM called 'Donald'), the Stasi was knocked off balance, even if only momentarily. Exhibiting the same skills as five years before, the dissidents realised that the regime's public rally in memory of the two dissident 'martyrs' of the Weimar era (killed because they had demanded peace and 'Socialism') offered the Berlin Group an opportunity of turning the regime's ideology into a weapon against itself. What could the SED do against 'Socialist dissidents' demonstrating in support of 'Socialist dissidents' alongside the SED itself? To do nothing would make the GDR look weak and insecure; to act against the Berlin Group would imply the regime refused to practise what it preached – which would make the GDR look weak and insecure. Caught between a rock and a hard place, the Stasi opted for damage limitation. They eschewed a pre-emptive strike as they had done in 1983 and arrested the group only after they had staged their demonstration. Yet this allowed the dissidents to make their point, and to make it before the eyes of the world, thanks to television. They had lost their freedom, but the group had won a significant fight in the struggle for civil rights.

Support from the west, and in particular support from Paul Oestreicher, enabled the dissidents to choose exile in the UK – as guests of the Archbishop of Canterbury – rather than gaol (a choice they found extremely hard to make since they feared that exile might isolate them from their followers). During this period, Oestreicher was at his most active – a real 'Scarlet Pimpernel'. Visiting the GDR now with great frequency, he counselled dissidents not to stage any further mass uprisings until it was certain that force would not be used against them. At the same time, he assured the apparatchiks in the SED that they would lose all credibility as a state committed to peace and freedom if they did not embark upon a serious dialogue with the dissidents. He then arranged for the dissidents to return to Berlin – to ensure that when the moment came they would be where they needed to be.[65] Once again, Oestreicher (viewed by the Stasi as a dangerous 'wolf'[66]) had outsmarted both SED and Stasi.

STASI POWER TURNS TO ASHES

Victim testimony, especially where it can be counterbalanced by the Stasi's own documentary evidence and witness testimony, provides an invaluable guide to the workings of the east German secret police in what Poppe rightly calls the 'second German dictatorship'. It shows that the Stasi's massive counter-measures were able to suppress open revolt for as long as the dissidents were not followed by the ordinary east German people, and the SED was supported by Soviet tanks. They were able, in addition, to subvert, from the inside, the dissident groups and their British lifelines. But the testimony also shows that *within* east German society there existed brave women and men who were prepared to stand up for human rights and risk terrible torture, prison and exile in order to make their stand. Their readiness to risk everything in their fight against the terror of the Stasi state had succeeded in making the GDR look vulnerable, and constituted one important nail in its coffin.

Even if it is true that the regime was brought down by a coming together of various factors, including the changes in Soviet thinking under Gorbachev and the mass emigration of ordinary east Germans in 1989, the dissidents acted as a real trigger to history. What is more, the mass demonstrations (which pushed communism from power) in every major

GDR city had sprung from a civic culture which the dissidents had chiefly constructed. The line that the dissidents somehow 'failed' is wholly unsustainable. What is more, they offered the people of the GDR a bridge linking the post-communist future to the west German *Rechtsstaat* – a bridge which the vast majority crossed with ease. The dissidents did not inhabit private 'niches' in which their oppositional thinking was tolerated by the Stasi. Rather, having tried to intimidate and steer these groups, the Stasi were obliged to look on as their own power turned to ashes. In the final analysis, they had not been able to steer dissidents: the dissidents had steered the Stasi.

Finally, victim testimony reveals, too, the depraved and corrupt nature of the east German secret police. It illustrates the need for judicial measures against those men and women who worked to maintain the hold of communism on east Germany and how misguided are those who call for an end to research in the Stasi files, or for an amnesty for human rights abuses more generally.[67] The use of terror and other means to suppress human rights, or to force humans who want liberty to flee their country require any *Rechtsstaat* worthy of the name to confront those who readily took part in this core dynamic of the GDR with the full force of German law. In this way, the free political culture of the Federal Republic will thrive – as will the legacy of civil values which the east German dissidents did so much to create.

NOTES

1. Thanks are due to the members of the ESRC, *Social Transformation Workshop,* and Eva Kolinksy in particular for help and encouragement in producing this study.
2. H. Weber, *Die DDR 1945–1986* (Munich: Oldenbourg, 1988), p. 105 (trans. A. Glees).
3. See, for example, C. S. Maier, *Dissolution: The Crisis of Communism and the End of East Germany* (Princeton: Princeton UP, 1997); M. Fulbrook, *Anatomy of a Dictatorship: Inside the GDR* (Oxford: Oxford University Press, 1995); C. Joppke, *East German Dissidents and the Revolution of 1989: Social Movement in a Leninist Regime* (London: Macmillan, 1995).
4. Joppke, *East German Dissidents*, p. 121.
5. Fulbrook, for example, concludes that the east Germans lived a 'symbiotic mode of life, a coming to terms with the parameters of the system and operating within often unwritten rules. Stability is predicated on a form of *Anpassung*, a preparedness to go through the motions' (*Anatomy*, p. 273). Elsewhere she is inclined to reject the view that the DDR was a vicious totalitarian state, or that any comparison between the GDR and the Third Reich could be 'appropriate', M. Fulbrook, *The Two Germanies: Problems of Interpretation* (Atlantic Highlands NJ: Humanities Press International, 1992), pp. 37, 38, 39, 42.
6. This is the official figure released in June 1999 by the *Bundesbeauftragte für die Unterlagen des Staatssicherheitsdienstes der ehemaligen DDR*, Berlin. See too L. Colitt, *Spymaster: The Exciting True Story of Markus Wolf – The Real-Life Carla* (London: Robson Books, 1996), p. 64; and D. Childs and R. Popplewell, *The Stasi: The East German Intelligence and Security Service* (London: Macmillan, 1996), p. 112. It is worth noting that the numbers of the secret police increased dramatically (rather than declined) as the regime aged. What is more, the large numbers of willing IMs enabled the Stasi to put vast numbers of people under surveillance.

7. Joppke, *East German Dissidents*, p. 95. Having stressed the major significance to be attached to the dissidents, he concludes, however, that the dissidents were not, in fact, dissidents, but 'revisionists' who wanted to reform communism and whose impact on the regime counted for less than those who sought to 'exit' the GDR.

8. This point is made in A. Glees, 'Social Transformation Studies and Human Rights Abuses in East Germany after 1945', in C. Flockton and E. Kolinsky (eds), *Recasting East Germany: Social Transformation after the GDR* (London: Cass, 1999).

9. Deep thanks are due to David Rose of BBC TV for his considerable assistance on this project, and to BBC Television for funding this research.

10. It is reasonable to argue that the Federal Republic of Germany, and its first Chancellor Konrad Adenauer, did seek to make restitution to the surviving Jewish victims of the Third Reich and to the State of Israel but preferred to draw a veil of silence over those Germans who had made themselves accomplices of the Nazis. See A. Glees, *Reinventing Germany: German Political Development Since 1945* (Oxford: Berg, 1996), pp. 82–4; N. Frei, *Vergangenheitspolitik: die Anfänge der Bundesrepublik und die NS-Vergangenheit* (Munich: Beck, 1996).

11. F. Werkentin, 'Zur Dimension politischer Inhaftierungen 1949–89', in Die Gedenkstätte für die Opfer politischer Gewalt (eds), *Die Vergangenheit lässt uns nicht los...' Haftbedingungen politischer Gefangener in der SBZ/DDR und deren gesundheitliche Folgen*, Erweiterte Berichte der gleichnamigen Fachtagung am 25.4.1997 in Hamburg für Aerzte, Psychologen, Gutachter, Juristen der Sozialgerichtsbarkeit und Mitarbeiter der Landesversorgunsämter (Magdeburg: Gedenkstätte für die Opfer politischer Gewalt, 1997), pp. 129–43.

12. See the chilling account by K. Behnke and J. Fuchs (eds), *Zersetzung der Seele: Psychologie und Psychiatrie im Dienste der Stasi* (Hamburg: Rotbuch Verlag, 1995). Joppke, *East German Dissidents*, writes 'Quite unique was the Stasi attempt to steer and manipulate the direction and agenda of opposition groups ... this political form of control became internally referred to as "Zersetzung"' (pp. 112–13). Psychological findings were intensively exploited by the Stasi. When it vacated its headquarters in the Normannenstrasse, dissidents discovered a book on Mielke's desk entitled *Forensic Psychology for Interrogators*. Information from Jörg Drieselmann in A. Glees and D. Rose, *Observer*, 4 July 1994.

13. Opinion stated by Manfred Kittlaus, Head of the *Zentrale Ermittlungsstelle für Regierungs- und Vereinigungskriminalität* in Berlin, 17 June 1997.

14. It has been estimated that to date some 22,000 allegations against individual Stasi and SED officials have been made and that some 24 former servants of the regime have been gaoled. Channel 4 News Bulletin, 17 January 1999.

15. Ibid.; also Joppke, *East German Dissidents*, p. 121.

16. Address to a conference entitled 'Burying the Past', St Antony's College, Oxford, 14–16 September 1998, unpublished manuscript.

17. Interviews with M. Kittlaus, Berlin, 12 June 1996, 17 June 1997, 24 September 1998.

18. Joppke, *East German Dissidents*, p. 92, writes: 'Some of the pivotal figures during the regime breakdown in 1989 such as Bärbel Bohley and Ulrike Poppe made their step from tacit disapproval to explicit opposition as members of the Women for Peace [Organisations] in 1982'. Also U. Thaysen, *Der Runde Tisch* (Opladen: Westdeutscher Verlag, 1990).

19. At www.h-net.msu.edu/~german/books/reviews/jarausch1.html. He speaks of the 'most interesting aspect of Stasi power, namely its *mythical* [my emphasis] character ... it would be interesting to analyse whether the Stasi was aware of the population's Angst and how far it consciously managed it in order to increase its control'. His use of the word 'mythical' is, however, unfortunate since it implies Stasi power was not real, something he clearly does not believe was the case.

20. The Stasi were particularly worried about the role played by the BBC and Reuters in publicising the call for civil rights and peace that they made. David Blow, the BBC's Berlin correspondent, was described accurately as a 'courier' for the dissidents. ZMAXX20585 Bd. 6–8, 6 December 1983. Interview with D. Blow, 11 November 1998.

21. Interview with Timothy Everard CMG, 27 August 1998. Everard was HM Ambassador to east Germany from 1984–88. He emphasised British foreign policy was to support dissidents in the Berlin area and concludes that he and his colleagues were 'very proud of our role in the bringing about of the end of the regime'. He maintained close links with Canon Paul Oestreicher, about which the Stasi knew, and of whom he held a very high opinion.

22. *New Yorker*, 16 February 1998, p. 52.

23. Unpublished documentary evidence from Bernd Lippmann, Berlin, August 1996; trans. A. Glees ('Wenn ich weiss, wo ich jemand am meisten treffen kann, wie ich jemanden kaputtmachen kann, und das ist psychisch meistens, dann mache ich es doch, wenn es mein Feind ist').

24. Unpublished documentary evidence supplied by B. Lippmann, August 1996. See also Behnke and Fuchs, *Zersetzung,* pp. 7–12, 27, 28–40, for further examples of *Zersetzung* including the fate of Templin; Joppke,who describes the attempted seduction of Ulrike Poppe by the Stasi in order to alienate her from her husband states: 'quite unique was the Stasi's attempt to steer and manipulate the direction and agenda of opposition groups', *East German Dissidents,* pp. 112–14.

25. This interpretation has been recently challenged in P. Cooke and N. Hubble, 'Die volkseigene Opposition? The Stasi and Alternative Culture in the GDR', in *German Politics,* Vol. 6, No. 2 (1997), pp. 117–38. They write that it is 'unbalanced' to portray the Stasi 'as an organisation of Orwellian Big Brother proportions' (p. 117) and that 'whilst the Stasi was successful in limiting the impact of the alternative culture and preventing it from becoming an organised political opposition, its influence was not total. The niches in which such groups were kept were also central to their existence: the octopus could not stretch its tentacles into every single nook and cranny. Although the fragmentation seemed to cause the end of the alternative culture's credibility after the end of the GDR, it would seem unfair [*sic*] to interpret this as a victory for the Stasi' (p. 130). While the authors regard it as being 'of great importance that the Stasi files are now open' they do not appear to have consulted the archives themselves.

26. Quoted frequently but see Joppke, *East German Dissidents,* p. 111.

27. Interviewed by Michael Buerk on BBC Radio 4, 24 November 1998.

28. This evidence has been presented on BBC Television in September and October 1999. IM Akten, Leipzig AIM.

29. The earlier phase is explored in A. Glees, 'Social Transformation and Human Rights Abuses'.

30. Interview with Frau Margret Bechler in Wedel near Bremen, 17 June 1997. See too her book *Warten auf Antwort: ein deutsches Schicksal* (Frankfurt am Main and Berlin: Ullstein, 1978 1st edn; 1993 18th edn).

31. Interviews with: Hermann Kreutzer, Günther Töpfer, Bernd Lippmann, Jörg Drieselmann, Mike Fröhnel, Heinz Gerull and E. Hellwig-Wilson in Berlin in May 1994, June 1996, June 1997 and autumn 1998. Extracts from these interviews published with D. Rose in the *Observer,* 4 July 1994 and 10 August 1997. See also A. Glees, 'Social Transformation Studies and Human Rights Abuses', pp. 165–89.

32. Childs and Popplewell, *The Stasi,* pp. 39–40, state that from 1948–50 there were 597 documented cases of CDU members being arrested. Probably the majority of them found their way into Soviet, not east German labour camps. The arrests were carried out by a prototype security organisation known as K5. It was 'scarcely more than an auxiliary of Soviet Intelligence ... in Saxony it handled 51,236 cases in 1948 ... It acquired a reputation just as bad as that of Stalin's secret police in the Soviet Union and worse than that of the Gestapo.' They add: 'the SED was following the Soviet example by gaoling political prisoners in its own labour camps. Here the new German regime was assisted by the Nazis who bequeathed to it their concentration camps. It is very difficult to estimate the number of Germans imprisoned at any one time ..., an official US survey .put the number of political prisoners in the eastern Zone at 25,000 for 1947. In 1949 on the eve of the creation of the east German state all but one of the camps were closed ... the inmates passed into the GDR's regular prisons instead.'

33. Interviews with G. Töpfer, Berlin, 12 June 1996 and 16 June 1997.

34. Interview with B. Lippmann, Berlin, 16 June 1998.

35. Interview with M. Fröhnel, Berlin, 13 June 1996.

36. Glees and Rose in the *Observer,* 1994.

37. The switch away from straightforward opposition to the 1982 military service law which permitted the drafting of women and to the introduction of militaristic activities into GDR kindergartens towards an insistence of fundamental human rights proved a seismic one. As Eberhard Kuhrt had noted at the time this shift had a 'system threatening potential'. E. Kuhrt, *Wider die Militisierung der Gesellschaft: Friedensbewegung und Kirche in der DDR* (Melle: Knoth Verlag, 1984), quoted from Joppke, *East German Dissidents,* p. 93.

38. Quoted from Joppke, *East German Dissidents,* p. 95.

39. See, for example, S. Wolle, *Die heile Welt der Diktatur: Alltag und Herrschaft in der DDR 1971–1989* (Berlin: C. H. Linkes, 1998); also Behnke and Fuchs, *Zersetzung.*

40. Interview with Ulrike Poppe, Oxford, 14 September 1998.

41. For an important contemporary account see J. Sandford, *The Sword and the Ploughshare – Autonomous Peace Initiatives in East Germany*, END Special Report (London: Merlin Press, 1983). Sandford wrote 'There are no "leading personalities" in the autonomous peace movement: there is no apparatus – nor for that matter the need or desire – for them to emerge. Some names are well known ... but it is above all a spontaneous movement of anonymous young people' (p. 23). Even in 1998, Poppe said she had never seen herself as a leader although the Stasi – and the historical record – state otherwise.

42. Honecker had himself apparently (and a little unwisely) at one stage said that the dissidents 'had the great advantage that they exist in a state that pursues the same goals'. Quoted from Joppke, *East German Dissidents*, p. 89.

43. 'Die DDR ist ein starker in der Welt geachteter Staat des Friedens und des Sozialismus ... Die DDR kämpft für Frieden, Fortschritt und Sozialismus in der Welt' ('The GDR is a strong state committed to peace and Socialism, respected throughout the world ... it fights for peace, progress and Socialism throughout the world').

44. ZMAXX20585, Vols 6–8, 'END'.

45. ZMAXX20585, Vols 6–8, 'END'.

46. Thompson was 'enigmatic' because he was a deeper thinker than some of his polemical writings could indicate and not the unilateralist he is often believed to have been; also because he was as opposed to communist missiles as to western ones, and, above all, quite unequivocal in his opposition to the communists' suppression of civic rights.

47. E. P. Thompson and D. Smith (eds), *Protest and Survive* (London: Penguin, 1980), pp. 9–62, 223–7.

48. See in particular the Reports of 11 April 1982, 14 November 1983 (prepared for Markus Wolf himself) and 6 December 1983, all in ZMAXX20585, Vols 6–8.

49. ZMAXX20585, Vols 6–8, 27 November 1981, 12 May 1982 (my emphasis).

50. ZMAXX20585, Vols 6–8, 9 June 1984.

51. Sandford, *The Sword*, p. 44, noted – with admirable caution – 'the issue of civil liberties is implicit in much that the autonomous peace movement has said and done: only occasionally has it become an explicit and specific theme in its own right. Civil liberties ... are inherent preconditions of any peace movement activity ... At the same time, curtailment of civil liberties is scarcely conducive to an atmosphere in which peace may flourish if it leads to resentment, disaffection, and tension within the population.'

52. The 1968 GDR constitution was not as liberal as that of 1949 but it guaranteed freedoms of speech, assembly and association (arts 27, 28, 29); freedom of conscience and belief was upheld in art 20 while the secrecy of post and telephone was guaranteed under art 31. Childs and Popplewell, *The Stasi*, p. 96.

53. Interview with U. Poppe, Oxford, 14 September 1998.

54. Interview with J. Sandford, Reading, 19 November 1998.

55. See the copious files, consisting of many thousands of pages, especially ZMAXX20585, Vols 1–8, ZMA XX 20585, Vols 6–8, but also HAXXZMA, MfSHAXX AKG 188 039321/947, all open to public scrutiny in the archive of the *Bundesbeauftragte für die Unterlagen* ... in Berlin.

56. MfS HAI Nr 1644, 10 November 1988.

57. Information from Bernd Zufelde, Luxemburg, 25 August 1998. Zufelde was a key member of the *Britain–GDR Friendship Society* from 1984–90, and its chief executive from 1987–90. He worked closely with his mentor Horst Brasch, a member of the Politbureau. He was succeeded by Dr Dieter Müller who confirmed much of Zufelde's information about those seen as the GDR's friends – and enemies – in the UK. Interview in Potsdam, 17 June 1998.

58. Information from David Rose, BBC TV.

59. MfS HAI Nr 1644, 10 November 1988 (trans. A. Glees); the Berlin Stasi report stated:

> 'In the operational area of the UK there exists a complex overall situation for agents. The Enemy has expanded the system of counter espionage. Especially the changes to the law, and the Security Service bill and Official Secrets Act demand from [us] that we act with great alertness, secrecy and conspiracy. Contact to colleagues in the state apparatus will become more complicated, their active involvement in defensive activities will be strengthened. This is especially true for those in the [UK] Foreign and Commonwealth Office and the Ministry of Defence.
>
> The strengthening of controls in public life (football identity cards, traffic checks, border controls) will result in more burdens. Those recognised as being representatives of the Socialist States will be targeted and more strongly controlled at border crossings. It is even more important

than ever to abide by traffic regulations since the British authorities will use offences as signals for expulsion. Driving after taking alcohol is to be decisively rejected. Every traffic rule must be obeyed. Operations in football stadiums must be avoided.

Due to the intensification of security in residential areas by so-called citizens' initiatives, police and security officials' cooperation with them will increase and the observation of those from the Socialist states will be heightened. For operative categories, no residential areas in the vicinity of military sites or especially monitored areas should be selected. Best places are suburbs with numerous tower blocks.

The question of identity cards is to be closely followed. If introduced, originals are to be obtained.

Recognised Enemy actions against the GDR collective in the UK have always concealed as criminal acts (break-ins). But as before it can be seen that the GDR representatives are not in the centre of the Enemy's attacks against Socialist states (the Soviet Union, CSSR, SRV and Cuba bear this burden).

The British secret services are the international leaders in the use of technical operations so that it must certainly be reckoned that conspiratorial operations, conducted by well-schooled operatives, may be either unrecognisable or barely recognisable.'

60. ZMAXX 20585, Vols 7–8, 25 November 1983, 5 January 1984. Thanks are due to Barbara Einhorn for confirming the details in the Stasi report upon her at an interview in Brighton on 4 December 1998.
61. Cited as A:

The Deputy of the Minister   Berlin, 14 November 1983
                                                              Diary No. 1664/83

PERSONAL!
TOP SECRET!
To Director Main Department XX
Comrade Major General (Generalmajor) Kienberg

As a result of further intelligence upon the cooperation of hostile forces within the Operational Area with oppositional groups inside the GDR, I am now sending you attached the following information: Contacts of 'European Nuclear Disarmament (END)' in Great Britain with Active Representatives of the 'Independent Peace Movement' in the GDR.
                                            Signed Wolf
                                            Colonel (Generaloberst)
Main Directorate A (Hauptverwaltung A)   Berlin, 1983
Department IX (Abteilung X)
(Translated by A. Glees)

Cited as B:

TOP SECRET!
SOURCE PROTECTION!
Contacts of 'European Nuclear Disarmament (END)' in Great Britain with Active Representatives of the 'Independent Peace Movement' in the GDR.

Unofficially, it has been reliably learned from the Operational Area that: Within the Organisation of END a special Women's Group is active which chiefly investigates problems concerning the role of women, their place in the State and the family, as well as the attitude of women to military conscription.

The members of this Women's Group have close ties to Westberlin and, via contacts in Westberlin, or directly, regular contacts to active representatives of the 'Independent Peace Groups' in the GDR. Via these contacts a regular exchange of information takes place, particularly about hostile-negative forces in the GDR and their activities. Part of this information serves the purpose of publicising hostile activities of these people in the Western media.

Particularly active members of the END Women's Group are the following:

BARBARA EINHORN 71 Hanover Street, Brighton, Member of the END Coordinating Committee and JANE DIBBLIN 227 Seven Sisters Road, London N4, Official of the Main Office of END.

Their contact partners in Westberlin are: [two names blacked out]. Active and regular contacts of these forces exist to the citizens of the GDR: Barbel Bohley, d.o.b 24.5.45, resident in Berlin and Ulrike Poppe, d.o.b 25.3.41, resident in Berlin, Einhorn plans to visit Bohley in the capital of the GDR, Berlin, on 3 December 1983.

ZMAXX20585 Bd 6–8, 14 November 1983. (Translated by A. Glees.)

62. The German term was 'landesverräterische Nachrichtenübermittlung'. Joppke, who did not have access to the Stasi files does not mention the Einhorn incident, assuming the charge of treason was triggered by the dissidents' desire to make contact with the west. In fact, it was the other way round – and much more serious as a result. Joppke, *East German Dissidents*, p. 92.

63. Interview with T. Everard, 27 August 1998.

64. This demonstration has often been described. See, for example, Joppke, *East German Dissidents*, p. 130.

65. HVAXXZMA 40354, 24 June 1988.

66. Information from Bernd Zufelde, Luxemburg, 25 August 1998: 'The Stasi told us: When Oestreicher is there beware! A wolf is in the room.'

67. See A. Glees, 'Social Transformation Studies and Human Rights Abuses'. For the arguments against legal investigations of the Stasi's activities and against research into the Stasi files see. A. McIlvoy, *The Saddled Cow: East Germany's Life and Legacy* (London: Faber & Faber, 1992), p. 107: 'To dissect the workings of the state security system, name the informers and look in horror at its methods and aims will not help Germany to come to terms with this chapter of its past ... overexposure and overpromotion of this topic will result in people drowning in a sea of ghastly detail rather than gaining any useful perspective on the Stasi and its legacy'; G. Shaw, 'Zeit für den Schlußstrich', in *German Life and Letters*, Vol. 50, No. 1 (1997), pp. 103–26, argues in favour of an amnesty.

Part III

Social Experiences and Attitude Change

10

Mother–Child Interactions at the Passage from Childhood to Youth: A Comparison of East and West German Families

Beate Schuster

CHANGES IN FAMILY LIFE

During the last three decades families in Germany have changed.[1] The external and internal structures of family life have become more liberal. Many children grow up with only one parent or with a new partner of their parent. Often further children enter the family as stepsisters or stepbrothers. But more characteristic of this liberalisation in the internal structures of families is the emphasis on equality, not only between parents but also between parents and children. Parents no longer simply permit or forbid things but in many domains are willing to negotiate rules with their children. Additionally, many parents conceive their role as being that of authority persons and their task as being to bring up their children very consciously. They organise their own life in a way that enables them to support their children's development optimally. Often this parental attitude is combined with high expectations of their children whose development thereby plays an important role in many parents' lives.

This social trend of liberalisation of the parent–child relationship has been described before 1989 for the Old Federal Republic and still today, ten years after the reunification, it seems to be stronger in the Old than in the New *Bundesländer*.[2] Studies of recent years have continually shown that parents in the New *Bundesländer* tend to control more and attach more importance to duties and obedience. Parents in the Old *Bundesländer* in contrast are more open and put more emphasis on their children's self-confidence and self-reliance.[3] Of course, parents from both the Old and the New *Bundesländer* claim that they intend to raise their children to be independent persons. However, their educational attitudes seem to be different, because they do not have the same idea of independence. Thus in the Old *Bundesländer* independence means that a child can decide things on the basis of his own judgement whereas parents from the New *Bundesländer* find that a child is independent when he manages his duties in the household reliably.

Krüger and colleagues in findings from a broad investigation of east and west German families conclude that changes of intergenerational relationships which have already been diagnosed for west German and western Europe families can also be tendentially recognised in their data; they nevertheless stress the fact that the educational practice of 'keeping children on a tight rein' characterises the second central pattern of interaction of east German families.[4] So all in all it seems still unclear whether ten years after the reunification a liberalisation of the parent–child relationship comparable to that in the Old *Bundesländer* is beginning to emerge in the New *Bundesländer* and if so how it is manifested in the reciprocal behaviours of parents and children.

Besides the general social trends of liberalisation it is important to consider that the relationship between parents and children begins to change at the end of middle childhood. The more children of about 10 to 12 years experience respect as equal partners and the more they learn to hold their own opinions in their interactions with peers, the more they strive for equality and respect in the relationship with their parents.[5] This change becomes apparent in the increase of conflicts between parents and children at the passage from childhood to youth.[6] In older, psychoanalytically oriented theories about youth this conflictual aspect of change was regarded as necessary for successful separation from the parents.[7] Newer research has increasingly taken into account the continuity of emotional connectedness between parents and children. This view suggests that families with pre-adolescent children are challenged to re-define their relationships. According to the psychological concept of 'individuation', parents and children have to negotiate a new balance between the possibility of offspring becoming more independent and developing their individuality, on the one hand, but simultaneously maintaining emotional attachment, on the other hand.[8] Different studies referring to the concept of individuation indicate that the more balanced the two domains of 'individuality' and 'connectedness' are in the relationship between parents and children, the more mature the adolescents are in their identity development.[9] Therefore to reach a newly balanced or 'individuated' relationship with parents is an important step in youth's development. It seems obvious that the process of individuation succeeds more easily in families in which parents try to orient their behaviour towards the modern model of being a negotiating and partnerlike parent. Because, as the above-mentioned differences show, parents in the New *Bundesländer* are not so strongly influenced by this model, we assume that differences between the Old and the New *Bundesländer* may exist with regard to individuation in parent–child relationships.

In a new study which refers to the concept of individuation, families with young people of nearly 15 years of age from Mannheim (Old *Bundesländer*) and from Leipzig (New *Bundesländer*) were compared. The comparison revealed only small differences in the two domains of the individuation concept, 'individuality' and 'connectedness', which, in addition, were different for girls and for boys. The male youths from Leipzig reported less connectedness with their parents than the male youths from Mannheim, who instead described less individuality. Among the girls the reported connectedness with parents was similarly high in both towns. In reference to individuality the girls from Mannheim had higher scores than the girls from Leipzig.[10] The three developmental patterns of the relation between individuality and connectedness, 'individuated', 'detached' and 'in process', which the researchers identified for the period from 15 to 18 years of age, stood in no relation to the youths' origin.[11] However, the authors discovered that the process of individuation in the families was influenced by experiences of social change such as 'dwindling purchasing power', 'job insecurity' and 'feelings of social insecurity'. The domain of individuality was independent from these three indicators of change. But the connectedness was higher in families with job insecurity and it increased over the three years (from 15 to 18 years of age) concomitantly with the feelings of social insecurity in the families. Both aspects, job insecurity and feelings of social insecurity, are more common in the New *Bundesländer*. The authors discuss their findings in connection with the newly described '*Nesthockerphänomen*'.[12] If the connectedness between youths and parents is over-developed, it encourages the youths to stay for too long in their parents' home. This jeopardising of the individuation process is probably higher for families in the New *Bundesländer* because of the social conditions there. By contrast, the transitional period between childhood and youth is rather characterised by an increase in the other domain. Observations of families with children of this age show that the conflict rate increases in this phase, because children begin to strive for more individuality in the relationship. Whether families in the New *Bundesländer* differ from families in the Old *Bundesländer* in this early phase of the individuation process has not been investigated up to now.

Our aim in this chapter is to investigate the intergenerational relationships in the family context during the status passage from childhood into youth. We refer not only to theoretical considerations of modernisation and social change as Krüger and colleagues do.[13] Like the research group of Noack, we also take into account the developmental perspective as it exists in the individuation concept. The following questions will be investigated in pursuit of the research aim:

1. How do children from the Old *Bundesländer* in comparison to children from the New *Bundesländer* strive for individuality in the relationship with their mothers?
2. How do mothers from the Old and the New *Bundesländer* shape their role as authority figures for and as educators of their children at the end of childhood?
3. Which patterns of reciprocal behaviour of mothers and children can be identified and are some of these patterns more frequent in the Old than in the New *Bundesländer*?

External structural aspects of the family, like size and household composition, have lost their significance as indicators for specific life-styles – in our case negotiating and partnership-like relationship between parents and children in the families.[14] At the centre of our analyses are therefore the observed interactional patterns of mothers and their approximately 8- to 12-year-old children from the Old and the New *Bundesländer*.

THE EMPIRICAL STUDY OF INTERACTIONS OF MOTHERS AND CHILDREN FROM FORMER WEST BERLIN AND FROM POTSDAM

The observations were conducted in the context of two single investigations.[15] The first investigation in which 50 mother–child pairs participated was performed in 1991/92 in former west Berlin. The children in this sample (22 boys and 28 girls) were between 8 and 12 years of age (mean: 10;9; standard deviation: 15.4). The second investigation took place in 1997 with 151 mothers and children from Potsdam, the capital city of Brandenburg, one of the New *Bundesländer*. The 71 boys and 80 girls were between 9 and 11 years old (mean: 10;9; standard deviation: 4.36). In both samples about one-third of the mothers finished school with the *'Abitur'* (matriculation examination). In the Brandenburg study only working mothers were asked to participate, whereas in west Berlin about 20 per cent of the mothers of the sample were not working.

The mothers and children of both samples were observed in a video laboratory. In both studies the setting was nearly the same. The mothers and children were seated at a table on which a game board was placed. This game required that they plan a one-week vacational trip together.[15] The game board therefore depicted eight activities which could be undertaken at the imaginary vacational place. The mothers and children were encouraged to choose different activities and try to convince each other of the merits of 'their' activities. The activities for the children were rather fun and consumer-oriented (an action movie, a video game hall, a fast-food restaurant and an attractive swimming pool to be visited). The activities for the mothers were cultural sites or things typically more liked by adults than by children (visiting an old cathedral, a museum of antique art, a sightseeing tour by bus and hiking in the woods). The faster and more effectively each of the players succeeded in persuading the other one to participate in his or her activities, the more points s/he could earn in the game. Moreover the payment of the activities had to be negotiated, because for each activity the players had to pay an entrance fee. The mothers were given more than enough money in the game whereas the children got only a small amount of pocket money. As a compensation for this disadvantage, the children were allowed to visit their attractions alone and to earn points for this if they could pay the entrance fee, whereas the mothers could only earn points if they succeeded in persuading their children to join them. So both partners were dependent on each other and had to negotiate their different interests.

It was not only because of the points to be won that the game occasioned negotiations. In order to understand the interaction, it is important to bear in mind that the mothers and children had different motives and aims in the observational situation. Most of the mothers of course aimed to present themselves as responsible and competent mothers. The children pursued the aim of presenting themselves as competent players who had understood the task involved in the game. The negotiations were therefore indeed stimulated by the game, but the game was not the actual subject of negotiation. The real subject of the negotiations was the differing types of self-definition and self-presentation which the mothers and children introduced into the interaction. Because the game sessions forced the mothers and offspring to reflect their 'selves' to each other, the game was well suited to observing the individuation process: that is to say, the balancing of desires for 'individuality' and 'connectedness' in the interaction.

Analyses of the Interactions

The analysis of the interactions between the mothers and children during the game sessions consisted of two aspects. On the one hand we looked at the formal aspects of how equally and symmetrically the interactions proceeded. The two categories in this area were: the proportion of words spoken by the child in relation to that of the mother, and the frequency of initiatives for a new decision in favour of one of the eight possible game activities by the child and by the mother. The second area referred to the attitudes the mothers and children adopted towards each other in the situation. For this area we developed from the video material five categories describing different attitudes of the children and five describing the attitudes of the mothers. In the next section these categories will be presented and explained.

Categories of Child Attitudes

'Competence'
This category was applied to utterances of the children which made clear that they were especially conscious of the demand to demonstrate their competence, such as when they tried to demonstrate that they understood the rules of the game perfectly and that they knew very well how to use them, for example, by teaching and correcting their mothers, by pointing to their own points gain or by using clever tactical arguments against the mothers' suggestions. By such behaviour, the children profiled themselves as relatively independent and self-reliant interaction partners.

'Challenge'
When it became apparent that the children construed the situation as an occasion to separate themselves from their mothers and to make clear their own point of view, the category 'challenge' was used. Examples for this category are: asking critical questions, being ironical towards the mother, not being prepared simply to believe her or to accept her proposals. This behaviour showed that the children felt secure and dared to try out a new, more equal position towards their mothers.

'Making concessions'
This category was used when the children's interactional behaviour indicated that they understood the situation and the relationship with their mothers as one which could only be satisfying for both of them if they were ready to respect each other's perspective, for example, by expressing insight into the mother's view or by suggesting compromises. The attitude shaped by this behaviour demonstrated that the children viewed mutuality as a fundamental principle of relationships.

'Internal conflict'
The category 'internal conflict' was applied when it became clear that the children recognised the demand of the game to hold their own view but simultaneously perceived this demand as a threat to the relationship with their mothers. Hints as to this category were when children did not dare to make efforts in order to earn points for themselves.

'Fun' (residual category)

A necessary residual category was called 'fun'. This category was applied for episodes of the interaction in which no hint as to a clear attitude of the children could be found. During these episodes the chidren simply seemed to enjoy dealing with the objects of the game (these were a game figure, their pocket money and stickers which indicated the points to be won).

Categories of Mother Attitudes

'Values'

Into this category all utterances of mothers were put which indicated that they adopted the attitude of an authority person and an educator. These mothers showed clearly that they understood the activities on the game board as important vehicles for education on which they had to state their opinions unambiguously. The values to which the mothers referred were: 'self-control', 'rationality', 'cultural interest', 'thriftiness', and 'good manners'.

'Fairness'

This category was applied when the mothers' utterances made clear that they were ready to construe the situation in the same way as their children did. So they conceived themselves as partners in a game in which 'fairness' as a virtue played an important role. But their attitude was not simply that of a game partner; the mothers seemed to want to develop a mutual and cooperative procedure with their children. Indicators for this category were, for example, 'suggesting procedures' (not activities), 'initiating compromises', 'talking about the meaning and the application of rules' and 'appeals to fairness'.

'Exercise'

In this category the mothers understood the situation as a kind of task. They seemed to have the idea that they had to support their children as well as possible so that the child could solve the task alone. Through this behaviour they struck the attitude of an expert and a teacher who has more knowledge than the child. The mothers did not want to take advantage of this knowledge but tried to use it for educational reasons. The utterances in this category referred not to the procedure but to the concrete requests of the game, like reading, counting, computing, remembering, and so on.

'Boycott'

This category was called 'boycott' because it included utterances of mothers which demonstrated that they disapproved of the whole situation and were not prepared to get involved in the game. They declared the game – mostly in an ironical form – as non-authentic and stated that it created differences between them and their children which did not occur in real life. Towards the children these utterances were often very authoritarian, because the mothers simply decided· which interests the children had or did not have in the situation.

'Clever play'

The utterances within the category 'clever play' had in common that they aimed at avoiding a conflict and showed a slightly lazy attitude on the part of the mothers. They used the possibilities which the game offered to circumvent the negotiations about the critical activities of the game like the action movie and the video game hall. Mostly they simply urged their children to pay for the activities from their pocket money. Thus, they did not have to state their opinion on these activities and were able to avoid possible conflicts. Although the mothers did seem to perceive an educational demand in the situation they felt free to choose the line of least resistance in dealing with it.

DEVELOPMENTAL CHANGES IN THE RELATIONSHIP BETWEEN
MOTHERS AND CHILDREN IN THE OLD AND THE NEW
BUNDESLÄNDER: EMPIRICAL RESULTS

Striving for Individuality in the Relationship with Mother – Differences Between Children from the Old and the New Bundesländer

In order to answer the first question – how do children from Old and New *Bundesländer* begin to strive for more individuality in the relationship with their mothers – the formal aspects of the interaction and the five attitudinal categories of the children were compared.

In relation to the formal aspects which describe how equally and symmetrically the children were involved in the interaction, the statistical comparisons showed that the children from the Old *Bundesländer* spoke rather more to their mothers than the children from the New *Bundesländer*. The relationships in both samples (Old and New *Bundesländer*) were asymmetrically organised: all children spoke and structured the interaction to a lesser degree than their mothers.[16]

The same was true for the different attitudes through which the children strove to demonstrate their individuality. No systematic differences were found between the mean frequencies of the five categories in the sample of the Old *Bundesländer* compared to that of the New

Bundesländer. The attitude most frequently adopted was to prove their 'competence'. Thus nearly all children tried to demonstrate their individuality by showing that they felt self-reliant and independent enough to stand up for their interests and to negotiate them with their mothers.[17] The effort to be not only a competent player but also to try to change the relationship to the mother directly by adopting a 'challenging' attitude occurred in children from both the Old and the New *Bundesländer* to a much smaller extent than 'competence'.[18] Also striving for individuality by demonstrating one's own readiness to 'make concessions' in order to get the mother to respect the child's interests as well was rarely used in both samples.[19] The different forms in which the children strove for individuality were distributed in the same way among the children from the Old and the New *Bundesländer*. Also, the frequency of conflictual attitudes (category 'internal conflict')[20] and the proportion of utterances in the remainder category 'fun',[21] which indicated that at that moment the children were not necessarily concerned with their self-presentation, showed no differences in mean between children from the Old and the New *Bundesländer*.

Shaping One's Role as Authority and Educational Person: Differences Between Mothers from the Old and the New Bundesländer

How the mothers from the Old and the New *Bundesländer* shaped their role as authority and educational figures was investigated by comparing the mean frequencies of the five categories of mother attitudes between the two samples.

Apart from the category 'boycott', which occurred in both samples, only in a few exceptional cases (both *Länder:* 1 per cent) were there clear differences in the mean frequencies of the other four categories.[22] Although all the five types of attitudes (five mother categories) could be observed in both samples, differences in frequency distributions indicated that the mothers from the Old *Bundesländer* preferred different attitudes to mothers in the New *Bundesländer*. The latter stated their definite opinions on the game activities and referred to clear 'values' much more frequently than the mothers from Old *Bundesländer* (category 'values', Old *Bundesländer*: 18 per cent; New *Bundesländer*: 41 per cent). In contrast, mothers from the Old *Bundesländer* were more strongly involved in playing the game together with their children (category 'fairness', Old *Bundesländer*: 34 per cent; New *Bundesländer*: 27 per cent) and they more often struck the attitude of an expert and a teacher supporting the child while s/he is trying to meet the requirements of the game (category 'exercise', Old *Bundesländer*: 39 per cent; New *Bundesländer*: 25 per cent).

An evading, conflict-avoiding and therefore slightly lazy attitude was seldom observed. In the sample of the New *Bundesländer* this attitude however was a little more frequent than in the other sample (category 'clever play', Old *Bundesländer*: 6 per cent; New *Bundesländer*: 9 per cent). Thus these differences revealed two tendencies: the mothers from the New *Bundesländer* very confidently dealt with their role as authority persons. They simply stated their educational point of view but when there was an occasion to evade the requirements connected with this role they felt free to choose this alternative. In contrast, the mothers of the Old *Bundesländer* dealt with their role as authority person more openly but also more insecurely. They could not simply state their opinions (and expect obedience) but were dependent on the child's compliance. Thus they had to try to obtain a mutually acceptable solution by working together with the child.

Patterns of Reciprocal Behaviour in the Mother–Child Pairs: Differences in Frequency Between the Old and the New Bundesländer

The mothers' behaviour in the interaction is contingent on the behaviour of their child and vice versa. In order to take into account this mutual dependency or 'reciprocity' we finally tried to identify patterns of reciprocal mother–child behaviour on the basis of our categorisations. We put the frequencies of all ten (mother + child) categories into a statistical grouping procedure. By means of this procedure four groups of mothers and children could be identified. The pairs within each of these groups had very similar patterns of behaviour concerning the frequencies of the single categories, whereas the differences between the groups were as large as possible. In order to answer the question as to which patterns are more frequent in the Old *Bundesländer* and which in the New, the distribution of the four patterns over the two samples was statistically examined. For all four patterns of behaviour statistically significant differences in the percentage of mother–child pairs from the Old and the New *Bundesländer* were found.

Descriptions of the Patterns of Behaviour of the Four Groups and Distribution of the Mother–Child Pairs from the Old and the New Bundesländer *in the Four Groups*

Group 1
The first group consisting of 22 pairs was mainly characterised by the highly apprehensive and insecure behaviour of the children of these pairs.

The mean frequency of the child-category 'internal conflict' was about five to ten times higher than in the three other groups. However, the mothers' behaviour in these groups did not reveal any remarkable respects in which they differed from the other mothers. This altogether rather exceptional pattern was seen equally seldom in the Old and the New *Bundesländer* (Old *Bundesländer*: 12 per cent; New *Bundesländer*: 11 per cent).

Group 2
Sixty-five pairs belonged to the second group. More than in any other group the mothers here had a clear idea of their educational goals and felt self-confident about them. The group showed the highest mean percentage of the mother-category 'value'. The children of this group as well as the children from the other groups (except those from Group 1) primarily tried to prove their 'competence', but they differed from all others because they challenged their mothers more often by criticising their attitudes. The percentage of pairs from the New *Bundesländer* (40 per cent) in this group was four times as high as the percentage of pairs in the Old *Bundesländer* (10 per cent).

Group 3
The 49 pairs in this group differed from the other groups in that the mothers' attitude was extremely fair and cooperatively-oriented. The children – besides demonstrating their own competence – were sensible and respectful. Relatively more pairs from the Old *Bundesländer* (36 per cent) belonged to this group than from the New *Bundesländer* (21 per cent).

Group 4
The fourth group consisted of 65 pairs. More than all others, these mothers behaved like experts and teachers. They interpreted the game as an exercise and tried to support their children as much as possible to complete it. The children though (here slightly more than in Groups 2 and 3) were characterised by the endeavour to demonstrate their competence as clever and strong-willed interaction partners towards their mothers. In contrast to the children in Groups 2 and 3 these children showed no further tendencies to express their individuality in the relationship with their mothers. This pattern was more frequent in the groups from the Old *Bundesländer* (42 per cent) than in the the New *Bundesländer* (29 per cent).

FINDINGS INTERPRETED AND ASSESSED

Considering the differences between the Old and the New *Bundesländer* on all three levels of comparison – children, mothers and pairs – the following tendencies become apparent:

(1) Children of the New *Bundesländer* do not use fundamentally different strategies to express their individuality in the relationship with their mothers than children from the Old *Bundesländer*. We found the same forms of child attitudes which we observed in the Old *Bundesländer* among the children from the New *Bundesländer*. Most frequently the children expressed their indidviduality by demonstrating their competence. This attitude showed that they already felt relatively self-reliant and independent from their mothers. Especially in middle childhood when children acquire most of the basic cultural skills, an important facet of a child's self consists of the self-concept of competence. This common developmental background may be the reason why we found this predominant attitude among children from the Old and the New *Bundesländer*. Thus the children from each part of Germany revealed no differences in their early endeavours towards individuality in the relationship.

(2) However, on the level of the mothers there were some differences. The mothers from both the Old and the New *Bundesländer* perceived educational demands in the situation and adopted the attitude of authority and educational figures. But they differed according to their orientations. While the mothers from the Old *Bundesländer* mainly focused on playing the game and cooperating with their children, the mothers from the New *Bundesländer* were much more oriented towards explaining their concepts of educational values in the interaction with their children.

The differences observed among the mothers also became evident in the patterns of the mother–child pairs. The four groups, which were characterised by specific behavioural patterns, also differed in respect of the mothers' educational orientations. The orientation towards values as predominantly observed in Group 2 was more frequent in the New *Bundesländer* whereas the orientation towards cooperation (Group 3) and solving tasks together (Group 4) was more often found among the pairs from the Old *Bundesländer*. In addition this third level revealed how the children (besides demonstrating their competence) reacted to different mother attitudes and how they tried to individualise. The children whose mothers were oriented towards values tended to individualise by being critical and challenging their mothers' position, whereas the children whose mothers were oriented towards cooperation tended to be sensible, respectful and willing to compromise. When looking at the children's behaviour we can conclude that there are no fundamental differences between the Old and the New *Bundesländer*. However, different tendencies become manifest in the different behaviour of the mothers from the two sets of *Länder*. According to our observations, in the New *Bundesländer* there is a stronger tendency to support a child's challenging attitude. In contrast, in the Old *Bundesländer* there was a stronger tendency to support an understanding and cooperative child.

Altogether our observations are in accordance with findings of other investigations in which parents and children were interviewed.[23] At the level of interactions it also becomes obvious that mothers from the Old *Bundesländer* are more strongly influenced by the new model of being like a partner who is – in certain domains – willing to negotiate rules with her children. Another indicator of this educational model was that the children from the Old *Bundesländer* spoke more and therefore their participation appeared more lively in the interaction than the children from the New *Bundesländer*. Similarly, our observations confirmed the difficulties which are connected with the willingness to negotiate. Mothers are on shaky ground when they try to meet this requirement, because despite the readiness to be like a partner it is sometimes necessary simply to ask the children to follow certain rules or agreements in order to offer them clear guidelines.[24] From other analyses of the mother–child interactions in the Old *Bundesländer*, we know that many mothers felt this dilemma. Some of them were open to negotiations and then had the experience of their children disregarding basic social rules in the interaction. Other mothers wanted to meet the requirements of the new model but were not really able to renounce their own idea about how their children should be.[25] The more socially competent the children were, the more they understood the insecurities and contradictions in their mothers' attitude and learned to use this knowledge in order to manipulate their mothers. Thus the negotiations were sometimes very tricky for the mothers.

Our observations also confirmed that the rather traditional educational attitude of 'keeping children on a tight rein' was more frequent in the New than in the Old *Bundesländer*.[26] The mothers from the New *Bundesländer* stated their position more naturally and clearly, and were more easily able to refuse things without getting involved in long discussions with their children. At first glance, from a new-*Länder* perspective this attitude seems to be very rigid and seems to suggest that the children of these mothers feel extremely controlled and therefore restrained or even impeded in their emerging desire for individuality. It was therefore quite astonishing to recognise that these children were on the one hand more reserved than their peers from the Old *Bundesländer*, but on the other that they nevertheless acted firmly and effectively towards their mothers. Thus we cannot conclude that the beginning of the individuation process is more complicated in the New *Bundesländer* although more mothers struck a rather traditional educational attitude towards their children.[27] Mothers from the Old and the New *Bundesländer* experienced different social conditions and therefore different forms of socialisation in their own childhood and youth, which prepared them for living in their particular social systems. We interpret our finding as an indicator for the assumption that this pre-conditioning still today influences their educational attitudes towards their children today. Thus, mothers from the Old *Bundesländer* more strongly tend to prepare their children for being able to find their own way in a social system which offers no clear options and or guarantees for adult life. Through the open and negotiative attitude of these mothers, the children get used to dealing with many different requirements because they learn to cooperate with other people and to try out different procedures. The secure and firm attitude of the mothers from the New *Bundesländer* seems rather to prepare the children – in keeping with the mothers' own experiences – to have a clear orientation and to take over responsibility for a certain domain in which the child is confronted with relatively clearly defined demands. Thus, although the social system of the former GDR was being brought into line with that of the former FRG ten years ago, we have to expect that differences in how children and youth deal with developmental or social requirements will still continue, because these ways have already been laid out one generation before.

NOTES

1. R. Nave-Herz, *Familie heute. Wandel der Familienstrukturen und Folgen für die Erziehung* (Darmstadt: Wissenschaftliche Buchgesellschaft, 1994).
2. H. Oswald, 'Sozialisation, Entwicklung und Erziehung im Kindesalter', *Zeitschrift für Pädagogik*, 36 (1997), pp. 51–75. Also Y. Schütze, *Die gute Mutter. Zur Geschichte des normativen Musters 'Mutterliebe'* (Bielefeld: Kleine Verlag, 1991).
3. M. du Bois-Reymond and K. Torrance, 'Die moderne Familie als Verhandlungshaushalt. Eltern-Kind-Beziehungen in West- und Ostdeutschland und in den Niederlanden', in M. du Bois-Reymond, P. Büchner, H.-H. Krüger, J. Ecarius and B. Fuhs (eds), *Kinderleben* (Opladen: Leske und Budrich), pp. 137–219. Also H.-H. Krüger, 'Kindheit im Umbruch. Zur aktuellen Lebenssituation von Kindern in den neuen Bundesländern', in H.-H. Krüger, M. Kühnel, S. Thomas (eds), *Transformationsprobleme in Ostdeutschland. Arbeit. Bildung. Sozialpolitik* (Opladen: Leske und Budrich, 1995), pp. 77–87; K. Pollmer and K. Hurrelmann, 'Familientraditionen und Erziehungsstile in Ost- und Westdeutschland', *Kind, Jugend und Gesellschaft*, 37 (1992), pp. 2–7; H. Reuband, 'Aushandeln statt Gehorsam? Erziehungsziele und Erziehungspraktiken in den alten und neuen Bundesländern im Wandel', in L. Bönisch, K. Lenz (eds), *Familien* (Weinheim: Juventa, 1997), pp. 129–53; H. Uhlendorff, L. Krappmann, and H. Oswald, 'Familie in Ost- und West-Berlin – Erziehungseinstellungen und Kinderfreundschaften', *Zeitschrift für Pädagogik*, 43

(1997), pp. 35–53; J. Zinnecker, 'Streßkinder und Glückskinder. Eltern als soziale Umwelt von Kindern', *Zeitschrift für Pädagogik*, 43, 1 (1997), pp. 7–34.

4. Krüger, 'Kindheit im Umbruch – zur aktuellen Lebenssituation von Kindern in den neuen Bundesländern', p. 83.

5. B. Schuster, H. Oswald, L. Krappmann, *Children's Social Integration and Negotiation Patterns in Mother–Child and Child–Peer Dyads*, paper presented at the 5th European Conference on Developmental Psychology, Sevilla, 1992). Also J. Youniss, 'Piaget und das in Beziehungen entstehende Selbst', in L. Krappmann and H. Oswald (eds), *Soziale Konstruktion und psychische Entwicklung* (Frankfurt am Main: Suhrkamp, 1994), p. 165.

6. B. Laursen, K. C. Coy, and W. A. Collins, 'Reconsidering Changes in Parent–Child–Conflict Across Adolescence: A Meta-Analysis', *Child Development*, 69, 3 (1998), pp. 817–32.

7. P. Blos, *The Adolescent Passage: Developmental Issues* (2nd edn, 1979) (New York: International University Press); also E. H. Erikson, *Identity: Youth and Crisis* (New York: Norton, 1968).

8. H. D. Grotevant and C. R. Cooper, 'Individuation in Family Relationships: A Perspective on Individual Differences in the Development of Identity and Role-taking Skill in Adolescence', *Human Development*, 29 (1986), pp. 82–100.

9. J. P. Allen, S. T. Hauser, K. L. Bell and T. G. O'Connor, 'Longitudinal Assessment of Autonomy and Relatedness in Adolescent-Family Interactions as Predictors of Adolescent Ego-Development and Self-Esteem', *Child Development*, 65 (1994), pp. 179–94; also H. D. Grotevant and C. R. Cooper, 'Patterns of Interaction in Family Relationships and the Development of Identity Exploration in Adolescence', *Child Development*, 56 (1985), pp. 415–28.

10. P. Noack, M. Oepke and K. Sassenberg, 'Individuation in ost- und westdeutschen Familien und Erfahrung sozialen Wandels', in H. Oswald (ed.), *Sozialisation und Entwicklung in den neuen Bundesländern – Ergebnisse empirischer Längsschnittforschung, Zeitschrift für Soziologie der Erziehung und Sozialisation*, Vol. 2 (1998), pp. 208–12.

11. B. Puschner, P. Noack, M. Hofer, B. Kracke, E. Wild and M. Buhl, 'Developmental Trajectories of Individuation and Psychosocial Adjustment of Adolescents in East and West Germany – A Longitudinal Study', paper presented at the 56th *Tagung der Arbeitsgsgemeinschaft für Empirische Pädagogische Forschung*, Mannheim, 1998.

12. C. Papastefanou, *Auszug aus dem Elternhaus. Aufbruch und Ablösung im Erleben von Eltern und Kindern* (Weinheim, München: Juventa, 1997). Also L. A. Vaskovics, 'Lebensläufe junger Erwachsener und elterliche Unterstützungsleistungen. Kontinuitäten und Diskontinuitäten', in H. Oswald (ed.), *Sozialisation und Entwicklung in den neuen Bundesländern – Ergebnisse empirischer Längsschnittforschung, Zeitschrift für Soziologie der Erziehung und Sozialisation*, Vol. 2 (1998), pp. 215–27.

13. Krüger, 'Kindheit im Umbruch'.

14. N. F. Schneider, *Familie und private Lebensführung in West- und Ostdeutschland. Eine vergleichende Analyse des Familienlebens 1970–1992* (Stuttgart: Enke, 1994), p. 105.

15. The west Berlin study was under direction of Prof. L. Krappmann (Max-Planck Institute for Human Development, Berlin) and Prof. H. Oswald (Free University of Berlin). The Brandenburg study was led by Prof. H. Oswald (University of Potsdam). Both studies were financed by grants from the *Deutsche Forschungsgemeinschaft* (DFG).

16. L. Krappmann, B. Schuster and J. Youniss, 'Can Mothers Win? The Transformation of Mother–Daughter Relationships in Late Childhood', in M. Hofer, J. Youniss and P. Noack (eds), *Verbal Interaction and Development in Families with Adolescents* (Stamford, CT: Ablex, 1998), p. 14. Also B. Schuster, *Interaktionen zwischen Müttern und Kindern. Die Konstruktion sozialer Wirklichkeit in Autoritätsbeziehungen* (Weinheim, München: Juventa, 1998), p. 62.

17. The mean differences between children from the Old and the New *Bundesländer* referring to the 'percentage of words spoken by the child in relation to his/her mother' are statistically significant as well as the difference between all mothers and all children referring to both categories of formal aspects.

18. In both samples about 60 per cent of the utterances of the children were subsumed under the category 'competence'.

19. The mean percentage of the category 'challenge' was about 10 per cent in both samples.

20. About 15 per cent of the utterances of the children of both samples were coded as 'making concessions'.

21. In the two samples about 10 per cent of the utterances of the children were subordinated under the category 'internal conflict'.

22. The mean percentage of the remainder category 'fun' was about 4 per cent in both samples.
23. Except for the category 'boycott', the differences in frequency of the other mother-categories were all statistically significant.
24. Du Bois-Reymond and Torrance, 'Die moderne Familie als Verhandlungshaushalt. Eltern-Kind-Beziehungen in West- und Ostdeutschland und in den Niederlanden'. Also Krüger, 'Kindheit im Umbruch – zur aktuellen Lebenssituation von Kindern in den neuen Bundesländern'; Pollmer and Hurrelmann, 'Familientraditionen und Erziehungsstile in Ost- und Westdeutschland'; Reuband, 'Aushandeln statt Gehorsam? Erziehungsziele und Erziehungspraktiken in den alten und neuen Bundesländern im Wandel'; Uhlendorff, Krappmann and Oswald, 'Familie in Ost- und West-Berlin – Erziehungseinstellungen und Kinderfreundschaften'; Zinnecker, 'Streßkinder und Glückskinder. Eltern als soziale Umwelt von Kindern'.
25. H. Lukesch, 'Leitbilder in der Familienerziehung', in L. A. Vaskovics and H. Lipinski (eds), *Familiale Lebenswelten und Bildungsarbeit: Interdisziplinäre Bestandaufnahme* (Opladen: Leske und Budrich, 1996), pp. 153–84.
26. B. Schuster, *Interaktionen zwischen Müttern und Kindern. Die Konstruktion sozialer Wirklichkeit in Autoritätsbeziehungen* (Weinheim, München: Juventa, 1998), pp. 151, 159.
27. For a comparison of relative degrees of traditionality one has to consider factors beyond that of whether the mother–child pairs are from the Old or the New *Bundesländer*; another relevant aspect is the size and the character of their places of residence. The mothers and children of the Old *Bundesländer* were from west Berlin, a very urban socially diverse region, whereas the pairs from the New *Bundesländer* lived in Potsdam which has a small-town character compared with Berlin.

11

Parenting in Times of Social Transformation

Harald Uhlendorff

UNIFICATION AND CHILDREN'S EDUCATION

In the German Democratic Republic (GDR), educational ideology was based on collectivist socialisation concepts. Conformity, the performance of one's duties, the observance of rules and norms, and the assumption of responsibility for others were seen by the state as prime educational goals.[1] By providing an extensive supply of childcare facilities, such as kindergartens and public after-school institutions (*Horte*), through a school system in which, in comparison to parents, teachers were granted considerable powers, as well as through the official child and youth organisations, the state had taken over much of the responsibility for the education of children.

Meyer and Schulze describe how, after unification, this public responsibility was given back into the hands of the parents.[2] Now parents are granted a greater say in school issues and especially in the choice of their children's schooling. Also, the organisation of the children's spare time cannot be left to state and school any longer, but has to be actively planned by parents and children. Parents, therefore, have had to adapt to their new role in the schooling process, and come to terms with the new school system. The new rights and duties they have to assume make many parents feel insecure. In the Federal Republic of Germany (FRG) the role of school and parents in child raising and education has long been a subject of public, and often controversial, debate. Thus east German parents and teachers do not have a clear set of guidelines to follow, and their feelings of insecurity are quite understandable.

The working life of east Germans has changed dramatically since unification. The threat of unemployment is palpable to all, many people work in positions less socially acknowledged than before, and long-distance commuting and work-related absences from home are commonplace. Meyer describes how the long absence from home of one parent because of work, leaving the other parent to cope with the new educational questions alone, has become a particular source of conflict within east German families.[3] The loss of occupational prestige can cause a shift in the power relations within the family, as Elder demonstrated for the period of economic breakdown in the 1930s in the USA.[4] Similar influences on familial education are to be expected also for east Germany. Single mothers are particularly affected by the changes in occupational life.[5] In the GDR, companies were, for example, aware of the fact that single mothers need more time for their children than other mothers. Now employers often do not take this into consideration, and single mothers are dependent on the help of other family members or friends when it comes to looking after the children.

To date, research has been scarce on the question of how parental experiences of unification affect educational attitudes towards children. In this chapter, some case studies will be presented which convey an impression of how, in times of fundamental social change, parents deal with the task of preparing a child for a society with which they themselves are not really familiar. What are the problems caused by unification with which they have to deal?

CASE STUDIES

On the basis of a large research project described in detail in Oswald and Krappmann, it was possible selectively to interview parents of 12- to 13-year-old children.[6] These parents differ from each other in many respects and thus mirror a broad spectrum of east German parents.[7]

Family A:
'We tell the truth and don't toe the line.'
Mrs A., 44 years old, works in the field of home nursing. She is a trained nurse and clerk. Her husband works as a locksmith. The family A. (father, mother, a 23-year-old son and a 13-year-old daughter) was determined to apply for an exit permit in 1990, when the son would have finished school. Mr A. and Mrs A. married because of the exit permit. Without marrying it easily might have happened that one of them was allowed to leave the country but the other not. 'You had to reckon with that kind of harassment', says Mrs A. today. Two sisters of Mrs A. had already emigrated to the FRG in the mid- and late 1980s. Mrs A. had refused to give up her contacts with the relatives in the west. 'From that very hour' she was no longer 'acceptable' as a clerk for her office. From the end of the 1980s, Mr and Mrs A. did not participate in the general elections any longer even though on election day they were personally called upon to do so and were supposed to be collected from home. Mrs A. never hid

her political opinions. She describes herself as 'stubborn and rebellious'. She did take care, however, not to end up in prison because of her utterances. In any case she knew 'I was a trained nurse, I was a trained clerk, my husband was a locksmith. We didn't have that much to lose.' Mrs A. describes unification as a mercy and a liberation. She is happy about the new opportunities and liberties. However, quarrels with employers do still happen. 'If you are the kind of person who likes to tell the truth, you are never really welcome anywhere. In the present system, too, it is better if you toe the line.'

Mrs A. believes that her views about child education basically have not changed: 'Children should hold their own views.' That was her opinion under the old system, too. Mrs A. expressly welcomes the fact that parents now have so much responsibility for the education of their children. 'I didn't want strangers to educate my children before, and I don't want it now. Well, the mistakes, I want to make them myself, but also the good things.' She is happy about the leisure activities on offer outside of school. She believes that they are better than the previous state-directed spare-time activities, even if now it is sometimes difficult to find a place in a sports team: her daughter came home from sports one day and said sadly that she had been 'fired'. But the family searched for and found something else for the daughter.

Mrs A. is sometimes worried about the effect of the financial consequences of unification on her children. Her younger daughter seems to take everything for granted now, the annual journeys abroad and expensive presents. Mrs A. tries to dampen such expectations somewhat. 'Sometimes one should think about the fact that other people don't have that much and that it is important not to think only of oneself.' That is why her daughter is supposed to give away some of her many toys to a good cause every now and again: 'A child has to learn to give away even something she values very much.' Mrs A. welcomes the new opportunities that are now open to her younger daughter. The whole world lies open before her now. It all depends on whether her daughter wants to do things and whether she 'commits herself' to them. The daughter wants to go to a good secondary school (*Gymnasium*) now. The family had some 'troubles' with this idea, they thought about it for a long time, also because the daughter's performance in mathematics was not that brilliant. Now they have organised extra tuition for her during the holidays, prior to her starting at the new school. At the same time Mrs A. emphasises that her daughter's performance is not so important for her. The daughter should try to achieve what she had planned but for Mrs A. it is more important that her daughter becomes a satisfied and happy person.

Wealth is not important to her, nor does she want her children to 'become some sort of geniuses, but completely fail in their daily life'.

ASSESSMENT

The identity of the parents as upright and rebellious people, which resulted from their opposition to the political system of the GDR, changed in the new social order of the FRG. However, this identity is still noticeable when it comes to quarrels with employers. The parents are happy about the new liberties and opportunities opening up for their children, but they have difficulties in supporting their daughter in her decision to go to the *Gymnasium*. This may be because of their GDR experiences, where higher education and the occupational prestige connected with it often indicated a degree of compliance with the state system, with a corresponding loss of independence. This is very understandable if one considers that their simple professions granted the family a living although they were politically conspicuous. The most important life aims defined by the parents for their daughter are happiness and satisfaction, and not individual performance, as is often demanded by the new system. Nor is wealth in itself worth striving for; as for the concept of 'genius', it seems to them that there is a real danger of not being able to cope with life in general. In spite of all their doubts, the parents decided to make it possible for their daughter to go to the *Gymnasium* and to support her from the beginning by extra tuition in her problem subject, mathematics.

Family E:

> **'Today you have to become active, to think for yourself, to decide yourself. This also applies to the children.'**
> Mrs E., 38 years old, cares for her 13-year-old son alone. During GDR times she actively participated in the Free German Youth (FDJ) which she enjoyed very much, and which was important to her. After secondary school she went to a technical college and became a technical employee in east Berlin. The company had to close down soon after unification and the job centre procured her a one-year 'electronic data processing and management' training course. After that she had to complete a three-month placement in Hamburg. In this period, it was mainly her parents who took care of her son. The company in Hamburg asked her to open up a branch in Berlin. At first she doubted her own ability, but everything went well. Soon, in fact, her job started to bore her. Now she works in another architectural office and is very happy about her 'dream job'. She can contribute her own ideas and decide many things herself.
> Mrs E. emphasises that as a single mother she has to count on her

son's autonomy. In his second year of primary school he was still attending the after-school institution in the afternoon. Mrs E. was very unhappy though with the care-giver, who did not appear interested in the children. Therefore, in the third grade, her son only went to the after-school institution for his lunch, and afterwards he went home, even though Mrs E. did not return from work until the evening. From the fifth grade on, the son prepared his meals at home on his own. After lunch he does his homework. Three times a week he goes to a sports club. After initial problems this daily schedule now runs smoothly. The son had always participated in hobby groups for children, first in a handicraft group, then he did swimming, now he plays handball. The school handball group has developed into a club. Mrs E. welcomes the way in which the club cares for the children because the coaches are very committed. Once, when the son was ill for a few days, the coach phoned and asked after the boy. Mrs E.'s educational ideas with regard to her son have changed notably since unification. In former times, she says, one was guided and directed. One had only to put a cross on a form to determine what a child was to do within or outside of school. Today one has to find one's own way, to make one's own plans, to think about it and organise it. Now, she tries to pass this mentality on to her son. When he did not want to go swimming any longer he had to help look for something new. He saw to it himself and considered what he could do, and what other children do in the afternoons. Mrs E. and her son were very well advised by the primary school about the forthcoming change of school. They organised special meetings where teachers of the different schools introduced themselves and also the class teacher of the primary school offered her services for counselling. But now in the *Gymnasium*, Mrs E. is not satisfied with her son's class teacher: 'If some children fail to come up to the required standards the teacher does nothing to help them; she does not even encourage the students to form working groups. She merely refers the parents to private tuition. During GDR times the school cared more for the children and the connection between teachers and parents was better.'

ASSESSMENT

Mrs E. pragmatically weighs up the advantages and disadvantages of personally coping with everyday life in the GDR and FRG. She compares things in a very differentiated manner, such as the situation in school, without taking an ideological stance. After some initial hesitation she now actively tests her abilities in new environments, and in doing so gathers positive experiences. She enjoys the fact that in her job she has to think and to decide for herself. As far as education is concerned, she wants to raise her son to be able to make independent decisions – for example, in actively planning his leisure time. From her point of view the demands on children for autonomy should be accompanied by personal attention on the part of teachers and educators. This new form of autonomy for children goes far beyond the reliable and competent completion of everyday life tasks which was the norm in GDR times.

Family D:

'In former times everything was straightforward and clear, today one has to fend for oneself.'

Mrs D., 42 years old, has to bring up her 12-year-old son alone. Her 20-year-old son recently left home. Mrs D. works full-time as a doctor in a hospital. She managed to keep her job in spite of some reorganising which was done because of unification. All in all, however, work has become a much greater burden. She complains about 'this idiocy. Either one has no work at all or one has too much of it. If you are fully employed they expect 300 per cent of you, eight hours a day are not enough any more. And this brings with it the usual consequences of overstrain.' She has less time to devote to her son than previously. The threat of possible redundancy is an additional worry, because 'who can say nowadays that unemployment does not concern them'.

Mrs D. reports that her moral standards for the education of her younger son have changed. 'During GDR times one taught one's child not to lie. Today, however, one has to fend for oneself and sometimes one has to resort to a white lie in order not to lose face.' As an example she tells the following story: her son was supposed to meet his class outside school for a basketball match. The boy did try to find the agreed meeting point, but could not locate it. Mrs D. comments on the situation as follows: 'And now he tells his teacher that he has a headache. Yes, I think this is okay. I don't think he has to admit that he was too stupid to find the place. In former times I might have thought differently about it. I would have insisted on more moral rectitude. Not that I would have squealed on him, but by myself I would have given a somewhat different judgement.' Mrs D. says that her son is now developing an antenna for obviously false promises made to him by adverts from shopping centres or in prize competitions, for example. Mrs D. compares these advertising methods with her experience from GDR times. Then 'the written word was a hundred per cent valid. It is something negative if one has to take it that not everything which is written in black and white is necessarily true. This does not speak well for the society in which it happens.' In school 'teachers explained to the parents that now, after unification, they have fewer rights than they used to have. Even if the children show obvious behavioural problems the teachers do not act on them.' Mrs D. does not want to blame the teachers for this: 'They too have to adapt to the new conditions.' Mrs D. considers the reports and judgements of teachers are more superficial than in former times, containing little of concrete value, particularly as the teachers are reluctant to write anything negative about the children. Towards the end of her son's primary school period Mrs D. was unsure as to which kind of secondary school would be best for him. She eventually decided after a private talk with her son's class teacher. The boy now goes to the same school as the teacher's daughter. Mrs D.'s older son finished the *Gymnasium* last year. At the moment he works casually. 'It is true that he can try out different things, but he does not have any job training or a university place.' Mrs D. believes 'this is thanks to the new conditions. In the GDR it would have been different; there, in the 10th or 11th grade, he would have had to write down what he wanted to be.' The sheets were signed by the parents and handed in. 'And in the senior classes almost everybody – 90 per cent or more – was assigned a university place or job training.'

ASSESSMENT

For Mrs D. the political change has no positive aspects. She judges the GDR life as straightforward, clear and orientated by definite moral value standards. Mrs D. experiences the FRG as a system in which it is difficult to orientate oneself. Value standards and responsibilities seem unclear and blurred. Thus teachers withdraw from their responsibilities because of new laws and regulations, and society allows, for example, fraudulent advertising, running the risk of confusing children. On the other hand, spare-time activities for children are not suitably provided. Education has become a more difficult task for Mrs D. since unification. A possible way out for her consists in the guidance of personally credible, specialised educators, such as her son's former class teacher.

Family B:
'We have to continue to talk to each other.'
Mr B., 52 years old, lives together with his 13-year-old son. His wife died about two years ago. During GDR times Mr B. worked in the diplomatic service. He spent a large part of the 1980s in Canada, together with his wife and son. He regarded the GDR as his 'retreat'. Unification entailed an enormous loss of prestige for him. Temporarily he worked as an insurance agent; now he works in shifts at a hostel for the homeless.

Mr B. often reflects about child education under the conditions of 'free-enterprise' in the FRG and makes comparisons with the GDR: 'During GDR times the whole school system was geared to the class as a unit, mutual help and support. It started with the teacher who operated according to the motto: "Here we have a weaker person, you are the stronger one. Now help the weaker". At that time it still used to be a negative point for the whole class if some of the students did not reach the required standard or if they repeatedly behaved out of line. If the others did not help it would have caused justified criticism against the class teacher as well as the subject teacher and the Collective of the class. "What kind of people are you that something like this is possible?" they would have asked. But today in the FRG everyone is responsible for his own actions. Now it is more important to assert oneself. Well, whereas at the time I would have criticised my son because of egoistic behaviour, I now say: "You have to learn to cope with it." In this society a sheep can't do anything against the wolves. He must be a wolf himself.'

Nowadays, teachers and students are very distant. During GDR times the teacher had to care more for the class, otherwise he would have been pressured by the Collective. In addition, Mr B. senses the arrogance of the teachers from west Germany who now teach in east German schools and who know little about the GDR and the former living conditions. His son's friendships are important to Mr B.: 'If he has a friend I try to establish contacts also with the friend's parents, so that we can exchange views.' Mr B. asks the teacher if the friendship of the two children has positive effects, if the friends 'pull each other up or if one pulls the other down'. He does not ask anymore, however, if the friendship is positive for the class as well. In spite of the family's difficult financial situation, Mr B. bought his son a good computer and a printer. He believes that this generation simply has to grow up with a computer. Mr B. finds the spare-time activities on offer to children 'lousy'. They immediately become a financial problem. Thus, his son was supposed to pay a large admission fee to join the football club and on top of that there are monthly subscription fees. Mr B. had to get used to his son's requests concerning his clothing – which has to be produced by certain companies: 'It is no longer enough to have a good pair of trainers. It has to be a leading brand.' His son does not want to wear other things any more. Last year, Mr B. for the first time bought his son a pair of designer jeans. His son was 'proud as a prince' when they left the shop. Now, the father no longer goes shopping without his son. Mr B. thinks that he has to bow to this situation if he does not want to discredit his son. Among the children this is a 'question of personal recognition. If children do not wear the proper clothing when playing football, it does not matter how well they play; if you want to be accepted you have to follow suit. Otherwise you become a laughing stock.' Mr B. emphasises that because of the great age difference he has to be 'extremely careful to stay trendy' and try not to push his personal views through, even though he thinks them right. Otherwise father and son would soon not be talking to each other any more. This must be prevented by every means. Mr B. fears that otherwise his son will one day say: 'My old man is crazy, totally not with it.' 'To struggle against material desires, to take up arms against them, does not get you anywhere. You can't change the situation by changing the individual, you have to change the outside conditions.' As a negative consequence of unification, Mr B. describes the following incident. His son reproached him some time ago: 'If you had learned something useful, you wouldn't be in this situation now.' Mr B. had 'put his hands in his pockets and said: "Son, you just can't understand this yet"'.

ASSESSMENT

The GDR gave Mr B. a feeling of security even when he lived abroad. The FRG conveys to him a completely different feeling. Here it is important to assert oneself, even to fight one's way through among the 'wolves'. Personal recognition is gained, at least among adolescents, through the possession of brand-name goods. If one does not have these things one is a lesser person. Mr B. believes that the school and the leisure time activities offered do not support the children as much as they used to in former times. Being away from home many hours a day because of his job, it is important to him to be well informed about his son's friends. Through talks with the friends' parents and teachers he tries to create a kind of security network around his son. Here he shows a protectively controlling attitude which, in part, is based on his feelings of mistrust about the new social conditions. It is very important to Mr B. to maintain a good relationship with his son. This relationship, however, seems to be somewhat endangered because of the father's loss of prestige and because of his political views. The father tries to contain his critical attitude towards the FRG in relations with his son and does not begrudge him his pleasure in consumption. On the other hand, however, he is dependent on his son's ability to deal with the father's GDR past in a gentle and non-deprecating manner.

COPING WITH THE CHALLENGES OF TRANSFORMATION: PARENTING
IN EASTERN GERMANY TODAY

This chapter addresses the question of how east German parents raise
their children in times of fundamental social transformation. Eight years
after the fall of the Wall there are still serious adaptive problems with
which people have to cope. It is striking how differently families reacted to
the challenges after unification. The case studies constitute exemplars of
how changed daily working routines affect parental educational ideas.
Owing to increased occupational pressures and absences from home
because of work, less time remains for the family and education. The
threat of unemployment also has an impact on education. Parents who are
threatened by unemployment are more ready to work overtime and have
less energy to deal with educational questions. For some parents,
unification was connected with a considerable loss of prestige. On the one
hand, these parents grieve over the loss of the old GDR conditions; on the
other, they have to adapt to the new social situation in the interest of their
children, otherwise they run the risk of not being taken seriously or
respected by them. If parents have experienced in their own work life that
personal initiative and the readiness to make decisions do pay, they also
encourage their children to become more active, to think about their
objectives, and not to be afraid of making decisions. In the presentation of
the case studies it was not possible, owing to lack of space, to consider the
interview passages where parents spoke of incidents of disappointment
and envy encountered at work. Parents would like their children to be
spared such experiences and therefore take care that the children stand up
for their own needs and do not easily let themselves be exploited by others.

The wide range of consumer goods on offer and the new possibilities of
consumption are experienced very differently by the interviewed families.
Some parents believe that children have to learn to deal with the
abundance of goods, and that they should not forget to share with others.
Other parents underline the quarrels within the family caused by the
discrepancy between the large number of goods on offer and the family's
financial limitations. Any discussion of brand names seems to be an
explosive matter, especially for parents who judge unification negatively.
Some parents are ready to buy their child a computer even if the financial
situation of the family is unfavourable. These parents believe that the
computer is a sensible investment for their children's future and might
even help the children cope better at school.

East German parents miss the former intensive personal relationships
between teachers and students, and deplore the fact that children who are
performing poorly are not supported enough by the teachers. They believe
that in former times the school, after-school institutions, and state child
and youth organisations were able to counterbalance any negligence within

the family. This is no longer an option. Such views are held by parents independently of any negative or positive change in their living conditions resulting from unification.

The spare-time activities on offer to children in east Berlin are described by the interviewed parents as variegated but expensive. In order to find interesting and affordable opportunities, parents and children have to become active themselves and look, for example, for appropriate clubs, hobby groups or other artistically oriented groups. It is no longer enough to rely on the school or other public organisations. The parents set a high value on their children being looked after by committed adults, because the children should profit not only from sport or artistic activities, but also from the personal relationships with coaches and educators.

Many east Germans are of the opinion that the state in the GDR often treated its citizens in a presumptuous way, and behaved patronisingly in educational matters as well. It is small wonder that many people heaved a sigh of relief after unification and enjoyed the new liberties available to themselves and their children. The case studies show, however, that these new liberties seem to have a completely different meaning for some of the parents. They believe, for example, that adults and children in the FRG have to fight as 'wolves among wolves', that lying is no longer regarded a problem in the relationship between teachers and children, and that adults and children may be cheated with impunity by aggressive advertising. These parents do not perceive the new opportunities for themselves and their children as a gain, but judge unification as having led to a regression in moral educational standards.

The interviewed parents' age seems to play an important role in the judgement of the consequences of unification. The cases presented in this chapter as well as families who could not be taken into consideration here convey the following impression: mothers and fathers who in 1989 were about 40 years old or older emphasised the political dimension of unification. For them, their personal and familial educational situation is closely linked with the general political conditions. Younger parents are more pragmatic, they engage more easily in the reality of the FRG, they search for a new way in the new system and very often encounter good experiences which they pass on to their children, without necessarily feeling ideologically committed to the new social system. This attitude might, on the one hand, be connected with the favourable occupational opportunities that opened up more for younger than for older people. On the other hand, younger parents had their political experiences mainly during the Honecker era (from 1971 on), a time in which GDR citizens could keep aloof from politics as long as they participated in the system's ideological rituals.[8] Private life could become a social niche, and even the reception of west German television programmes was permitted.

Compared with the era of Stalinist influence, or the period of the erection of the Berlin Wall, it was easier to define oneself as unpolitical. Older people have experienced the earlier GDR phases in which the individual could not avoid being involved in politics. Maybe this is why the political dimension plays a greater role in their reflections on unification and education than it does with younger parents.

NOTES

1. L. Ahnert, S. Krätzig, T. Meischner and A. Schmidt, 'Sozialisationskonzepte für Kleinkinder: Wirkungen tradierter Erziehungsvorstellungen und staatssozialistischer Erziehungsdoktrinen im intra- und interkulturellen Ost-West-Vergleich', in G. Trommsdorff (ed.), *Psychologische Aspekte des sozio-politischen Wandels in Ostdeutschland* (Berlin: de Gruyter, 1994), p. 97. See also G. Trommsdorff and P. Chakkarath, 'Kindheit im Transformationsprozeß', in S. E. Hormuth, W. R. Heinz, H.-J. Kornadt, H. Sydow and G. Trommsdorff (eds), *Individuelle Entwicklung, Bildung und Berufsverläufe* (Opladen: Leske und Budrich, 1996), p. 31.
2. S. Meyer and E. Schulze, *Familie im Umbruch: Zur Lage der Familien in der ehemaligen DDR* (Stuttgart: Kohlhammer, 1992), p. 120.
3. D. Meyer, 'Eltern-Kind-Beziehungen in den neuen Bundesländern nach der Wende', in P. Büchner, M. Grundmann, J. Huinink, L. Krappmann, B. Nauck, D. Meyer and S. Rothe (eds), *Kindliche Lebenswelten, Bildung und innerfamiliale Beziehungen* (Weinheim: Juventa, 1994), p .149.
4. G. H. Elder, *Children of the Great Depression* (Chicago: University of Chicago Press, 1974).
5. E. Kolinsky, 'Women, Work and Family in the New Länder: Conflicts and Experiences', in E. Kolinsky and C. Flockton (eds), *Recasting East Germany: Social Transformation after the GDR* (London: Frank Cass, 1999), p. 108.
6. H. Oswald and L. Krappmann, 'Social Life in a Former Bipartite City', in P. Noack, M. Hofer and J. Youniss (eds), *Psychological Responses to Social Change* (Berlin: de Gruyter, 1995), p. 170.
7. In 1997 about 40 parents living in east Berlin were asked by letter to participate in an interview about their parenting behaviour and attitudes after the fall of the Wall. These parents had taken part in a larger research project in 1992/93 and were selected according to the following criteria. Parents were contacted who judged the changes in their personal living conditions after unification clearly positively (according to various scales), as well as parents who showed an obviously negative judgement. A complementary goal was to interview single parents as well as two-parent families. Thirdly, parents with higher and lower educational levels were to be sampled. Eight parents in all gave an affirmative answer and were personally interviewed; four of these interviews which were productive (illuminating) and not redundant were selected for the case studies described here.
8. T. Gensicke, *Die neuen Bundesbürger* (Opladen: Westdeutscher Verlag, 1998), p. 157.

12

Investigating Change in the Way Children Deal with Time

Dieter Kirchhöfer

THE AIM OF THE STUDY

Against the backdrop of the dramatic changes taking place in east Germany in autumn 1989, the idea arose in both east and west Germany of documenting the anticipated change in the life-style patterns of children. Initially, the intention was simply to compare the daily life of children in the two social systems, but it soon became evident that a deeper process of transformation could be expected, and that here was an opportunity not simply to record after the event, but to monitor development over a number of years. The premise of the study was that the changes would be discernible not only in the changing conditions of childhood, but above all in the activities and processes of the children's daily lives. Thus the project concentrated on the analysis of changes in the way children in east Berlin led their everyday lives. The aim was to explore, from a child-centred perspective, the relations between the changed conditions, the type of activity engaged in daily by children and their patterns of behaviour. Assuming space, time, social relations and resources as the vital components of a life-style, this chapter will focus on *organisation of time* and attempt to identify those features where change is in evidence.

RESEARCH METHODS: ACCESS TO EMPIRICAL DATA

The study set out to make a qualitative analysis of the daily routine of children. To obtain the requisite empirical data, a method of charting the course of a day was used which had been successfully employed in ethnology, socioecology, psychology and linguistics. From the beginning of 1990, researchers monitored 10-year-old children in districts of east Berlin for a week at a time. Following a procedure described by Barker and Wright,[1] seven days in the life of each child, from getting up in the morning to going to bed at night, were recorded. Further sets of data were obtained for the same children in 1992 and 1994. New groups of 10-year-olds were brought into the study in both these years and, as for the first cohort, three sets of data were obtained for each, at two-yearly intervals. In addition, for the group born in 1980, seven days of a typical week in 1989 were reconstructed to permit analysis of their life before the fall of the Berlin Wall. During each monitored week, the children recorded their activities, as well as the relevant times and associated places and people.[2] The information could thus be subsequently represented as an activity sequence in a spatiotemporal framework. The focal interest, both in the study and in this chapter, was not the time spent on individual activities, but the time structures. Thus the activity switches were of particular significance, the points at which the children made decisions regarding their next activity, having to call up or form corresponding intentions. These changes of activity are the points at which interpretation begins. The following vignettes of examples of situations are intended to demonstrate the procedure adopted; they are not intended as exemplars or even as a data basis for the subsequent treatment of general changes in the time organisation of east German children.

SITUATION I

1990
Analysis of activity switch

12th activity switch, a Tuesday in October:
Ten-year-old Mark goes home straight from school, arriving at 13.40 hours. He has two hours before his mother comes home from work, thus giving him a first contact which will also free him for the afternoon.
Possible activities open to him:

1. Watch television.
2. Make a sandwich for lunch.
3. Relax.
4. Read.
5. Do homework.

Decision: Mark begins his homework, working his way through quickly and finishing in 20 minutes.

His decision to begin his homework at once and to complete it in one sitting could have been prompted by any of the following plausible intentions:

Assumption 1.   His parents had instructed him to do so.

Assumption 2.   Mark is used to this routine from the childcare group
                     he attended when younger.

Assumption 3.   Mark has adopted a disciplined approach, in which he
                     first completes the less pleasurable tasks as quickly as
                     possible.

The very next activity switch increases the credibility of the third
assumption.

13th activity switch: Mark empties the bin before making himself
                         some lunch.

Other activity switches during the day, in which similar decisions are
evident, indicate that Mark's use of time involves advance planning,
control and discipline.

18th activity switch: Upon his return from a sports session, Mark
                         deposits his sports gear and towel in the bathroom
                         before joining his sister who is watching television.

Analysis of changes in time organisation

1992

Situation: Mark has now changed schools and has further
                         to travel. He goes straight home from school,
                         arriving at 14.00, and is alone in the flat. The
                         possibilities open to him are virtually
                         unchanged.

Decision: He has a break and watches television.

Subsequent decisions: He watches television for a short time only, then
                         begins his homework, which he interrupts after
                         ten minutes to telephone a friend, after which he
                         resumes his homework.

1994

Situation: Mark comes straight home from school, arriving
                         at 14.05. His mother is at home.

Decision: Mark lies down on his sofa-bed and rests for
                         half an hour.

Subsequent decisions: He switches on the computer, but leaves it after
                         15 minutes to begin his homework which he
                         interrupts after another 15 minutes, when his
                         mother brings him something to eat.

The comments on change refer to the same basic facts: Mark has broken up the activity sequence which was dominant in 1990 (return from school followed by uninterrupted completion of homework); the other days included in the 1994 study show a similar breaking-up of the sequence (return–relaxation–play–homework with interruptions).

These changes may be explained as follows:

Interpretation 1.	Mark has reduced the rules and routines of self-disciplined timing.
Interpretation 2.	Hedonistic elements are now part of Mark's lifestyle.
Interpretation 3.	The amount of homework given at the secondary school necessitates a different organisation of work time.

Other situations during the day indicate that Interpretations 1 and 2 are plausible: Mark has reduced the elements of self-discipline and is now more open to relaxation activities. A footnote to this comment, however, is the fact that Mark still completes his homework *before* his leisure activities and thus still subjects himself to a certain time discipline. The explanation of the changes identified implies age as a factor affecting time discipline: children as they get older distance themselves from previous routines and rules. At the same time, however, Mark has retained elements which give daily life a certain order – elements which were also observed among 10-year-olds in 1994 and 1996.

SITUATION 2

1990
Analysis of activity switch

14th activity switch, a Wednesday in October.

Situation:	Ten-year-old Adina comes home from school, arriving at 13.30. She is alone in the house. She begins her homework, throws together some lunch, changes out of her 'school clothes' and at 14.15 switches on the television. Five minutes later, she stops watching television and returns to her homework, which she finishes at 14.45. At 16.00 she is due for a training session at a sportscentre. The journey there, as she knows, usually takes 35 minutes by bus.

Possible variations on these activities:

                        1. Watch television again.
                        2. Telephone a friend (which she often does).
                        3. Leave for the sports centre.
                        4. Read.

Decision:	Adina packs her sports bag and leaves the apartment. Her decision to leave early could be explained by the following intentions:
Assumption 1.	Adina always allows plenty of time to ensure that she will not be late.
Assumption 2.	Adina cannot judge how much time she needs.
Assumption 3.	Adina is bored at home.

The decision was preceded by two situations which indicate that the first assumption would be most plausible. In the morning, Adina left the apartment 40–50 minutes before school was due to begin, although she only has a five-minute walk to school. She had also checked the bus timetable on her way home from school, to be quite sure that she knew what time the bus was due. This would suggest a pattern which seeks to avoid risks and ensure punctuality.

Analysis of changes in time organisation

1992
Adina has kept her morning routine. Although she has changed schools and has further to go, she still leaves the apartment with around 50 minutes to spare, and has altered the time she gets up accordingly. She allows similar reserves of time for other activities such as choir practice.

1994
Adina continues to leave the apartment with plenty of time to spare. She now explains that she does not like to rush, does not enjoy hectic situations and does not want stress. She applies the same behaviour to meetings with friends and reports that she does not sleep properly if an early appointment the following day alters the time she gets up. These points indicate a consistency of behaviour in which time risks are to be avoided and punctuality ensured. Further details about the method are given in the report of the longitudinal study.[3]

The reconstructed routines of 462 days in children's lives, evidencing 20–30 activity switches each, provided a set of data which allowed conclusions to be drawn about where change had taken place. The focus here should not be on the quantity of data, however, but on the opportunity it affords to explore examples and patterns of behaviour beyond the individual day and the individual child. Thus no attempt was made to formulate a universal statement about the age-group, but to obtain evidence from within the age-group to the effect that there had or had not been changes. In contrast to other projects, which inferred changes in individual life-styles from changes in the social system, this investigation focused on individual activities, seeking from this to identify how conditions in society had changed.

CHANGES IN GIVEN DAILY TIME STRUCTURES FOR CHILDREN IN EAST GERMANY

Societal changes in east Germany since the fall of the communist government have already been widely discussed, and the transformation process has been documented in a range of studies.[4] In the study presented here, features such as the restructuring of the labour market and changes in the content and organisation of adult work could be clearly identified. Some changes were because of the introduction of the west Berlin school system and the paring back of school's role in coordinating and regulating the public behaviour of children. Also, in many districts, particularly in areas of new housing, retail outlets, services and amenities began to cluster outside residential areas, separating what had been geographically integrated domains. The network of institutions providing childcare and community education free of charge, which had developed in the GDR, was reduced and commercialised and no longer formed part of the state school system. The children's scope of activities was affected by the families' changing material conditions, the reduction in the time needed for meeting basic needs and the opening up of new areas for travel. These changes generated new time structures to which children needed to adapt, which is why we referred above to changes in *given* time structures. The timing of parents' work, the organisation of weekends by institutions, school timetables, public transport systems, the opening times of shops and restaurants – all these factors influenced the children's daily time frameworks, offering possibilities or regulating them, opening up new options or barring previous ones. Children in the GDR lived in an environment in which the daily organisation of time was, to a large extent, predictable (constant) and functionally transparent. In terms of timing, many activities in which the children took part were coordinated and optimised. The exploitation of opportunities and compliance with prescribed routines was thus – as in other societies – not only an issue of individual willingness, but was directed by institutional scheduling. The institutionalisation of time had created an anonymous time structure, which also sustained dependencies.[5] These institutionalised and rationalised structures dissolved in united Germany. A large number of changes in given time structures were recorded, including the following examples.[6]

1. Separation of individual routines within families. The assumption that the new situation, bringing so many uncertainties with respect to the future, would cause families to move closer together proved incorrect. In fact, individual routines separated out in spatiotemporal terms. In all of the samples, the time children and parents spent together decreased: some meals which had been taken together were now taken separately, shopping together declined, and in the evenings less time was spent together, because the children chose to eat, watch television or play on their computers in their own rooms.

2. Growing unpredictability of time structures in the child's environment. The changes in employment resulted in a more flexible organisation of working hours, and some parents had also taken on additional jobs or started retraining programmes; and in cases where mothers were unemployed for a time, their commitment to temporary jobs, trips to the employment office, interviews and meetings with friends still contributed to a growing unpredictability in work-day timing. Leisure time, too, became more unpredictable. Formerly, institutionalised activities had been assigned to certain days of the week, and on these days no homework was given. The institutions themselves had had regulated days and times of opening, and the children were also aware of the times they would spend within the social networks of their families. Societal change brought an end to this coordination of school and out-of-school schedules: the institutions began to open as required and desired. Colleagues saw less of each other; relations and friends were more tied to their own commitments, or less prepared to commit themselves. There was also a greater degree of unpredictability among peers. The unity of group identity created by neighbourhoods, school classes and leisure activities dissolved and children could no longer be certain that their acquaintances would be available for shared activity in their spare time.

3. Destructuring of daily routines: functional interlacing of activities. The standard days of the 10-year-olds recorded in 1990 evidenced a fixed structure which we termed phase structure. This featured a morning phase of preparation for school and a school phase, followed by a midday phase in which the children were alone at home and during which they did their homework and/or their household chores. This was followed either by an institutionally organised phase or a free-play phase, usually commencing around 15.00, when one or both parents (usually the mother) arrived home, and finishing around 18.00. After this would be time for communication before and during the family dinner. The short after-dinner phase was used for relaxation, watching television and personal hygiene.

This functionally determined structure began to break up. Television before school became more common. The midday phase was used more for relaxation, particularly television. The parents' return from work varied or was not predictable. The boundaries between midday and afternoon phases became blurred, homework was done at arbitrary times throughout the rest of the day, and the evening meal lost its structuring role. New media also had a destructuring influence: videos and computer games provided diversions at any point during the day.

4. Changes in public social control. The reduction of institutional coordination and control, that is, by school and particularly by class teachers, led to changes in prestructured activity. Formerly, school had not only constantly demanded, monitored and regulated individual academic achievement, but in terms of time, space and human contacts had also guided the children's out-of-school activities, their political participation and their social peer inter-action. Now the children were faced with a number of separate areas of life, for which they themselves had to take responsibility The various centres, clubs, organisations and groups began to plan their programmes independently, leaving the children to strike the balance of timing. The network of informal social control which had existed in the residential areas – through the parents' acquaintance with the parents of classmates, with the people who worked in the local shops and with the members of local committees – was diminished. Often, the children no longer attended the same class or school, and the parents began to observe a tacit rule not to interfere. This reduction in public control was accompanied by new modalities of parental control in relation to children's behaviour in public, towards adults or towards money and property.

CONTINUITY AND CHANGE IN EAST GERMAN CHILDREN'S MANAGEMENT OF TIME

Changing conditions for children's actions do not necessarily lead to changes in the time management associated with the actions, and it is in fact an aim of this contribution to question such an assumption of linear causality. It is true that children in the GDR had acquired, with respect to time management, significant constraints which also disciplined and formed adult society, and had adapted to the various other-determined structures and thus experienced heteronomy. However, they had not just fitted into these structures, but had also formed them to suit themselves; outwitting the power of given time structures, they had created their own, which proved, however, equally stringent. In terms of time they had acquired a certain level of competence which had become a prerequisite of their own existence as subjects dealing with time and thus with their environment, and the practice continued, even though the conditions had changed. In our study we encountered a high level of stability with respect to individual life-styles in families and among children. At the end of the 1990s, parents and children reacted to daily situations with patterns and intentions which they had acquired in the course of their lives, short though these were in the children's case. The new situations were perceived as unchanged or familiar, and the strategies and rule systems used to cope with the situations were the old ones. This was all the more astonishing considering that at the time the changes were taking place in east German society, the children were at an age when they were just beginning to develop ways of leading their lives and managing their time, and the process was subject to the dynamics of age.[7] Virtually all of the children acted with a high level of competence when dealing with time. They made realistic estimates of required time, were able to cope with various demands on their time, kept a constant check on time during the day and sought regularity.

This evident stability, however, conceals the fact that even for children the living out of daily life was a balancing act in which either the situations requiring action or the alternative courses of action had to be evaluated. The arrangements with respect to time which the children had developed in the course of their dealings with the environment were constantly disturbed by new demands. In the long run, the time management strategies could not withstand the tension between the changed (conditions and given structures) and the constant (patterns and rules). Daily confrontation with the changed conditions required the children, for example, to find different ways of coordinating the new choice of activities open to them and the new pluralist nature of the demands upon them. The circumstances in which decisions needed to be made had become less predictable. The children were required to work out new intentions and refer to changed sets of values within frameworks which had become more complex.

In the GDR they had been called upon to demonstrate independence in coordinating various demands for action, but now they were required not just to fulfil the coordination expectations of others, but also to make their own agreements and arrangements. In the past they had been forced to make decisions as independent actors in changing situations; after the *Wende*, they not only had to assure the disciplined and effective implementation of such decision making, but also needed to relate this to certain objectives. Naturally, children in the GDR had learnt to reflect on their actions, the conditions for these actions and, above all, on the results of these actions. A whole series of educational procedures and rituals had engendered a high level of self-reflection. In the new system, the children also learned to reflect on their own self-interest, and to explore the utilitarian relationship between the interests of others and their own. Whereas previously they had operated within a closed and largely homogeneous framework of intent, they now had to orient themselves within a spectrum which was being eroded and fragmented. A thorough analysis of daily lifestyles therefore revealed, among many consistent features, a whole range of inconsistencies and new features. A gradual and even contradictory erosion of time management was and is still taking place, which throws up contradictions in behaviour. Here we focus on a small number of selected features which had developed in the GDR and which can be subsumed under the heading 'time regime': time planning, discipline, thrift, cooperativeness, orientation to purpose.[8]

Variability in Planning

The organisation of life inside and outside the family in the GDR made planning both necessary and possible. Children planned the times for their homework, as well as their household and community tasks. Each class at school had a workplan for the year with feedback schedules and report deadlines. Study and work brigades in the class acted in accordance with workplans or 'operational plans' encompassing tasks with individual responsibility. At many schools, individual plans requiring self-commitment and the pursuit of personal goals were in place for years at a time. The principle of strict time planning that governed the production process was, at least in the 1950s and 1960s, also an organising principle of school work, most consistently expressed in the demand for syllabus fulfilment within the appointed periods. As the teachers made students aware of the time constraints in syllabus fulfilment, time was a major factor in the students' experience of school discipline. After 1989, the pressure stemming from a given, anonymous timeframe was removed; the plan as an abstract, anonymous determiner of time lost its influence, at least in school. As many of the functions of life within families and also at school remained stable, however, the regulated nature of time organisation remained. Children continued to aim to give their lives a certain rhythmic time-scheduling, to seek fixed points for meeting friends, to make appointments. In this respect, children also continued to plan their activities. If they had arranged to do something with friends, the date would provide a point of orientation and a focus of planning, over weeks in some cases (such as concerts). But the planning referred primarily to the arrangements the children had made themselves, and only to a lesser extent to externally determined timing. Less time was allocated to the heteronomously determined periods; possible infringements were no longer a source of worry. It was the aims and the contents of planning that shifted, rather than the planning procedure. Outside the structures they had created themselves, the children waited to see what external arrangements were on offer and only then decided the degree to which they would pursue these possibilities or fulfil these requirements.

Erosion of Time Discipline

As early as 1990, it was apparent that the children displayed remarkable competence with respect to time and evidenced coordination achievements comparable with those of adults (for example, afternoons involving collection of younger siblings, shopping, homework, playtime with friends, punctual return, household chores); this required initiative, flexibility and a willingness to make decisions. This kind of autonomous initiative applied in particular to the assurance of task completion. The competent management of time included the skills of estimating and checking time, or coordinating parallel demands, and generated a certain degree of discipline and self-discipline, often associated with the secondary virtues of punctuality and reliability. The observance of time constraints functioned as a principle of organisation in families, and as an element of public discipline. A developed form of time discipline emerged in the production-based school subject *Polytechnischer Unterricht*, in which the children were familiarised with the terms associated with timing in the industrial production process, such as machining times, cycle times, lead times, etc. The regulated nature of family and school life and the familiarity with self-determined planning meant that discipline with respect to time management was retained under the new system.

However, children no longer exercised this discipline as a duty, or out of obedience, or because they wished to please adults, but as a useful tool. Keeping to the regulated routine was less bother than the resulting confrontations if the external time requirements were flouted. If infringements still took place, the children adopted a strategy of 'keeping cool' and putting up with adults' reproaches. Time discipline continued to be highly valued among peers. Meetings and dates within the peer group took unqualified precedence over all other commitments. The level of time control required in these cases was high, and criticism in case of failure to comply was sharp.

Lessening of Time Pressure

In the GDR, children experienced a permanent shortage of time, stemming from the large number of activities in which they were expected to engage, their institutionalisation and the manner of organisation of family life. In particular the time patterns of working parents forced the children to accelerate their home-based activities and thus affected children's daily time management. The shortage of time and thus the need to save time became a basic feature of individual behaviour regulation that corresponded to a socially desired and required pattern of time rationalisation. This economic approach to time applied on the one hand to the gaining of time for autonomous activity with friends, and on the other to possibilities for sharing time with the family. The functionally determined division of labour in families not only highlighted the serious nature of the work done by the children, but also created an awareness that the completion of these tasks enabled the family members to spend time together. Time for tea in the afternoon, a game on a weekday evening, television on a Saturday evening or an outing at the weekend were only possible if household tasks and homework were finished and the spare time therefore 'earned'. Thrift as an attitude to work was also propagated in more concrete terms, and the propaganda slogans such as 'Save every gram, every second, every penny' were compulsory educational maxims for children's work in schools and factories. Waste of material (or time) counted as a misdemeanour.

This thriftiness underwent an erosion. In the years following the *Wende*, children's leisure time increased and not only was there more time available, but that time was to be filled by self-determined activity. In the past, children had always needed time for the activities which were possible. Now they needed activities to fill the time at their disposal. Admittedly children still used phrases such as 'I haven't got time', but these were more likely to be defence mechanisms against requirements from outside, rather than a reflection of a true shortage. In the daily routines of 10- to 12-year-olds, many phases were observed which the children described as 'boredom'. In this context we observed a phenomenon which could be termed 'fragmentation of activity'. Whereas in 1990 the children had engaged in longer term projects during their free time, some of which might last for days, in 1994 and 1996 they chose spontaneously from among the opportunities on offer in the environment. They now switched activities, moving from television to computer games and back, from toy cars or electro-mechanical toys to relaxation and back, whereby some of the activities were carried out in parallel. This changing, spontaneous approach to activity heightened the dependence on available objects and external resources.

Relinquishing of Collective Time

Work processes in school and in the production sector had given the children experience of *collective time organisation*. Study Collectives had the objective that their members would complete certain preparations in a certain time. Mutual help was organised with the goal of allowing everyone to attain the learning goal or task completion at a particular time. Each individual member of the brigade carried the responsibility of ensuring that no disturbances came from the Collective which could restrict the common learning process. The aim of this social learning process was to guide children within their Collectives towards responsible time-keeping, by others as well as themselves. Within the Collective approach, a culture of cooperative time developed in which the predictability and reliability of the individual became a precondition of group task completion, and where a relationship of mutual responsibility was required: on the part of the Collective for the work of the individual, and on the part of the individual for the achievement of the Collective. It cannot be denied that this system also created control and self-control mechanisms which generated conditions of personal dependence.

The continuing discipline of time-related behaviour still operating in the peer group indicated in surveys of the 1990s that former time norms persisted in the new society, but without shaping *cooperative* time management. Individual division and control of time no longer occurred with respect to a goal set externally for the community, and the community was no longer judged in terms of the amount of time spent communally and the contribution which the individual had made to it. Time lost its capacity to be a means of discipline in the community. This led to a situation in which the individual could no longer dispose of another's time if the latter did not expressly give permission. The use of one's time now lay to a large extent in one's *own* hands.

Decline of Time as Source of Meaning

Education in the GDR, organised primarily in and through school, was embedded in the concept of a labour society which legitimised its goals and provided its sense of purpose. Work was not only a source of meaning, but a channel through which insights into political and economic frameworks could be developed and corresponding values, including attitudes to time, acquired. Wholly in keeping with the Protestant work ethic, the individual could and should demonstrate his or her moral worth in disciplined labour and make maximum use of the time available. Children and their parents agreed, at least partially, with this ideological guide. Parental patterns included, for example, the idea that time should not be wasted in inactivity. Children should always be busy with something, should always have something meaningful to do, whereby 'meaningful' was always equated with 'something useful'. Lazing, day-dreaming, doing nothing were considered a waste of time. Thus time, in the everyday understanding of families, was always 'time for something'. Adages such as 'Never put off till tomorrow what you can do today' or 'First work then pleasure' became well practised routines for everyday organisation. Although the emphasis lay more on a self-imposed, voluntary exercise of work than on a passive submission to timetables and routines, the exercise was still geared to attaining a more efficient, i.e. more disciplined, more intensive fulfilment of work tasks and the organisation of time they required.

The maxim of holding children to a meaningful use of time was largely retained, although the interpretation of what was to be understood as 'meaningful' expanded. Computer games were included in the definition in many families, as well as occasional Internet surfing; reading continued to be highly rated by parents; sport did not relinquish any of its standing. Television was perceived as a less valuable pastime. However, across the board it could be observed that parents were now more likely to accept phases of relaxation and dreaming, justified by the children as a need for a break, a time of relaxation, or an escape from stress. Lazing, doing nothing, 'hanging around' gained in status. The children had assimilated these phases into their personal time-schemes and the parents not only accepted but even approved the development.

A BRIEF CONTRIBUTION TO THE TRANSFORMATION DEBATE

The principle of time economy had permeated all areas of east German society. As in other industrial societies, a network of interdependencies had built up around features of timing, which had taken on a dynamic of their own.[9] Time had become an element of discipline. The changes in society taking place after 1989 did not topple the dominance of time, but did reduce its orientation to the work process and put its role as a maxim of education into perspective. There is evidence to suggest that, inasmuch as time regimes characteristic of different societies exist simultaneously in the lives of east German children, changes in time management strategies are moving in different directions and time patterns appear ambivalent in children's development. An assertion of this nature allows critical comments to be made with regard to the current debate on the transformation of east German society:

(1) Discussions and studies repeatedly reflect a conception that changes in objective conditions have a linear effect in changing lifestyles and patterns of thought. Thus it is said, for example,[10] that the experience of crisis in the wake of the sociopolitical upheaval of reunification would lead to a heightened perception of anomie and a – perhaps short-term – lack of individual orientation. Journalists express surprise that the increase in buying power and the increase in the range of commodities on the market have not led to greater social satisfaction, yet also comment that widespread long-term unemployment has not led to greater social conflict. Our study findings indicate that children in east Germany are confronted with vastly differing processes of change in conditions and given structures, as well as in life-style, patterns and values, and that these changes cannot be said to be directly linked or mutually determining. It would thus appear that in the case of current developments in east Germany, there cannot be said to be *one* process of change, but a variety of transformations of differing intensity, depth and speed.

(2) Literature in the field[11] frequently marvels at the slowness of the adaptation to western patterns in east Germany, and at the differences evident between the generations. A 'new wall' is considered to be developing in people's minds. Our analysis gives cause to doubt that the changes can be construed as linear in the sense of adaptation to western patterns. Instead, we might suggest a multi-dimensionality in which adaptation and harmonisation processes are taking place while at the same time new structures are developing. It could be conceivable that over a longer period even younger generations will cultivate a way of life which can be seen as specifically east German, in which biography and history, adaptation and constancy, integration and differentiation are united without giving rise to debate about a moral struggle between two collective identities.[12]

(3) Politically determined discussions in particular have recently focused on the new deficits in childhood (child poverty, childcare, deviancy) and

re-evaluate GDR childhood, either upgrading[13] or condemning.[14] Our study confirmed the assumption that the changes are ambivalent and defy moral evaluation as a story of loss or progress, as improvement or collapse, as the liberation or restriction of childhood. In this respect, any statements would be inadequate which suggest that a lost generation is developing in east Germany, characterised by apathy and exhaustion, with a lesser sense of happiness.[15] This manner of interpretation of present developments pursues *ad absurdum* certain lines of thought which postulate that certain developments could be stopped or reintroduced. Quite apart from the wishes and desires of some of the actors, processes in childhood are historically irreversible; even if the desire to do so were present, childhoods cannot be recovered.

NOTES

1. R. G. Barker and H. F. Wright, *One Boy's Day: A Specimen Record of Behavior* (New York: Row and Peterson, 1951); R. G. Barker and H. F. Wright, *Midwest and its Children: The Psychological Ecology of an American Town* (New York: Row and Peterson, 1955).
2. H. Zeiher, 'Verselbständigte Zeit – selbständigere Kinder?', *Neue Sammlung*, 28, 1 (1988), pp. 75–92; H. J. Zeiher and H. Zeiher, *Orte und Zeiten der Kinder* (Weinheim und München: Juventa, 1994).
3. D. Kirchhöfer, *Aufwachsen in Ostdeutschland* (Weinheim und München: Juventa, 1998).
4. M. Bois-Reymond, P. Büchner, H. Krüger, H.-H. Hermann, J. Ecarius and B. Fuhs (eds), *Kinderleben* (Opladen: Leske und Budrich, 1994); H. Oswald and L. Krappmann, 'Social Life of Children in a Former Bipartite City', in P. Noack, M. Hofer and J. Youniss (eds), *Psychological Responses to Social Change* (Berlin and New York: Walter de Gruyter, 1995), pp. 163–86; P. Büchner, B. Fuhs, H. Krüger, H.-H. Hermann (eds), *Wege aus der Kindheit in Ost- und Westdeutschland* (Opladen: Leske und Budrich, 1996); G. Trommsdorff (ed.), *Sozialisation und Entwicklung von Kindern vor und nach der Vereinigung* (Opladen: Leske und Budrich, 1996); J. Zinnecker, R. K. Silbereisen, *Kindheit in Deutchland: Aktueller Survey über Kinder und ihre Eltern* (Weinheim und München: Juventa, 1996); H. Oswald, 'Young People and the Family', in E. Kolinsky (ed.), *Social Transformation and the Family in Post-Communist Germany* (Basingstoke: Macmillan, 1998), pp. 164–79; H. Oswald, 'Sozialisation und Entwicklung in den neuen Bundesländern. Ergebnisse empirischer Längsschnittforschung', *Zeitschrift für Soziologie der Erziehung und Sozialisation (ZSE)*, Beiheft 2 (1998), pp. 4–16.
5. J. Ennew, 'Time for Children or Time for Adults', in J. Qvortup, M. Badry, G. Sgritta and H. Wintersberger (eds), *Childhood Matters: Social Theory, Practice and Politics* (Aldershot: Avebury, 1994), pp. 125–45.
6. *Aufwachsen in Ostdeutschland*.
7. J. Youniss, P. Noack and M. Hofer, 'Human Development Under Conditions of Social Change', in J. Youniss, P. Noack and M. Hofer (eds), *Psychological Responses to Social Change* (Berlin and New York: Walter de Gruyter, 1995), pp. 1–9.
8. D. Kirchhöfer, 'Kinderarbeit und die Ökonomie der Zeit in der DDR. Eine Betrachtung zur Rationalität des Kinderalltages in der DDR', *Sozialwissenschaftliche Informationen (SOWI)*, 27, 2 (1999), in press.
9. 'Verselbständigte Zeit – selbständigere Kinder?'.
10. M. Grundmann, T. Binder, W. Edelstein and T. Krettenauer, 'Soziale Krisenerfahrung und die Wahrnehmung sozialer Anomie bei Ost- und Westberliner Jugendlichen: Ergebnisse einer Kohorten- und Längsschnittanalyse', *Zeitschrift für Soziologie der Erziehung und Sozialisation*,

Beiheft 2 (1998), pp. 171–87.

11. K. Biedenkopff, 'Die Einheit: eine einzigartige Leistung', *Die Zeit*, 9 September 1995; W. Schluchter, *Neubeginn durch Anpassung. Studien zum ostdeutschen Übergang* (Frankfurt: Suhrkamp, 1996); R. Finke, 'Zukunftsvorstellungen ostdeutscher Jugendlicher' (Berlin: Institut für angewandte Demographie (IFAD), 1998).

12. L. Ensel,*'Warum wir uns nicht leiden mögen...'* *Was Ossis und Wessis voneinander halten* (Münster: Agenda, 1993).

13. Emnid-Studie, 'Die Ostdeutschen', *Berliner Zeitung*, 1 August 1995.

14. R. Wald, *Kindheit in der Wende – Wende der Kindheitt* (Opladen: Leske und Budrich, 1998); C. Pfeiffer, 'Die letzte Bastion der DDR', *Berliner Zeitung*, 12 March 1999.

15. A. Hessel, M. Geyer, J. Würz and E. Brähler, 'Psychische Befindlichkeiten in Ost- und Westdeutschland im siebten Jahr nach der Wende', *Aus Politik und Zeitgeschichte*, B13 (1997).

13

Managing Unemployment: Experiences and Strategies of Women in the New *Bundesländer*

Vanessa Beck

The whole of unified Germany is currently facing the problem of mass unemployment but in the New Bundesländer the experience is even more painful than in the west, and unemployment figures for women are still higher than those for men. The profundity of the experience is due, partly, to the socialist heritage and partly to the gender divisions in the formerly west German tradition. Findings of previous research on unemployment were drawn on to design research questions and expectations, but also to compare and contrast them with east German women's responses to unemployment, an experience virtually unknown in the GDR. Employment was not only the basis for financial security but also the link to social activities, health and childcare provisions – work equalled societal integration. The empirical research introduced here focuses on the responses to unemployment as well as the impact for individual women. How do women cope with losing a fundamental aspect of their lives? How do they react to this very basic threat? In looking for answers, 22 in-depth interviews were conducted with unemployed women in Magdeburg, Saxony-Anhalt, in April 1998. The very small sample made it possible to concentrate on individual experiences and coping strategies and therefore responses to unemployment.[1] The underlying framework for the interviews was derived from previous, traditional research on unemployment.[2] The empirical research at stake here indicates east German women to be flexible and active and, therefore, not using traditional patterns of reactions to unemployment. These indicative results should be used to reflect on (and reconsider) both general and representative reactions to unemployment.

EAST GERMAN WOMEN SINCE THE *WENDE*

East German women's background socialisation in the GDR was one in which full employment, as well as its compatibility with family and motherhood, was possible and even enforced. Although these opportunities provided by the state no longer exist, it must be recognised that the past has had a lasting influence on these women's life plans, patterns and current expectations. The continuous work motivation, which has been widely documented, proves their distinctiveness.[3] They are not merely accepting the changes but are attempting to continue their life plans by adjusting to the changed environment and circumstances. Ultimately, this is an attempt to influence the political agenda in their favour.

In addition, it must be considered that united Germany is continuing the western trend of the male breadwinner model which, although currently being eroded, is nevertheless a shock for east German women. The mere fact that this model is still a basis of the social security system and, even more importantly, is still ingrained in popular perception, is alienating. Eastern women thus perceive the move towards what Beck[4] has called the 'risk society' as far stronger. In this, the family-based social security system[5] is being replaced by a more individualised approach that – albeit threatening to women – is also opening new opportunities. Consequential discontinuity in occupational biographies can ultimately lead to financial hardship; and mass unemployment, the main issue at stake here, heightens these dangers.

The new German *Bundesländer* have moreover had to adjust to the western system. Institutional transition is completed but the process of social transformation continues as norms, values and milieus are also transferred. The latter is proving to be more difficult and lengthier than expected. The fact that a significant element of the east German population feels second-class citizens and voices discontent with the implementation of democracy is a strong indicator that the east is maintaining a distinct identity.[6] Statistically, it could be argued that east German women are attempting to minimise the risks by recasting their biographies.[7] Marriage, divorce and childbirth patterns have all changed dramatically since German Democratic Republic (GDR) times, giving rise to terms such as the 'birth-strike'.[8] While the figures for marriages and births stabilised at about half the GDR's rate, divorces quickly surged and have exceeded even the high figures of the GDR.[9] Increases in single households are in part due to an ageing population but it could also be suggested that women prefer to stay or become single and refrain from having children until an ever-later age to ensure their independence, for example in pension benefits. Similar strategies would thus also be possible in east German women's responses to unemployment.

UNEMPLOYMENT AND THE LABOUR MARKET
IN SAXONY-ANHALT

Saxony-Anhalt shows a typical development for the New *Bundesländer* in that its unemployment rates have been persistently high, and difficult economic changes have complicated the situation. The region formerly relied mainly on three sectors – the chemical industry, mechanical engineering/lignite mining and agriculture – all of which have experienced a drastic decline since the *Wende*. In Magdeburg it was especially the splitting up of well-known firms such as SKET (*Maschinen- und Anlagenbau AG*) and SKL (*Motoren- und Systemtechnik AG*) that created problems. The small enterprises formed out of branches of these big firms might well be prospering but that does not compensate for previous mass redundancies. Moreover, it was not only easier for the *Treuhandanstalt* (Trustee Institution charged with the restitution, privatisation and restructuring of GDR state assets) to privatise male-dominated sectors, such as building, but the idea of *Sozialverträglichkeit* (socially-acceptable change), making privatisation socially manageable, was usually based on the male breadwinner model introduced from the west, so that women would lose out on the few jobs that did remain.

In Saxony-Anhalt, as in most of the New *Bundesländer*, unemployment has given the second labour market great importance. The most frequently subsidised measures are work creation schemes and further education and retraining. Although active labour market policies are, in the short term, a financial benefit and offer psychological relief, their long-term effect must be questioned. The interviews showed that any time spent out of employment generally, and specifically out of an occupational field for which the individual has trained, can lead to a loss of human capital, stigmatisation and exclusion from the first labour market.[10] Moreover, despite securing a continuation of entitlement to unemployment benefits, the measures do not halt a possible decline into poverty as badly paid work creation schemes will form the basis for subsequent unemployment benefits. In this context, criticism of the federal government's implementation of active labour market measures should be mentioned, as this has been seen as a manipulation of (un-)employment statistics. Women in Saxony-Anhalt are thus in a situation in which their secure life-style from GDR times has been replaced by risk. Exclusion from the institutional level and the consequential importance of the second labour market add to these insecurities.

INSTITUTIONAL VERSUS INDIVIDUAL LEVEL

What will be proposed here is a Three-Phase Model of reactions to unemployment rather than the four phases of most previous research on unemployment which have apathy as their final outcome. The first two phases, in which the individual is at first very optimistic and active in a search for re-employment but sinks later into depression if these attempts are futile, were detectable in the interviewees. The consequential withdrawal from society, loss of time structure and final apathy were not observed. Instead, a stabilisation occurred at the individual level. The term 'individual' or private sphere depicts a continuation of the niche society and is therefore not limited to the unemployed women themselves, as they must be seen in the context of their direct environment, where they look for help and support. This contrasts strongly with the rejection they experience at the institutional level and from which they consequently retreat. In this context, the term 'retreat' is used to signify that official institutions are no longer relied on to solve the problems encountered in unemployment and it should not be confused with the possibility of retreat from society and into isolation, as traditional research outlines. There were very few direct statements regarding the exact time it took to reach this period of stabilisation but it became obvious that this differed within a range from a few weeks to half a year.

In general, most women stated that their social environment had not changed and that pre-*Wende* contacts had been maintained. It is interesting to see that former work colleagues are also part of their contacts as this reinforces the point that such contacts were an important aspect of employment. As for the family, the general impression[11] conveyed is that these women had formerly not spent enough time with their partners and children and were now enjoying more balanced relationships.

> Ja, mit meinem Mann nutze ich das mehr. Wie gesagt, der Tobias, der Kleine, der ist ja ganz viel mit seinem Sport unterwegs und da passiert nicht mehr so viel gemeinsam, aber mit meinem Mann genieße ich das schon. Wenn er nach Hause kommt, bin ich im Grunde genommen fertig. Ich mach auch sehr viel mehr im Garten, so daß er da nicht so viel mithelfen muß und da ist das schon schöner. Da haben wir abends ganz viel Zeit zum Radfahren und Spazieren gehen.[12]

Although this woman spends more time with her husband there is no indication of an excessive development. It should nevertheless be mentioned that this increase in mutual leisure time does seem to depend on the establishment of gender-specific roles. However, at the individual level the women interviewed had vital relationships that supported them in their coping strategies. Both family and friends, whether they were old ones or newly established post-*Wende* ones, provided resources for the majority of women, although it was more important for some to cope on their own. Marriages and partnerships were considered to be based on an equal contribution by both partners and this situation extended to the sharing of household duties. Despite this there were examples (such as the above quotation) of a genderisation of tasks as well as a return to a traditional gender role.

Nevertheless, all interviewees attached great meaning and importance to work. The experience of unemployment included a sense of uselessness, especially as most women had liked their jobs. The social aspects attached to work in the GDR were also relevant so that the women missed social contacts, being challenged and having the feeling that they were contributing to society. Despite this, there was no attribution of fault to themselves as none of the interviewees felt guilty for being unemployed. This is important because feelings of guilt can heighten the psychological impacts.[13] If the failure can be attributed to others, rather than to the individual concerned, it makes coping with the process easier.

This held for all interviewees, but they were also aware of the general situation and environment and many women stated that, in times of mass unemployment, it is futile to blame the individual. In this context the picture of the average citizen, *'der kleine Mann auf der Straße'*, was a recurring theme in many of the interviews, thus also reinforcing an often mentioned sense of helplessness. The individual was thus not seen as having any influence or power, all of which was ascribed to the state, sometimes in combination with industry. The women thus indicated that they did not feel part of, or at least had no influence on, society. This is in line not only with previous research[14] but also mirrors the commonly voiced, profound criticism of help structures, especially of the employment offices. There are indications that personnel within these bureaucratic structures have not changed from GDR times.[15] This explains the strength of what could almost be called hostility towards the employment offices. It also helps explain why individuals perceive them as ineffective:

> Denn das Arbeitsamt das können'se vergessen (lacht). Können'se vergessen. Wenn'se nicht wollen, wollen'se nicht. Und so wie ich das gesehen habe jetzt, und ich kann mir wohl ein kleines Urteil erlauben da, da wird sehr viel geschoben, mit ABM-Stellen und so weiter und so fort … Und ich könnte manchmal, wenn ich zum Arbeitsamt gehe

oder die Leute sehe von früher – ich liebe Offenheit, Ehrlichkeit, ich kann keine Ungerechtigkeit ertragen – und wenn ich die sehe, daß die alle wieder da sind. Nee![16]

A spokesperson from the employment office in Magdeburg stated the reason for non-acceptance to be that these institutions are new and, consequently, need time to be accepted. In addition, active labour market measures had been seen as a temporary bridge and a preparation of the population for the competitive labour market. This had raised hopes of a fast transfer into stable employment which did not take place and therefore merely added to the mistrust.

Although they may be correct, these statements consider only one aspect of the problems and, according to the interviews, much of the distrust is due to individual encounters rather than general changes. Most women do not consider the employment offices to be helpful in any way. Ultimately, this results in a lack of official channels for any re-integration into the job market, especially as the inability of employment offices to deliver actual jobs could have reinforced old patterns of withdrawing to the individual level for solutions. The offices are not perceived as providing access but are seen as mechanisms of exclusion. Statements on how the employment offices are undermined by informal networks indicated this. The results of the interviews show that these women depend virtually exclusively on informal networks and channels, similar to those in the GDR. Although this maintenance of old habits may make it easier for some to get by in the new system, this at the same time disadvantages those without these effective networks. Overall, women withdraw individually because they feel forced out of the institutional structures.

RESPONSES TO UNEMPLOYMENT

Although the first reaction to unemployment was often extreme, usually shock or relief, this was unlikely to be sustained for a long period of time. As indicated in the Three-Phase Model of Reactions to Unemployment, the women did demonstrate a process of stabilisation, reached by what has been termed a retreat to the individual level. The most common response to questions regarding the current situation within unemployment was one of acceptance. The women were 'getting by' despite problems. These seemed to have moved into the background. The interviewees conveyed a sense of having come to terms with and arranged their lives in accordance with their redundancy. Within this, it should be mentioned that general feelings and attitudes were not unambiguous but varied on a regular basis between optimism and pessimism. The mood swings, though, were no longer as strong as during the initial phase.

This stability is maintained by different means as each woman finds an individual solution of how to get by. One very common tactic seems to be a repression of any thoughts about unemployment. Any activities or contacts described as part of the individual level must therefore be seen as vitally important as they primarily repress negative feelings established by unemployment and, secondly, fulfil functions formerly filled by the workplace. The point to be made is that an equilibrium has been established which enables these women to lead a reasonably normal life.

> Die jungen Frauen, die jetzt in den Beruf gehen, die haben von ihren Müttern noch was anderes mitbekommen. Ich mach mir um unsere Tochter weniger Sorgen als um unseren Sohn. Es gibt eine andere Haltung zur Arbeit und die Ostfrauen identifizieren sich mit der Arbeit. Und jetzt wo sie keine Arbeit haben, denke ich ist diese Identifikation noch viel größer. Weil ich jetzt auch merke, wie wichtig mir das war. Das hat einfach mit dem Verlust zu tun ... Ich denke auch, wenn man aufgibt, dann hat man verloren ... Also ich füge mich nicht dem Schicksal und das bringt mir dann irgendwo auch Spaß.[17]

Although the developments are seen as fate this does not mean these women resign to them. The attitude of not wanting to give up (and even to enjoy battling against fate) shows a strong resilience and determination which is explained by the identification with the workplace as well as the painful loss of it. Attempts to return into the labour market thus continued, although most women conveyed the impression that they had integrated their search for employment into their daily routine and were searching constantly but 'on the side'. This continued work motivation is significant because it indicates that the retreat to the individual level is not irreversible but is merely considered to be a phase which will bridge the time until re-integration into employment. Although there are, objectively, few chances of this happening, these women have not given up hope altogether. Due to the activities and social contacts they maintain, it could be hypothesised though, that were re-integration to occur, it would be easier for the individual herself to accomplish.

The financial situation is important because it has an enhancing or mitigating effect on the jobless. Flockton[18] states female wage rates to be relatively high as there has been a positive income development in the east of Germany, but at the same time predicts that income poverty might increase. He argues that due to the expiration of transitional arrangements after unification, the increase in income differentiation could accelerate. It should also be mentioned, though, that the earnings gap is narrowest in the new German *Länder* when compared within Europe.[19] Nevertheless, the shift from unemployment benefits to social assistance, which usually only applies to the long-term unemployed (and thus a large proportion of the sample in this study), bears an even higher risk of poverty. If the interviewees are not currently poor they are threatened by poverty. The results of the interviews regarding this aspect were not clear-cut. In part this is due to a variety of situations: some husbands were still in work, thus giving financial security, and benefits can offer broad coverage. Not only is there an important difference between unemployment benefits and social benefits but the rates also depend on the last wage that was paid to the individual. In some cases this was paid during GDR times and was consequently very low. The GDR as a background is also important as it pre-conditions the individual's attitude to money and materialism. A typical, perhaps even stereotypical, response was that although less money was available during GDR times, this had been enough to ensure a decent life. Often this depended on two incomes so that this is an area where women have now lost out in their independence – partly due to unemployment and partly to a gender gap in wages which translates into a gap in unemployment benefits.

> Also, so lang mein Mann gearbeitet hat da war's so, daß es ausgereicht hat. Und da konnte man auch sich mal einiges leisten. Aber jetzt wo er 'ne Rente bekommt, ich Arbeitslosengeld, das auch mal aufhört, also, da muß ich sagen, sehe ich doch mit Bedenken in die Zukunft.[20]

Although more money was the norm after the *Wende*, most women were only just coping. They stated they had enough but only if they planned carefully and did not spend on any extras such as holidays, expensive clothing or meals out. Different evaluations of the financial situation by the various interviewees suggested correspondence to the length of unemployment, thus reinforcing the point that second labour market measures are not necessarily beneficial in the long term. A similar diversity was noticeable in the influence of financial situations on individual lives. The responses included fear and worries, nightmares and nervousness as well as a perceived threat of social exclusion and lack of social contacts.

A key theme of previous research on unemployment has been its effect on health. The severe shock and trauma experienced upon unemployment has been linked to illness. In responding to a shock experience such as unemployment, mind and body can be regarded as linked. Psychosomatic reactions are thus also a possible side effect of unemployment. As already stated, the final conclusions of traditional research cannot be supported by the present findings. Although most women in this study underwent a phase of depression, they did not, at the time of the interview, give any indications that giving up was even a possibility for them: they thus showed signs of a *Durchhalte-Ideologie* (a 'seeing it through' mindset) . One women even stated that she did not know depression because she was so optimistic:

> (A)m Anfang habe ich plötzlich tausend Wehwehchen gehabt, die ich vorher nicht kannte, aber das hatte sich denn – ließ das auch wieder nach ... Und ich sag mir immer, irgendwie wird's schon weitergehen und ich mach denn eben was mir Spaß macht und dadurch bin ich nicht so 'n Typ, der dann gleich verzweifelt oder sowas, aber das ist wahrscheinlich von der Mentalität abhängig.[21]

This optimism cannot be taken for granted, however, as the following quotation shows. In her reply to whether being ill was a direct result of unemployment, this women nevertheless shows an ironic sense of humour:

> Ja, ja, daß macht einen irgendwie krank. Ah, das ist so das Gefühl, ich möchte bald sagen, das ist ein seelisches Gefühl des nicht mehr gebraucht und nicht mehr gefördert zu sein ... Ja, ich meine psychisch – das legt sich dann ja auch alles auf den Körper irgendwie ab. Manchmal, so dunkele Tage, da sind Sie richtig deprimiert und dann vielleicht noch sowas schönes, wenn der Herr Kohl dann sagt, wir sollen doch endlich mal die Arbeitslosen an die Arbeit bringen. Das ist doch deprimierend. Wenn der Herr Kohl soviel gearbeitet hätte wie unsere Leute in der DDR, dann würde er auch einen Zentner dünner sein. Es ist so.[22]

It must be mentioned that the majority of the participants were reluctant to go into any depth on this issue. Nevertheless, the psychological aspect seemed to predominate and within this, anxiety seemed to be far more common than severe depressions. Even if the women did not state it themselves, the fact that many of these worries were related to unemployment suggests that the effects of job loss may be more severe than most would admit. Despite amounting to a suppression of emotions, this can be expected to assist coping strategies.

These strategies are especially important considering that some women spoke of social stigmatisation. This seemed to take three different forms. Firstly, a belief that in the public's opinion, the unemployed do not want to work and secondly, that this view does not differentiate between individual situations; thirdly, that obligatory visits to the employment office are considered to be stigmatising. The employment offices were mentioned frequently in this context, thus reinforcing their above-mentioned bad reputation. The cushioning effect of the collective experience of mass unemployment is disturbed via stigmatisation, especially as the allocation of work was described as arbitrary. The only possible solution is therefore individual. This is a description of a divided society in which employment is the determining factor of influence, integration and possession.

A further strategy of managing daily life within unemployment is the relation to time and the structuring of a typical day. Traditional research would point to loss of time structure in daily life. Within the second phase of the responses to unemployment the results of traditional research seem to be applicable as the depressed phase often included a withdrawal from society and a loss of interests and activities. As soon as the women entered the third phase and retreated to the individual level this no longer seemed to be the case. There was a problem evaluating time management, though, as activities mentioned in interviews were not necessarily day filling, despite being considered to be so by the interviewees. In some cases it was difficult to distinguish clearly between the depressed phase and the retreat to the individual level, as many women stated that they still have temporary depressions within the latter. It could also be that the women did not consider all daily activities worth mentioning, as most of them gave a general overview rather than in-depth descriptions. The main statement by the women was, nevertheless that they knew how to occupy themselves. Hobbies, for example, were often mentioned. In some cases this almost took the form of a justification as some women insisted on an overabundance of things to do. This corresponded with an awareness of the danger of 'letting go' as many had experienced this temporarily. It has been suggested that the second phase of unemployment is a depressive one, during which activities decline and any interest in the environment can terminate. Due to this, a structure or time plan was often, consciously or unconsciously, imposed on daily life.

Although many of the interviewed women stated they felt helpless in respect of unemployment or politics in general, their individual responses and daily structures showed a high level of activity and thus resilience. Most knew they had few, if any chances on the labour market and, due to the importance they attached to work, considered this a depressing fact. This did not stop them from continuing their search for employment but they did not seem to consider the institutional level worth 'wasting their energy on'. The opposite was found to be the case for the individual level.

POTENTIAL AND OUTLOOK

The results of the interviews conducted for this study showed a very differentiated picture of the responses to unemployment by the women in Magdeburg. The two main findings are that these women demonstrate strong signs of distress similar to those found in men in previous studies, while they also have a remarkable resilience and individual potential to cope.

The women participating felt the institutional level had let them down. Most of them were fully aware of the fact that they have few chances in the labour market and that this is, to a large extent, due to their gender. Nevertheless, attempts to remain in the labour market emerged as a key strategy of coping with unemployment. Despite the lack of employment these women have not given up hope and continue their active search for re-employment and thus re-integration into the labour market, even if only on the second labour market. These second labour market measures are nevertheless not considered as an end to or even a break in unemployment. They are a temporary relief, in both financial and psychological respects, but are not a structural solution and can even be seen as a dead end. Despite their beneficial effects in the short term, their low status and, often, their inadequacy in relation to the first labour market they can work out to be further disadvantages.

As a consequence of the situation in both the first and the second labour market, women have been forced out of the institutional structures. The responses of the interviewees were, almost obstinately, to get by despite the disadvantages; they attempted to continue life patterns and plans. Functions formerly satisfied by employment are replaced by activities at the individual level. Despite all the difficulties, such as the length of unemployment or the depressive phases these women experience, they quite clearly did not give up. Thus, the ultimate results of previous research on unemployment in which the responses finally led to apathy cannot be confirmed.

Due to the limited scope of this study and its particular focus, some more general questions remain unanswered. On the basis of the individual responses to unemployment presented here it has been possible, to some extent, to generalise the reactions, but no clear-cut typology has been established. This should be determined by broader based research. Within this, factors such as age, familial status, qualification, existence of children (and their age) would have to be considered.

Women's perception of institutional support, or rather the lack of such help, highlights the mismatch between the services of the employment offices and actual needs. Voicing this dissatisfaction could pressurise the employment offices into being more responsive to women's needs. In addition, the establishment, for example, of unemployment or women's groups and the activities of the equal opportunities representatives are already active steps in the direction of exerting influence and pressure. Women have made their non-acceptance of unemployment public and have begun to articulate their dissatisfaction with existing institutional provisions. In doing so, their voices may change the political agenda in two ways. Firstly, they could influence institutions to be more 'user' friendly, especially towards women. Secondly, they force a reconsideration of women's (un-)employment, as they wish it to be recognised that the 'alternative' role of housewife and mother no longer has validity. Consequently, the agendas of institutional support should be reset towards accepting women's entitlement to labour market opportunities. These possibilities would then have to be weighed against problems such as the lack of integration of women into the political decision-making process, which amounts to a lack of future influence. The practical implementation of this issue of integration as well as development of women's activities to influence the process should be the subject of further research.

In focusing on coping strategies, the importance of women's interests and reintegration into the labour market has been established. These cannot be neglected, in the light of the interviewees' life plans and patterns. This study has shown that women have a certain ability to cope with unemployment, despite its profound and negative impact, but this should not suggest that they be denied employment opportunities and limited to the roles of housewife and mother.

The research presented here indicates that east German women's response to unemployment is an individualised but normal experience; they do not however sink into exclusion and failure. Representative research must show whether this is actually the case. The abilities, levels of resilience and patterns of activity found among the Magdeburg interviewees suggest that the potential of these women has not been realised, especially considering the qualifications and experience most of them display. This potential should not be wasted, especially when one considers that the abilities demonstrated by the interviewed women do seem to fit the requirements of the new 'risk society'.

NOTES

1. The sample consisted of 22 unemployed women. Some of them were currently – and all of them had been in the past – on labour market measures. On average, the women were 46·8 years old and their age was reflected in the fact that over half were married and with adult children. The average length of unemployment was 4·2 years. Qualifications varied strongly and it was noticeable that

over a third of the sample had more than one qualification, most of which had been achieved during GDR times.

2. The term 'traditional' research is used because few studies are explicitly on women's unemployment. Alternatively, they are based on the presumptions of the male breadwinner model, which skews the perception and reinforces bias. See, for example, Klaus Heinemann *et al.*, *Arbeitslose Frauen – Zwischen Erwerbstätigkeit und Hausfrauenrolle* (Weinheim: Beltz, 1983). Nevertheless, valuable findings can be highlighted. Prolonged unemployment has been found to have a severe social and psychological impact on the individual, which can lead to withdrawal and exclusion from society, isolation and depression.

3. See, for example, E. Kolinsky, 'Women in the New Germany', in G. Smith, W. E. Paterson and S. Padgett (eds), *Developments in German Politics 2* (Basingstoke: Macmillan, 1996), pp. 267–85; Hildegard Maria Nickel, 'Der Transformationsprozeß in Ost- und Westdeutschland und seine Folgen für das Geschlechterverhältnis', *Aus Politik und Zeitgeschichte*, B51 (1997), pp. 20–9; and S. Schenk and U. Schlegel, 'Frauen in den neuen Bundesländern – Zurück in eine andere Moderne?', *Berliner Journal für Soziologie*, 3, 3 (1993), pp. 369–84.

4. U. Beck, *Risikogesellschaft* (Frankfurt: Suhrkamp, 1986).

5. This existed in both German states although the changes are likely to be more threatening when compared with the secure situation in the GDR, in which individuals could and even had to plan ahead for a whole lifetime.

6. Dieter Fuchs *et al.*, 'Die Akzeptanz der Demokratie des vereinigten Deutschlands', *Aus Politik und Zeitgeschichte*, B 51 (1997), pp. 3–12.

7. E. Kolinsky, 'Recasting Biographies: Bestandsaufnahme einer problematischen Normalisierung', unpublished paper presented at the *Social Transformation and the Family* ESRC Seminar (Potsdam: University of Potsdam, 13–15 February 1998).

8. Reinhard Liebscher *et al.*, 'Bevölkerungsentwicklung und Bevölkerungsstrukturen', in Gunnar Winkler (ed.), *Sozialreport 1995* (Berlin: Gam Media, 1995), pp. 48–80.

9. The demographic developments described here are based on data provided by the *Statistisches Bundesamt* under http://www.statistik-bund.de.

10. M. Eichler, 'Arbeitsbeschaffungsmaßnahmen in Sachsen-Anhalt', *Forschungsbeiträge zum Arbeitsmarkt in Sachsen-Anhalt* (Gelbe Reihe), 10 (1997), pp. 25–56.

11. This is supported by other studies; see, for example, B. Bütow *et al.*, *Frauen in Sachsen: Zwischen Betroffenheit und Hoffnung* (Leipzig: Rosa-Luxemburg-Verein, 1992).

12. Yes, with my husband I do make more use of it [free time together]. As I've already said, Tobias, the little one, is often out and about with his sports and we don't do that much together any more. But with my husband I do appreciate it. I've done [all the housework] when he gets home. I also do a lot more in the garden so that he doesn't have to help and that improves matters. We then have plenty of time in the evenings to go cycling and for walks.

13. David Klein *et al.*, 'Learned Helplessness, Depression and the Attribution of Failure', *Journal of Personality and Social Psychology*, 33 (1976), pp. 508–16.

14. D. Walz and W. Brunner, 'Das Sein bestimmt das Bewußtsein', *Aus Politik und Zeitgeschichte*, B51 (1997), pp. 13–19.

15. J. Glaeßner, 'Regime Change and Public Administration in East Germany', *German Politics*, 5, 2 (1996), pp. 185–200.

16. Forget about the employment office (laughs). Just forget it. If they don't want to help, they just don't want to. And the way I see it – and I think I've the right to make some sort of judgement – there's a lot of wheeling and dealing with work creation schemes and all that … Sometimes at the employment office or when I see people from the past [all still in the same job] – I love openness, honesty and I can't stand injustice – and when I see those ones who're still in the same places, I just think, Oh no!

17. There are still young women entering the labour market now who learned different things from their mothers. I'm less worried about my daughter than about my son. There are different attitudes towards work, and women from the east identify with work. And now that they've no work, I believe this identification has become even stronger. Because I now realise how important it was to me. It's something to do with loss … I think too if you give up, you're finished … I don't bow to fate and somehow that gives me satisfaction.

18. C. Flockton, 'Economic Transformation and Income Change', in E. Kolinsky (ed.), *Social Transformation and the Family in Post-Communist Germany* (Basingstoke: Macmillan, 1998), pp. 99–117.

19. According to a handout distributed at a Women's Committee Meeting of the European Trade Union Confederation (http://www.etuc.org) in February 1999 the wage gap in the New *Bundesländer* was narrowest (at 12 per cent), which is significantly less than in the member state with the smallest difference: Sweden at 17 per cent.
20. Well, as long as my husband was working, it was enough. And we could afford things now and again. But now he's on his pension and I'm on unemployment benefits and that'll stop sooner or later, well, I must say, I have my doubts about the future.
21. At first I had a thousand aches and pains that I never had before – but they went away again … And I always say to myself that somehow or other things will be all right, and then I just do what I like doing and so I'm not the kind of person to give up or anything like that. But it probably just depends on your outlook.
22. Yes, it does make you ill somehow. It's a feeling, I'd almost say a really emotional feeling, of not being needed or supported any more … Well, psychologically, I think it has a sort of impact on the body too. Sometimes on dark days, you feel depressed and then 'nice' things happen like Mr Kohl saying jobs should be found for the unemployed. It's depressing. If Mr Kohl had worked as much as our people in the GDR, he would weigh 100 kg less. That's the way it is.

14

Violence Against Women: Sexual Offences and Victim Support in Saxony-Anhalt

Ingrid Hölzler

VIOLENCE AND GENDER RELATIONS

As a theme for discussion and research, violence has gained prominence in recent years. Several studies have shown how violence against women manifests itself, examined its origins and causes and evaluated the help available to its victims.[1] Laws have been amended in favour of women, notably the law of 26 January 1998, the law to combat sexual offences and other dangerous acts of violence.[2] Since then, rape inside marriage has been placed on a par with rape generally and classified as a criminal act. In fact, in the Federal Republic as a whole, no more than 10,000 cases of sexual violence a year are reported to the police. Only one-fifth of these ever goes to court and there most end in acquittal of the accused. It has been estimated that between 50,000 and 300,000 such offences go unreported every year. There can be no doubt that efforts have to be targeted on prevention, drawing on the support of all existing social institutions.[3] On the one hand, women and children have to be protected from violence; on the other hand, stringent social sanctions are required to deter potential offenders from committing acts of violence.

At present, there is little public awareness of the fact that violence against women and children goes beyond attacks against the physical and emotional integrity of a person. It also extends to less apparent forms of force such as behaving in a manner designed to intimidate or deter the expression of an independent will by women and children, and generally riding rough-shod over their needs and wishes. Violence extends from harassment in the street or at work to various forms of misrespect, such as treating individuals as objects, assault and sexual abuse inside and outside the family, as well as rape, the illegal trade in women, forced prostitution or murder. Published findings on the manifestations of violence against women and children and the complex reasons for such violence show that sexual violence can be traced to gender inequalities and the historically uneven power positions of men and women.[4] As in the past, violence against women has been boosted by indifference and a tendency to treat it as a taboo.

Views about violence in gender relations continue to be shaped by the distinctly different discourses in east and west on this issue. Because women in the GDR were 'to some extent less dependent on their husbands since they enjoyed financial independence',[5] official women's studies as well as practical approaches in social work did not acknowledge rape of women and the sexual abuse of children as viable topics. In the Federal Republic, on the other hand, the activities of the new women's movement put violence against women on the agenda as an urgent theme for public discussion.

Despite such different approaches to the issues in the two Germanies, similar practices prevailed. In western and eastern Germany, it was commonplace to let the perpetrators go free while accusing the victims. This arises from the fact that violence against women and also against children is committed in the immediate social environment. The closer the relation between perpetrator and victim, the more difficult it is to press charges. Often, the victims themselves are not convinced that the crime against them would be punished.[6] Thus, it has been observed for both eastern and western Germany, that certain offences, notably sexual abuse and rape, militate against the victims receiving justice; often, women who press charges are ostracised in their neighbourhood or by the authorities. Not least since they are ashamed of what happened to them, most female victims of sexual violence do not come forward.[7] In the German legal system, it is up to the victim to provide evidence and to prove that she is honest (*Glaubwürdigkeitsgutachten*) and of good character. Often, the victim is suspected of telling an untruth, in particular if the accused does not have a criminal record. Sometimes, the crime itself is portrayed as minimal and women are suspected of having encouraged the offender by their appearance or by a lack of resistance.[8]

After the collapse of the GDR, it became evident that 'in the GDR, the theme "violence against women" had not been discussed much'.[9] Encouraged by the successes of the women's movement in the west, east German women now found the courage to acknowledge that sexual violence and rape had existed in the GDR and even reached significant proportions. In confronting the GDR past, it emerged that the official treatment of women as equals had constituted an obstacle to admitting that sexual violence occurred. To highlight such offences was regarded as a critique of the social order. Pressing charges did not get off the ground, since arbitration commissions or the commissions of the Sozialistische

Einheitspartei Deutschlands (Socialist Unity Party of Germany (SED)) or the trade union organisation tended to insist that such a matter was settled 'peacefully'. It is, however, impossible to provide hard evidence for this procedure, but equal opportunity commissioners in east German communities and employees of family and marriage counselling bureaux reported on these problems in conversation.

After unification, it appears that violence against women in the family and sexual violence generally had increased in the wake of high unemployment, an increased economic dependency of women upon their husbands as well changed values and stronger media influences. This, however, cannot be proven, since there are no comparable data for the period before 1989 and any comparison would be unreliable. The academic evaluation of violence is further complicated by conflicting theories. For the purposes of this discussion, the definition of violence formulated by the peace researcher Galtung is the most useful: 'Violence exists when human beings are influenced in such a way that their physical and mental self-actualisation is lower than their potential.'[10] Thus, violence can be divided into two main types: direct or personal violence and indirect or structural violence. While personal violence includes physical assault and all forms of psychological or verbal humiliation, structural violence is 'built into the system through evident inequalities of power relations and the life chances resulting from them'.[11] Both types of violence are closely linked and influence one another. 'Violence is the structural component of a patriarchal society which uses it to secure its hierarchy of power.'[12] Violence manifests itself at a variety of levels such as gender-specific socialisation, employment chances, role expectations and perceived identities.[13]

'Social violence' exists if individuals lack independence as social beings and are denied responsibility by having to seek permission at every turn. Women risk punishment if they do not obey. Ultimately, social violence results in social isolation, loneliness and a loss of identity. Such women feel that nobody would believe their story and are afraid of exposing the actions of their male partners. Often they experience extreme helplessness and powerlessness which may lead to depression, a sense of hopelessness and thoughts of suicide.[14] Women are rarely able to free themselves from this situation since they are ashamed of the violence they suffer and because they fear that nobody will believe them.

'Economic violence' may be defined as financial dependence on a partner who does not allow access to bank accounts and exercises strict control over all economic resources. Especially discriminatory, however, is sexual violence. It exists when the man takes no notice of the individual wishes of the woman by committing coercion, rape, unwanted sexual advances in public life, at work or in the family. The humiliation arising from coercion and rape is the worst of its kind, since it inflicts physical and psychological harm. Contemporary statistics show that beatings occur in all social strata and at all educational levels. It has been suggested that no less than 50 per cent of all women have been subjected to violent treatment at some point in their lives. In the Federal Republic, some four million women a year are assaulted by their husbands; violence, it seems, mars one in three marriages.[15] Commonly held views of marriage and the family and, no less important, the legislation governing them, are framed in such a way as to allow one partner to dominate the other. Suffering, including suffering violence, has even been praised as the pinnacle of femininity. Only the recent changes in the law which recognise violence inside marriage as an offence, have put the spotlight on these problems and clarified the rights of individuals. Today, sexual violence inside the family against women and children has clearly been defined as a crime and is no longer condoned or treated as excusable.

Sexual Violence in Saxony-Anhalt before and after 1989

Notwithstanding the promise of gender equality in the Basic Law, Saxony-Anhalt remains dominated by patriarchal social structures. Men occupy the key positions and receive the higher incomes. In Saxony-Anhalt, just 10 per cent of top management posts are held by women.[16] Such continuing inequalities militate against open discussion of sexual violence and make it impossible to trace its development before and since unification. Taking the GDR statistics of 1986 and 1988 (Table 14.1) reveals that sex offences constituted a relatively small proportion of recorded offences. The data for 1989 (Table 14.2) show the situation for the districts of Halle and Magdeburg. In 1989, 20 per cent of the GDR population lived in Saxony-Anhalt; comparing the data for the GDR in Table 14.1 with the regional data in Table 14.2 suggests that 12 per cent of all rapes and 23 per cent of other sexual assault occurred in the region.[17]

There is, however, a severe shortage of information on the situation in the former GDR. The 1991 Statistical Yearbook records data for Germany since unification but does not cover the former GDR. Even several years later, data remain incomplete. Thus the 1997 *Datenreport* notes that 'since there are no comprehensive crime statistics for the new *Länder* we cannot present results for Germany as a whole'.[18] Data on the old *Länder*, by contrast, are much more comprehensive. Thus, in 1988, 4,843 of a total of 693,499 were 'criminal offences against sexual self-determination'.[19]

In the course of post-communist social transformation, two factors in particular impacted on violence against women in Saxony-Anhalt. The

TABLE 14.1
VICTIMS OF SEXUALLY-ORIENTED CRIME IN THE GDR, 1986–88

Type of criminal offence	1986	1987	1988
Killing with intent	112	136	113
Physical assault	9,842	10,304	10,134
Rape	518	563	530
Sexual assault	402	377	445
Sexual abuse of children	491	560	481

Source: Statistical Yearbook of the GDR, 1989 (Berlin: Staatsverlag, 1989), p. 396.

TABLE 14.2
VICTIMS OF SEXUALLY-ORIENTED CRIME IN THE DISTRICTS OF HALLE
AND MAGDEBURG, 1989

Type of criminal offence	Halle	Magdeburg	Total
Killing with intent	22	7	29
Physical assault	1,241	966	2,207
Rape	16	44	60
Sexual assault	54	66	120
Sexual abuse of children	141	74	215

Source: Statistical Yearbook of the GDR, 1990 (Berlin: Staatsverlag, 1990), pp. 440-1.

first of these was an increasing glorification and radicalisation of male power and strength in the media[20] which are likely to encourage discriminatory or aggressive behaviour towards women. In films, aggressive behaviour, some of it destructive in character, goes together with a male role. Children who spend a significant part of their leisure time watching television absorb gender-specific behaviour patterns linking aggression and resistance with boys, while girls learn that men are in charge or protecting women.[21]

On the other hand, an increasing willingness among women to talk about violence has tended to boost their self-confidence. In direct consequence of this development, women are more likely to press charges than they had been in the past. The statistical records for Saxony-Anhalt show that in 1996, 758 women were victims of physical assaults and grievous bodily harm, 201 women were raped, 167 sexually assaulted, while 108 girls suffered sexual abuse. It can be assumed that the actual number of cases was much higher than the number recorded in the crime statistics, since, as mentioned earlier, many women do not press charges and shun the publicity and shame associated with a court case. In 1996, 0.5 per cent of recorded offences were crimes against 'sexual self-determination'.

While constituting a small proportion of all criminal acts, the number of

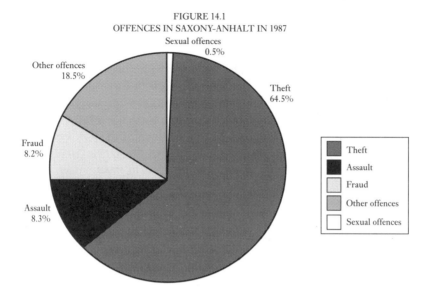

FIGURE 14.1
OFFENCES IN SAXONY-ANHALT IN 1987

Source: Volksstimme, Magdeburg: Lokalanzeiger (25 February 1989), p. 5.

sexual offences increased by 14.5 per cent between 1996 and 1997 (Table 14.3). The increase was particularly marked in relation to rape and sexual abuse of children. In the region as a whole recorded crime fell from 319,665 in 1995 to 294,202 in 1997 while a larger number of crimes was solved and their perpetrators apprehended.[22] A focused publicity campaign and a growing confidence in the police succeeded in reducing the reluctance to report crimes and in encouraging victims to press charges.[23]

The Gendered Context of Violence against Women

When asked to explain why they resorted to using violence, men frequently refer to their childhood and the violence they experienced and learned early in life. Wölfel points out that men 'hardly express any sense

TABLE 14.3
VICTIMS OF CRIMES AGAINST SEXUAL SELF-DETERMINATION IN SAXONY-ANHALT, 1995–97

Criminal offence	1995	1996	1997
Offences against sexual self-determination	1,318	1,430	1,639
of which rape	147	201	205
of which sexual abuse of children	529	525	582

Source: Unpublished material provided to the author by the Ministry of the Interior, *Land* Saxony-Anhalt (6 February 1998).

of doing wrong. Most feel they are innocent and provoked. They describe how they lost control of their senses when they beat their wife or children. Some stress that they had learned during their childhood to react to conflict by using violence.'[24] The main reason for brutal behaviour rests in the traditional role model which men absorb in early childhood. 'A man always has to be strong and "cool". The father is perceived as dominant and able to get his way, as someone who is always active, never cries and never shows emotion. There was no need for him to show emotion since this was the domain of the woman, the mother, the female partner.'[25] These expectations, however, are impossible for men to meet. After the *Wende*, when personal uncertainties and the pressures to achieve and succeed had increased, men felt even more strongly that they had to cope and had to prove that they were irreplaceable.

Research into violence against women further identifies social inequalities between men and women and patriarchal social structures as decisive causes in addition to traditional notions of gender roles and a gender-specific division of labour.[26] No less important are the tendency to belittle and tolerate the use of violence and the male claim of owning the wife or partner. Even language can promote violence against women: 'language may be designed to offend, vilify, accuse, discredit, besmirch, disregard, ignore, ridicule, humiliate or libel and in this way advocates violence'.[27] Trömel-Plötz notes that women suffer violence in conversation through sexist language.[28] Such language permeates dictionaries, school books, newspapers, magazines, joke books and, above all, television. Women are portrayed as stupid and reduced to sex objects. Violence is committed because this image turns into reality in the heads of men.[29] In the final analysis, this type of communication implies that even the dullest and most limited man is, by virtue of his gender, superior to any woman. In everyday life, economic and social hardship, stress at work, lack of self-worth, alcoholism, drug dependency, fear and jealousy can activate the violent potential of men. Men often regard the use of violence as a last-ditch attempt to salvage a relationship. Violence, then, is applied to hide a fear of failure, disappointment, helplessness and feelings of isolation.[30]

Aggressive behaviour is not innate but learned behaviour. It is wrong to assume that aggression is a natural force designed to create or restore order. Rather, the roots of violent behaviour can be traced to childhood experiences where men themselves may have been victims of violence, and to assumptions about women and gender roles they developed in the course of their socialisation. The use of violence 'is more than just an individual act of a man against a women; it is rooted in society and culture and the gender relations – the images of men and women – prevailing in them'.[31] The existence of male violence can only be explained 'with reference to our image of the dominant, conquering male and the related image of women enduring men's violent behaviour.'[32]

Support Services for Women in Saxony-Anhalt: A Case Study

At the request of the section for women's policy at the regional Ministry for Employment, Women, Health and Social Affairs, the author collected information in 1997 and 1998 about support services for women and in particular for victims of sexual violence in the *Land*. The survey draws on written questionnaires[33] and on structured interviews with officials in the police headquarters at Dessau and Magdeburg, the Equal Opportunity Offices at Madgeburg, Dessau and Wittenberg and other social centres in the Magdeburg area, in Naumburg, Weißenfels and Zeitz. The survey revealed positive developments as well as gaps: 'Since 1991, 28 women's houses have been created in Saxony-Anhalt, offering refuge to 240 women and 330 children throughout the region. In 1996, 1,127 women and 1,385 children made use of them in order to escape from violent situations, cope with the trauma associated with these experiences and reorganise their lives.'[34] Yet, there are not enough carers with specific psychology qualifications to assist victims of sexual violence. Existing refuges are inadequate for children and young people and lack specific programmes for rape victims. Moreover, most centres report that they have to refer women and children in need of help to other institutions, since they lack the relevant support services. Women's refuges are publicly funded and rely on staff in work creation schemes. This is unsatisfactory since such employment is insecure and temporary, and entails frequent changes of personnel and a lack of experienced staff. Despite these obstacles, much has been learned from similar institutions in the old *Länder* and a number of effective support measures are in place which will be discussed below:

- *Provision and quality of advice.* Offers of advice for those in need of it, including assistance with finding safe accommodation.

- *Victim support.* Victim support by social workers during interviews with the police and assistance with arranging appointments with doctors and therapists. The involvement of psychiatric social workers also shields witnesses from traumatic consequences of their experience.

- *Individuals accompanying victims.* Individuals who accompany victims of sexual violence or perpetrators of such violence may receive counselling support.

Provision and quality of advice

Our survey showed that 77.8 per cent of all institutions contacted offer a broad range of advisory services for women, including special support for victims of sexual violence.[35] Of the various support programmes on offer, advice is the most fundamental since it provides a first opportunity to communicate specific problems and obtain assistance about the next step. We found that 35 per cent of respondents regarded this first port of call as the most important element of women's support. All conurbations in Saxony-Anhalt have institutions offering such advice. Special emergency telephone numbers allow women and girls to make contact. In 1997, 311 women who had been subjected to sexual violence sought help in this way. Among the reasons for these emergency calls acute sexual violence (30 per cent), psychological violence (13 per cent) and physical violence (10 per cent) were the most frequent. The type of problem determines to which institution or support agency a woman is referred. In the first instance, it is important to give women the feeling that they are not alone with their troubles and that steps can be taken to help. The *Leitstelle für Frauenpolitik* (Policy and Coordination Centre for Women's Issues) of the *Land* also prepared an information booklet, *Help Network for Sexual Violence*, which lists relevant centres and institutions and facilitates contacting them. Moreover, in nine cities in the region special working groups focus on sexual violence and the prevention of sexual abuse.

Our survey of advisory centres revealed that girls and boys rarely sought help from educational or church-affiliated institutions or from the Equal Opportunities Offices in their locality, but turned to helplines. A child-line telephone – *Kinderkummertelefon* – operated from Magdeburg for the region as a whole and on a 24-hour basis. Its telephone number was displayed in schools, care homes and other relevant institutions enabling children from the *Land* as a whole to seek help when they need it. In 1997, 3,381 children called the *Kinderkummertelephone* of whom 1,411 received further personal advice. By far the largest group seeking help are girls aged between 7 and 13. Experiences of violence ranked third among the callers' problems.

Our survey also showed that 40 per cent of the victims of sexual violence seeking advice were transferred to other agencies. The interviews revealed, however, that being transferred to another agency, although intended to be supportive, was experienced as negative and discouraged many from seeking further help. There are signs that some institutions have begun to work more closely together in order to deliver support more effectively. This cooperation should benefit those in need of help.

Significant problems remain in the case of female drug addicts who are also victims of sexual violence since advisory centres for addiction do not cover problems of sexual violence. This void is all the more surprising since researchers and practitioners have provided powerful evidence that experiences of violence and drug additions often go together.[36] The close link between drug consumption, including alcohol and prostitution, highlights the risk of sexual violence in this area.[37]

Today, Saxony-Anhalt operates 28 safe houses which, in accordance with their charter, offer advice and refuge to maltreated and threatened women and children. Of the women residents, 15 per cent had been raped inside a marriage or partnership.[38] Advisory centres operated by Equal Opportunities Offices do not have facilities for providing needy women with accommodation; even self-help groups can only in exceptional circumstances provide housing and a refuge to individual women.

Victim support
One of the most important aspects of victim support concerns support for victims of sexual violence in pressing charges. Here, social workers play a pivotal role in counselling women, young people and children on the consequences of pressing charges and on the processes this will set in motion. At the same time, they direct victims towards therapy and similar programmes.

Between May 1995 and April 1996, 284 individuals received support from a social worker during their contacts with the police. A women police officer stressed during her interview 'that a women who has just been raped by a man should not be put in a situation where she has to face a male police officer at the station all by herself. She should be accompanied by a woman in order make her to feel less vulnerable and more secure.'[39]

The involvement of psychiatric social workers at court is no less

TABLE 14.4
WITNESS SUPPORT DURING CRIMINAL PROCEEDINGS, BY TYPE OF OFFENCE
(1996, in %)

Type of offence to which witness testified	%
Sexual abuse	34.5
Rape	18.7
Sexual assault	11.7
Other sexual offences	15.8
Grievous bodily harm	5.8
Theft	1.8
Reporting a missing person	2.9
Other	8.8
TOTAL	100

Source: Final Report of the research team 'Magdeburger Interventionsprojekt' for the victims of sexual violence see B. Kavemann (Magdeburg and Berlin: Leitstelle für Frauenpolitik des Ländes Sachsen-Anhalt, 1996), p. 13.

important. After charges have been pressed, the victims – women and children – should receive support until the case comes to court and during court proceedings. The practice of accompanying witnesses has also been most beneficial. As Table 14.4 shows, witness support has been particularly significant in cases of sexual abuse (34.5 per cent) and rape (18.7 per cent).

In order to reduce stress during court proceedings and also protect women and children from further abuse, courts have set aside special safe rooms for witnesses. The protective and support measures outlined above are of special relevance in cases involving sexual offences, since social and psychological support during police interviews and in the deposition procedure may impact positively upon the conduct of the main trial.

Individuals accompanying victims
Victims do not normally go to the police or appear in court on their own but in the company of another person. In the case of children, the accompanying person is normally the mother. It has often been overlooked that these accompanying persons also need support. They are expected to strengthen and console the victims, but they often lack the resources to do so. They have been sucked into the crisis consuming the family. Indeed their very presence often makes matters more difficult for the victims since they become impatient when matters do not move quickly enough, notably after the interview with the police. A programme of counselling and of sharing experiences for family members of victims or for accompanying professional helpers can contribute significantly to avoiding stress, generating a sense of stability and counteracting a sense of stigmatisation and isolation.

Similar support measures can and should be offered to individuals accompanying perpetrators but constitute only a very small proportion of support programmes at present. However, extending services to include men seems absolutely necessary. Such services should include advice, therapy and group discussions. Our survey revealed that the virtual absence of such support services for those having committed sexual violence is seen as a shortcoming in the overall provisions within the region.

IMPROVING SUPPORT FOR VICTIMS OF SEXUAL VIOLENCE

By way of conclusion, we should like to detail a number of concrete steps which would improve provisions and their effectiveness for victims of sexual violence.

- In the short term, existing institutions should work more closely together, establishing networks of care which could respond flexibly and appropriately to the problems of sexual violence as experienced by women, young people and children. A model project could prepare the ground for a resource centre of the type already proposed for Madgeburg by the research team on sexual violence in the city.[40]

- In the medium term, an educational programme for the *Land* Saxony-Anhalt could reduce sexual harassment at work. Information should be targeted at occupational sectors and disseminated in special introductory and interdisciplinary seminars. Among the participants, nursery nurses, teachers and social workers, police officers and social psychologists would feature prominently. Such an educational programme would include basic instruction on how to recognise child abuse and child neglect and how to develop concepts of intervention. It would also focus on detecting violence in gender relations, notably rape. Above all, it would provide information on the consequences of violence, the fears and uncertainties of the victims of such violence and suitable support for partners and family members. In order to conquer the dread of legal institutions, the educational programmes should also cover the impact of trials on witnesses and explain the protection available for plaintiffs in criminal proceedings.

- In the longer term, a further step could be taken. In conjunction with an educational programme, guidelines could be developed on how to support the family members of perpetrators and defendants, the professionals accompanying them, and define what therapy might consist of. The *Land* North Rhine-Westphalia has already recorded a favourable outcome from implementing such guidelines. In Saxony-Anhalt, any guidelines should refer specifically to development and problems in that particular region. Support services in Saxony-Anhalt remain less coordinated and patchier than in the western *Länder*. It is evident that public awareness and activity have begun only recently. Before unification, there was no tradition of social work in Saxony-Anhalt and structures for such work had to be created since then. That the *Land* is constantly short of money means that none of the new social institutions is financially secure and the social care work which has been accomplished may be jeopardised or even dismantled at any time.

- Two aspects, it seems, are particularly important in reducing the risk of violence against women. The first concerns the self-confidence of women and girls, and the need to strengthen it. The second concerns public awareness of discrimination against women, an awareness which needs to be sharpened in all walks of life. In order to reduce the risk of violence by men against women, women's social position generally needs to be enhanced. Rendering the glorification of violence in the media unacceptable may be one way of assisting this process.

NOTES

1. See M. Baurmann, 'Positionen, Entwicklungen und Perspektiven bei der Arbeit zum Abbau der Männergewalt: Ein Beitrag aus Männersicht', in Ministerium für die Gleichstellung von Mann und Frau des Landes Nordrhein-Westfalen (ed.), *Gewalt gegen Frauen. 'Was tun mit den Tätern?'* (Düsseldorf: Ministerium für die Gleichstellung von Mann und Frau des Landes Nordrhein-Westfalen, Dokumente und Berichte 24, 1993); K. Frerks, 'Dokumentation Frauen sagen Nein: Bei aller Liebe keine Gewalt' (Hannover und Hamburg: Niedersächsisches Frauenministerium, 1992); A. Minssen and U. Müller, 'Wann wird ein Mann zum Täter?' (Düsseldorf: Ministerium für die Gleichstellung von Mann und Frau des Landes Nordrhein-Westfalen, Dokumentation und Berichte 35, 1995).
2. *Bundesgesetzblatt 1998,* 1, 6 (Bonn, 30 January 1998).
3. I. Hölzler, 'Abschlußbericht zum Forschungsprojekt: Bestandsaufnahme von Angeboten für Frauen und Kinder im Land Sachsen-Anhalt, die Opfer sexualisierter Gewalt geworden sind' (Magdeburg: Leitstelle für Frauenpolitik des Landes Sachsen-Anhalt, unpublished report, 1999), p. 64.
4. Details in C. Hagemann-White, *Strategien gegen Gewalt im Geschlechterverhältnis* (Pfaffenweiler: Centaurus, 1992); E. Ringel and L. Rosenmayr, *Ursachen und Folgen von Gewaltanwendung gegenüber Frauen und Kindern* (Vienna: Bundesregierung Österreichs, unpublished report, 1992).
5. A. Schwarzer, 'Der Mann schlägt immer wieder, wenn...', *Bild der Frau* (25 January 1999), p. 36.
6. 'Innere Sicherheit beginnt daheim', *Neues Deutschland* (24 February 1998), p. 6.
7. Amt für Gleichstellungsfragen der Landeshauptstadt Magdeburg and other institutions (ed.), *Frauendschungelbuch, Wege und Auswege von Frauen für Frauen in Sachsen-Anhalt* (Magdeburg: Amt für Gleichstellungsfragen der Landeshauptstadt Magdeburg, April 1997), p. 201.
8. *Frauen sagen Nein,* pp. 12–13, 57–9; Frerks, *Bei aller Liebe keine Gewalt.*
9. *Frauendschungelbuch,* p. 202.
10. J. Galtung, *Strukturelle Gewalt* (Reinbek: Rowohlt, 1975), p. 15.
11. Ibid., p. 14.
12. D. Kampf, 'Gewalt gegen Frauen in Recht und Rechtsprechung', in Ministerium des Landes Nordrhein-Westfalen für die Gleichstellung von Mann und Frau (ed.), *Dokumentation der Frauengleichstellungsstelle der Landeshauptstadt Düsseldorf* (Düsseldorf: Ministerium des Landes Nordrhein-Westfalen für die Gleichstellung von Mann und Frau, 1990), p. 48.
13. H.-C. Harten, *Sexualität, Mißbrauch, Gewalt* (Opladen: Westdeutscher Verlag, 1995), p. 174; see also Kampf, *Gewalt gegen Frauen,* p. 61.
14. See in particular Emile Durkheim and his work on the interrelationship between social conditions and suicide: E. Durkheim, *Der Selbstmord* (Neuwied: Luchterhand, 1973), reprint.
15. C. Elsner, *'Mit mir nicht': Gewalt in der Partnerschaft* (Munich: Rasch and Röhring, 1995), pp. 14, 388–9.
16. Interview with G. Kuppe, *Mitteldeutscher Rundfunk* (6 October 1998).
17. Staatliche Zentralverwaltung für Statistik (ed.), *Statistisches Jahrbuch 1990 der DDR* (Berlin: Staatsverlag, 1990), pp. 440–1.
18. Statistisches Bundesamt (ed.), *Datenreport 1997* (Bonn: Bundeszentrale für politische Bildung, 1997), p. 231.
19. Statistisches Jahrbuch 1991 für das vereinigte Deutschland (Wiesbaden: Metzler and Poeschel, 1991), p. 373.
20. J. Röser and C. Kroll, *Was Frauen und Mädchen vor dem Bildschirm erleben: Rezeption von Sexismus und Gewalt* (Düsseldorf: Ministerium des Landes Nordrhein-Westfalen für die Gleichstellung von Frau und Mann, June 1995).

21. Harten, *Sexualität, Mißbrauch, Gewalt*, p. 175; R. Luca, *Zwischen Ohnmacht und Allmacht: Unterschiede im Erleben medialer Gewalt von Mädchen und Jungen* (Frankfurt and New York: Campus, 1993); also Rösner and Kroll, *Was Frauen und Mädchen vor dem Bildschirm erleben*, p. 2.
22. T. Wischnewski, 'Staftaten rutschten unter 300000', *Magdeburger Sonntag*, 8 February 1998, p. 3.
23. Information provided to the author by the Ministry of the Interior for the *Land* Saxony-Anhalt (6 February 1998).
24. Interview with H. Wölfel; C. Sperlich, 'Wohin mit der Wut?', *Neues Deutschland*, 8 April 1998, p. 6.
25. Ibid.
26. See I. Dröge-Modelmog and G. Merner, *Orte der Gewalt. Herrschaft und Macht im Geschlechterverhältnis* (Opladen: Westdeutscher Verlag, 1987).
27. S. Trömel-Plötz, *Gewalt durch Sprache* (Frankfurt am Main: Fischer, 1985), p. 50.
28. Ibid., p. 53.
29. Ibid., p. 54.
30. Sperlich, 'Wohin mit der Wut?'.
31. M. Brückner, 'Einbettung von Gewalt in die kulturellen Bilder von Männlichkeit und Weiblichkeit', *Zeitschrift für Frauenforschung*, 1–2 (1993), p. 47.
32. Brückner, 'Einbettung von Gewalt', p. 47.
33. In total, 266 questionnaires were sent out, of which 99 could be included in the analysis – a response rate of 30 per cent.
34. 'Innere Sicherheit beginnt daheim'.
35. Provisions in the region were as follows: general advice was offered by so-called 'Wildwasser Centres' in Magdeburg, Halle and Dessau; specialist advice for victims in Magdeburg, Halle, Dessau, Halberstadt and Stendal; support for victims of sexual violence in Magdeburg and at the advisory centre *Mißmut* in Stendal. Assistance during interviews with the police could be obtained at the police headquarters in Magdeburg and at the district courts in Madgeburg, Halle, Dessau and Stendal, the Crown Court in Magdeburg as well as in the Children's and Youth Court in Magdeburg. The Children's and Youth Protection Centre in Halle also offered programmes in the support of witnesses.
36. A. Flügel and Ch. Merfert-Deite, 'Frauenspezifische Therapie', in Deutsche Hauptstelle gegen die Suchtgefahren (ed.), *Jahrbuch Sucht* (Geesthacht: Deutsche Hauptstelle gegen die Suchtgefahren, 1994); U. Kreyssig, 'Zum Zusammenhang von sexuellem Mißbrauch', in G. Amann and R. Wipplinger (eds), *Sexueller Mißbrauch* (Tübingen: Deutsche Gesellschaft für Verhaltenstherapie, 1997).
37. B. Leopold, and E. Steffan, 'Eva Projekt: Evaluierung unterstützender Maßnahmen beim Ausstieg aus der Prostitution' (Berlin: SPI-Forschung, 1997); B. Kavemann, 'Abschlußbericht der wissenschaftlichen Begleitung des Magdeburger Interventionsprojektes für die Opfer sexueller Gewalt (Magdeburg and Berlin: Leitstelle für Frauenpolitik des Ländes Sachsen-Anhalt, July 1996), p. 86.
38. C. Hagemann-White and B. Kavemann, 'Hilfen für mißhandelte Frauen. Abschlußbericht der wissenschaftlichen Begleitung des Modellprojektes Frauenhaus Berlin', Vol. 124 (Stuttgart: Schriftenreihe des Bundesministeriums für Jugend, Familie und Gesundheit, 1981); Hagemann-White, *Strategien gegen Gewalt im Geschlechterverhältnis*.
39. Hölzler, 'Abschlußbericht zum Forschungsprojekt', p. 86.
40. See Kavemann, 'Abschlußbericht des Magdeburger Interventionsprojektes'.

15

Recasting Civil Society in East Germany

Jonathan Grix

NOTIONS OF 'CIVIL SOCIETY' IN EAST AND WEST GERMAN CONTEXTS

The question of whether there has been some convergence in forms of civil society between east and west Germany over the decade since 1990 is of considerable interest, since it could point to an increasing similarity in structures and modes of associational participation throughout unified Germany. However, the question itself raises the problematic of what is civil society, and whether a universal form can be found for contemporary democracies: this is, in essence, the problem of cross-cultural comparison.

In an east–west setting in Germany, it is obvious that the radically different political, economic and social structures of state centralism and liberal democracy will have had profound impacts on the shaping of modes of voluntary association, and in spite of the flourishing of spontaneous, organic, oppositional forms of participation during the pre-*Wende* (fall of the Wall) period, east German society still retains a distinctiveness of its own and follows a somewhat different path in associational development. While modes of association and participation flourish in the west, easterners still look to the state for much social provision,[1] and a significant section, in supporting the Partei des Demokratischen Sozialismus (Party of Democratic Socialism (PDS)), remain wedded to the solidarity and economic security of the previous regime. It is therefore problematic to assume that both parts of Germany are following the same trajectory in the evolution of civic participation, an activity considered here as central to the development of civil society. This chapter discusses the type of civil society that has emerged in east Germany since the collapse of communist rule. By drawing on pre-unity developments of civil society in the German Democratic Republic (GDR) and by revisiting the post-unity transformation process in the east, it seeks to trace both the distinctiveness and commonalities of civic participation as it exists in east and west.

The definition of the concept of civil society can be extremely broad and presents difficulties in a cross-cultural context. The analytical approach here focuses on civic association and participation, and is informed by the notions of 'Civic Community' and 'Social Capital', in particular those applied in Robert Putnam's study of *Making Democracy Work*.[2] For Putnam, a civic community is one which is characterised and bound together by 'horizontal relations of reciprocity and cooperation, not by vertical relations of authority and dependency', one in which a healthy stock of social capital – that is informal and formal social networks, societal cooperation, norms and above all trust – has been able to develop.[3] Social capital is productive 'like other forms of capital ... making possible the achievement of certain ends that would not be attainable in its absence'.[4] Social capital also further promotes social trust,[5] something obviously in need of rebuilding following GDR citizens' past experience of a society in which trust was a rare commodity and had been systematically violated by the state. Putnam's concepts help sharpen the focus of this chapter on the participatory elements of civil society and on the informal relations that underpin them.

In an east–west comparison, the Putnam concept is far from unproblematical, since it appears to be rooted in a liberal democracy, with what could be taken to be American features. Clearly, and this is a point developed below, the state centralism of the GDR was inimical to the development of independent, formal types of association, but the GDR society was characterised by dense informal networks, in a significant way as a reaction and individual defence against the attempts of the regime to incorporate and coordinate social groupings. Informal networks and relations, prevalent and essential for survival in the GDR, are less easy to measure than formal membership of intermediary associations. Yet, it is these very networks, according to Putnam, that are closely related to and important for civic participation in a democracy.

In contrast, the Bonn Republic developed further the established forms of economic employers' associations, industry and trade union associations which had developed under the Weimar Republic. It also displayed, through the environmental movement among others, the growth of certain forms of post-materialist association to a greater degree than in many other advanced democracies. A further difficulty with the Putnam definition lies in the question of which forms of association and participation are more important for a civic community. Throughout the west, participation in trade unions, in political parties and at elections, in formal associations and so forth is in decline: how do we assess this in terms of the strength of civic culture?

In any east–west German comparison, the analysis must address the historical antecedents, the growth of a public oppositional culture in the GDR in the second half of the 1980s, the survival (or not) of oppositional groups and parties into a unified Germany, and the evolution throughout the 1990s in the new and old *Länder*. The focus in this text is devoted expressly to the new *Länder* with the result that limited reference will be made to associational behaviour and structures in the west. However, to set in context the discussion of the problematic character of (informal) civil society under state centralism, the following brief points can be made of its evolution in the west.

The Bonn Republic had been able to cultivate its own social capital and with it a growing associational culture over a period of some 40 years. The so-called 1968 and post-materialist generations helped shape the nature of political culture in the west, contributing considerably to the experience of open, public articulation of interests. Both 'New Politics' and social movements, which are located at the core of civil society, had a huge influence on the west German political landscape from the 1980s onwards. Their emergence can be traced to dissatisfaction with traditional forms of representative democracy in a mature democratic state.[6] No such evolutionary process was allowed to take place in the GDR.

The thesis in this chapter concerning the uncertain evolution of civil society in east Germany is that, under state centralism, informal modes of association played a central role and the deliberate erosion of the public sphere in the GDR by the authorities determined to consolidate the leading role of the party led to the enforced retreat of citizens into what has been termed a *Nischengesellschaft* (society of niches).[7] It was within this sphere that relationships, informal networks and contacts between citizens were forged. In the second half of the 1980s there was a burgeoning of mass civic activity culminating in the events of autumn 1989, but, significantly, these failed to continue beyond unification. Given the nature of the social, psychological, political and economic transformation processes in east Germany since 1990, one may interpret these as important obstacles to the growth of civil society and trust in the east, such that the two halves of Germany may not necessarily be drawing closely together. In particular, the social values of easterners, which strongly favour state provision, solidarity, an all-encompassing welfare system and, for example, social discipline in the schools and training system, exhibit a view of society which is more centrally directed and ordered than the more individualistic, free associational form implicit in the Putnam conception of civic community. After an overview of the development of societal participation in east Germany in recent years (in which there has been a dramatic decline in membership of secondary associations particularly in the period immediately after unification), the chapter concludes by suggesting that a paradoxical situation in east Germany exists, whereby the widespread existence of strong informal networks does not necessarily result in strong forms of civic participation, and hence a thriving 'Civic Culture'.[8] Differing pasts, frames of reference, socialisation processes and political cultures continue to shape distinct civil societies in east and west Germany today.

'CIVIC COMMUNITY' IN PRE-UNITY EAST GERMANY

We begin then with the question of whether, in a Putnam sense, civic community could exist in the GDR. According to Putnam, 'vertical bonds of clientelism restrain civic involvement and inhibit voluntary, horizontally organized manifestations of social solidarity'.[9]

The process of consolidation of communist control and the coordination of almost all areas of life according to Marxist–Leninist principles characterised the formative stages of the GDR's existence. The economic, political and public spheres were effectively conflated together by the fledgling authorities. Tasks previously carried out by the traditional family, church and civil social organisations were now taken over by the state; for example, in 1955 the *Jugendweihe* – the initiation into young adulthood at the age of 12 – began replacing confirmation in the church.

Broadly speaking GDR society was characterised by a distinct lack of independent social and political associations and vehicles for interest representation. Channels that existed for articulating interests were either extended arms of the Sozialistische Einheitspartei Deutschlands (Socialist Unity Party of Germany (SED)), for example, the mass organisations FDGB (Confederation of Free German Trade Unions), FDJ (Free German Youth) and the DSF (Gesellschaft für Deutsch-Sowjetische Freundschaft), or constitutionally enshrined 'safety-valves' such as *Eingaben* (petitions) or readers' letters to local newspapers. The east German regime was sustained to a great degree by integrating the population into its structures and organisations essential for its functioning. For example, almost all of the workforce were members of the FDGB, through which practically all holidays, rest cures, shopping and many other services were distributed 'top-down'.[10] Almost all citizens over 14 years of age were members of at least three mass organisations or political parties,[11] for example, youth movements, women's culture leagues and so forth, in addition to the work brigade and collective.[12] This led to the population directing demands upwards, to the state, to the party and politicians, especially when seeking answers concerning their personal welfare and the economic performance of the economy.[13] Furthermore, privileges were traded for loyalty between rulers and ruled in vertical fashion (very much like southern Italy's tradition of patronage and clientelism). Such a system resulted in a stark hierarchy in GDR society between the ruling elite and the masses and to vertical relations of authority and dependency, with citizens 'programmed to think in terms of vertical structures'.[14]

The Society of Niches and Informal Networks

Communist rule in east Germany eventually turned public opinion into private opinion. Civil society was substituted by 'face to face primary groups'.[15] The society of niches, which embodied the ultimate in retreatism from state politics, was made up of atomised individuals who had close, trusting relations with family members, relatives, friends, work colleagues and other acquaintances.[16] The niche society had the function of a safety-valve with the majority of east Germans using their niches to escape and retreat from the tedious party propaganda and over-politicised daily life of communist society to pursue activities that made their lives more bearable. The concept of niches in a dictatorship is not restricted to the private sphere alone. There were also many types of professional niches, allowing citizens an amount of limited personal freedom. These ranged from school teachers[17] through to the position of church pastor.[18] The externally enforced *Anpassung* (that is, the recognition of and adherence to the parameters of the dictatorship) did not result in total conformity but rather the appearance of such. Both those citizens in private and professional niches had learned how best to come to terms with the conditions of the dictatorship without actually endorsing the powers in charge. With the various techniques developed to survive life under a dictatorship and make it more bearable, individuals were able to achieve a certain intellectual independence. The majority in the GDR seemed to be able to live a dual existence between the 'lie' in the official discourse and their normal discourse within the niche society.[19] This *Doppelzüngigkeit* became the norm without people noticing it.[20] Thus under GDR authoritarianism, in which force and the family provided a 'primitive substitute for the civic community',[21] there existed little chance of public free expression, no sphere outside the niche society in which civic values free from party ideology and indoctrination could prosper. The horizontal relations of reciprocity and cooperation which bind a civic community together were 'ordered' from above and not allowed to grow organically. The centralist 'top-down' nature of GDR society was not conducive to the growth of civic virtue, for associationalism – which lies at the heart of the civic community – was arranged by the elite through the workplace, a microcosm of society and the centre of social life under east German socialism.[22] However, in common with other Soviet satellite states, the enforced retreatism actually encouraged the creation of both strong informal social networks built around families, friends, acquaintances and so forth, on the one hand, and networks and patron–client connections in the barter economy, on the other, through which scarce goods/services could be procured. Solidarity among citizens was shaped in the *Mangelgesellschaft*, in which reciprocity was the only answer to overcoming seemingly insurmountable problems, for example, the acquisition of building materials to construct a house.

East Germans were extremely good at 'making do' in a society with scarce resources. By utilising contacts within the shadow economy, where barter, under-the-counter sales, black-market goods and even contraband goods were commonplace, citizens developed complex informal networks parallel to and outside of the official sphere,[23] thereby creating their own social capital. Both types of informal network were based on trust – the lubricator of social relations. This dual society was underpinned by the existence of a *Lauben* culture, a community of garden plots whose number swelled from 940,000 in 1965 to 1.5 million in 1988.[24] The relatively low mobility of citizens in the GDR probably assisted in the maintenance and deepening of such informal networks, in which the GDR's equivalent to the western concept of civic community was to develop.

Civic Activity: Mid to Late 1980s

In addition to the informal networks described above, civic activity from the mid to late 1980s was driven by groups of would-be emigrants, dissident groups and citizens, all intent on developing and expanding a replacement public sphere (*Ersatzöffentlichkeit*) within the closed GDR society. Among the wider citizenry this ranged from a huge rise in critical and usually unpublished or unanswered *Eingaben* and readers' letters to the increased use of companies'/factories' 'wall newspaper', incidents of graffiti, anonymous telephone calls and the burgeoning growth of critical discussions at the workplace – all of these represented a break with the previous *Anpassung* of the masses and constituted a common desire for a public sphere in which dialogue could take place.[25] This broad trend coincided and often overlapped with another increasing phenomenon: exit to the west, real or imagined. The exit 'movement' contributed considerably to the establishment of a replacement public sphere in and around the church by politicising meetings and focusing on topics such as human rights and freedom of travel which were of a political nature in the GDR. Would-be emigrants, who had filed an application to leave the country, had to suffer disadvantages in the GDR, something that brought them together in loose groups of like-minded people.[26] The shift from the individual act of applying to leave to the collective frustration of having to remain assisted the formation and networking of 'exit' groups throughout the republic. These groups often set precedents by undertaking public action to draw attention to their cause which was then emulated by so-called dissidents' groups, whose relationship to the would-be emigrants remained strained until autumn 1989.

The churches, in particular the Protestant church, gradually became the only quasi-independent institution in the GDR. For dissident grass-roots groups such as 'New Forum', 'Democracy Now' and 'Democratic Awakening', which sprang up in 1989 on the back of years of latent oppositional activity, the church offered a forum for meetings and discussions. The year saw a strengthening of organisational structures and previous loose networks, all of which assisted in channelling the pressure from 'below' in the factories, firms and so forth by offering dissemination of information and a focal point for the articulation of interests. These focal points, in combination with the influence of would-be emigrants, who greatly assisted in politicising church meetings, soon spilled over into full-scale demonstrations, which took place in some 511 different villages, towns and cities throughout the republic.[27] Common to all participants were a desire for change and the need to create a public sphere in society. Beyond this, the diversity of political orientations gathered under the umbrella of New Forum and the others was wide. Protestant dissidents demonstrated beside Conservative Catholics and manual workers. Once the Berlin Wall had been breached and the GDR effectively imploded, the theme binding many participants and compelling them to undertake public action no longer existed, clearly shown by the huge drop in the numbers at demonstrations at the end of 1989 and the beginning of 1990. The majority of *Bürgerrechtler* (civil rights activists) and alternative groups, it should not be forgotten, were neither the initiators of the mass demonstrations nor did they organise them.[28] In fact, before the tumultuous events of 1989 the small groups of intellectual dissidents did not enjoy any widespread support from the masses,[29] whose opinions of and attitudes toward the state were nearer to those of the would-be emigrants.

In no way can this flurry of civic activity in the late 1980s be compared to a traditional organic associational culture developed from years of interest conflict as has happened in west Germany. The situation in east Germany in late 1989 was far removed from the high levels of corporatism and rich associational culture of the west. East Germany could not have inherited a 'substantial stock of social capital in the form of norms of reciprocity and networks of civic engagement'[30] necessary for facilitating social unity with west Germany, because of the distinct lack of modes of association free from the state's influence. The burgeoning of civic activity, contingent upon the specific conditions of the late 1980s, was then unable to survive unification because of two core factors: the nature of the transformation process itself and because it was not embedded in a long tradition of established social norms and networks that had emerged as outcomes of prolonged historical processes. The revolution of 1989, while to a great extent the result of a long evolutionary process of *decreasing* loyalty of the population toward the state and *increasing* attempts at creating an open public sphere by would-be emigrants, dissidents and the masses, was still only contingent civic mobilisation. Equally, as discussed above, there was no east German '1968' or post-materialist generation and no history of free public interest articulation via civil society organisations to shape the political culture as in the west.

CIVIC COMMUNITY IN EAST GERMANY SINCE UNIFICATION

The communist system left a double legacy which directly affects the vibrancy of civil society: 'individuals are likely to have a high degree of trust in their immediate social network, and a high degree of distrust in the formal institutions of the state'.[31] The civic mobilisation of the late 1980s was not robust enough both to dispel citizens' distrust in formal institutions and to withstand rapid systemic transformation, because of its failure to secure lasting horizontal societal relations in east German society. Additionally, several factors have inhibited the organic growth of civil society in east Germany since unification. First and foremost, many of the former channels of interest articulation and mobilisation discussed above have vanished with state socialism. Second, the speed and extent of the unprecedented transformation process itself brought with it a number of unforeseen social, economical and psychological problems for former GDR citizens.

Above all the difficult economic restructuring process has had a profound effect on people's attitudes towards the unified state. In the paternalistic GDR citizens entered an unspoken *Sozialvertrag* (social contract) with the leadership, whereby social welfare, full employment, subsidised foodstuffs were guaranteed by the state in exchange for outward conformity (*Anpassung*), lip service to state ideology and recognition of the SED's leading role. Thus the incumbent government was and is seen to be responsible for the state of the economy. The uncompromising manner in which the GDR's state sector was privatised following unification, the devaluing of skills and qualifications gained under socialism and the onset of mass unemployment bolstered east German citizens' existing distrust of politicians and institutions and solidified the deep misunderstandings between east and west Germans. The loss of employment, especially, has had a devastating effect on many citizens, who had been socialised in a society with one of the highest employment rates in the world,[32] and who had become used to the social role of the workplace. The net result for the process of interest articulation and civic participation – core ingredients of a flourishing civil society – has been a renewed retreat into the private sphere and a partial relapse into the vertical relationships of the past. East German citizens make less use than westerners of established (west German) mechanisms of civic participation – including their right to vote[33] – and interest intermediation, and feel themselves to be 'second class citizens' and strangers in their own country.[34] And at a more general level, they display a sense of alienation from the political system[35] which dwarfs even that of a western German population long noted for its *Politikverdrossenheit* (sullenness about politics and politicians). All in all, one can suggest that citizens' attention since the *Wende* has been focused on surviving in the unified state's parameters 'rather than on associational activity'.[36]

As we have seen, the past plays an important role in the perceptions and behaviour of east Germans in the post-unity period. While the institutional framework extended to east Germany in 1990 was the result of 40 years of west German stable democracy, it will take time to erode the socialist legacy of distrust in politicians and institutions alike. The unforgiving transformation process and, above all, the accompanying mass unemployment have added to citizens' scepticism of the new state. It is also important to remember that regional variations exist within east Germany itself. One of the most striking cases with a wide variety of factors fuelling distrust and scepticism of the new system among the population is that of Mecklenburg-Western Pommerania (M-V). While many of M-V's problems are symptomatic of those experienced by the other new *Länder*, one must bear in mind that M-V is agricultural and therefore the patterns of associational activity and participation and the levels of employment will be somewhat particular to the region, although unemployment has hit the former state and collective farms very badly. The north of the former GDR, known as the country's 'larder' because of its predominantly agricultural nature, had little industry apart from shipbuilding on the coast and has always been Germany's most economically backward region. As discussed, the growth of civic community in east Germany has not been facilitated by mass unemployment in the post-unity period. The number of people in employment (*Erwerbstätige*) in M-V has dropped dramatically from 1,168,500 in 1989 to only 712,672 in 1998.[37] Mecklenburg also suffers from a continuous 'brain-drain' of citizens and in 1998 outward migration of mostly younger citizens from the *Land* continued to outweigh inward migration by some 3,737 (and where female migrants were twice as numerous as male).[38] Additionally, M-V registered over 53,000 commuters with jobs in other *Länder* for 1997, around 75 per cent of whom worked in the Old *Bundesländer*, a further sign of economic dependency on the west. Many of the citizens who exit Mecklenburg are the very people needed to build the foundations of a civic community. All of these developments are detrimental to the growth of an organic associational culture and have had a profound effect on the social fabric of society. Even those *in* employment in the east today have lost the hitherto 'top-down' network of intermediary structures. These structures could have provided citizens with coping strategies and mechanisms for coming to terms with the unknown phenomenon of unemployment. This is compounded by the lack of a *Verein* tradition (that is, one based on a history of clubs and associations) especially in rural areas, which can be instrumental in assisting communities in coping with transitional adjustments.

SOCIETAL PARTICIPATION IN CONTEMPORARY EAST GERMANY

Taking the participation in clubs, associations and political parties as one benchmark for the development of civil society and therefore for the exercise of democratic rights is fraught with problems. Firstly, one needs to ascertain which clubs, associations and so forth foster civic engagement among their members. Secondly, one has to be wary of measuring an emerging east German political culture with the tools of mature democratic western states. Lastly, falling rates of associational participation and the collapse in party affiliation along traditional class or religious boundaries is a worldwide phenomenon of late capitalist societies, yet democracy *per se* is not seen to be in danger in these countries. It is within this broader context that statistics regarding east German levels of participation are to be analysed.

There is evidence of forms of self-organisation springing up on the local, regional and even east German-wide levels.[39] A wide variety of clubs and associations have been set up since the collapse of one-party rule, something that is looked upon by east Germans as one of the most positive aspects of unification.[40] East Germans are very familiar with membership of organisations due to their experience with the 80 or so in operation in the GDR. According to analyses of citizens' 'willingness to participate in organisations with varying tasks' for the period 1992–97, levels have remained relatively stable. While in 1992, 34 per cent of citizens were prepared to participate in organisations classified as 'social and voluntary', the proportion had dropped only slightly to 30 per cent by 1997. Interestingly, among those citizens with a higher education, the proportion went from 45 per cent in 1992 to 37 per cent in 1997, possibly as a result of a change of values or of the increasing trend to retreat into the spheres of private life and leisure.[41] The upward trend toward undertaking leisure activities has continued strongly year-on-year from 1992–97.[42]

As always, citizens' willingness to participate in organisations, parties, associations and voluntary associations is not matched by the actual number of members. Active participation in groups with a more political character (political parties/citizens' initiatives) has declined rapidly from the early 1990s.[43] Many citizens involved in citizens' initiatives were disillusioned by unification and the dominance of west German political parties in the political process. Equally, membership of the main parties fell in line with the rise in dissatisfaction with the transformation process outlined above. Between 1991 and 1997 membership in clubs, associations and voluntary associations fell dramatically from 42 per cent to 30 per cent of the east German population, although the last three years of this period saw hardly any change.[44] Union membership, however, has suffered the most among all organisations in the east. With many of the privileges of the former regime no longer applicable, rising unemployment and the general dissatisfaction with their situation, membership declined from 42 per cent in 1992 to just 19 per cent in 1997.[45]

The long and traditional associational culture of west Germany is reflected in the number of participants in sport clubs, choirs, church associations, political parties and citizens' initiatives. In all of these cases west membership far outstrips that of the east. The most outstanding examples are sports clubs (27.6 per cent compared to 9.8 per cent), choirs (6.3 per cent compared to 1.2 per cent) and general clubs and organisations (19.2 per cent compared to 13.6 per cent). Finally, 52.9 per cent of east Germans and 43.9 per cent of west Germans do not belong to any type of club at all.[46]

Thus if one quantifies 'civic community' by taking numbers of active citizens in organisations and clubs, it would appear that east Germany still has some way to go in reaching west German levels. However, a decrease in civic participation has to be both qualified and placed in a wider context. Does trade union membership reflect the vibrancy of civil society? Does falling membership of political and civic parties and associations herald the demise of democratic principles? Or are the developments in east Germany simply falling into line with civic participation in mature democracies around the world? There is a case for arguing that east

Germany is by-passing many of the phases of development of a normal 'modern' state, by virtue of its being thrust from a low productivity, state centralist economy and society towards a high productivity, market economy and liberal society today. In the same way as state of the art infrastructure and technology are replacing their obsolescent socialist equivalents, it might be argued that civic participation has leapfrogged the evolutionary developments experienced in the west and arrived at the current *Politikverdrossenheit* that characterises many democracies. However, perhaps more likely is that east Germany may be following a trajectory of development of its own, reflecting the past and the deeply painful restructuring. This trajectory combines the unusual mixture of low civic participation, a well-developed sector of non-profit organisations (mostly state-dependent),[47] and a heavy reliance on informal networks consisting of friends and family. Almost by definition, social change and geographical mobility in the new *Länder* has been very high 'with virtually all individuals having experienced a change in occupation, status, and/or residence', while simultaneously having 'lost the loci of social interaction' (mass organisations/socialist work collectives/cultural institutions) present in the GDR.[48] All of these factors taken together point to the emergence of an east German distinctiveness and are reflected in people's behaviour, values and attitudes.

The president of the Federal Constitutional Court, Jutta Limbach, and the Federal Commissioner for the Stasi Documents, Joachim Gauck, recently caused a storm by proclaiming a decreasing support for democratic principles among east Germans. Gauck, a former pastor and New Forum member, suggests that decades of living under dictatorial conditions (effectively the beginning of the Third Reich in 1933 to the end of the GDR in 1989) had prevented his countrymen from seizing the chances offered by a democratic and free system.[49] Furthermore, it is alleged that east Germans have a 'fear of freedom', are not used to responsibility and were never trained for autonomy.[50] Both Gauck and Limbach have been criticised for their statements. According to the *Leipziger Volkszeitung*, the introduction of democracy in west Germany was connected to the positive experience of the 'Economic Miracle', while, as we have seen, in the east democracy and freedom were accompanied by the loss of jobs, social security and abrupt systemic change.[51]

In contrast, Manfred Stolpe cites the east Germans' lack of support for and open criticism of the Nato bombing in Kosovo and their expectations of the welfare state as examples of the 'freedom of opinion' in east Germany.[52] The Germans' reactions to the Kosovo war are indicative of the deep-rooted divisions that run through east and west. The Kosovo war fault line between east and west was evident with around 56 per cent of easterners and 38 per cent of westerners opposed to the Nato bombing.[53] For some, this shows 'freedom of opinion'; others explain it by the fact that the west can look back on 50 years of democratic rule and ever closer ties to western Europe and Nato, while the east has experienced just 10 years of pluralism and witnessed decades of anti-Americanism.[54] This division in public opinion reflects the differing political party dynamics in both sides of the same country, differing values and historical experiences and differing public opinions on a range of topics including the role of the welfare state (east Germans look positively upon the GDR's social welfare provision).[55] To be sure, one can speak of an emerging east German identity as distinct from the west, one which has been created *following* the collapse of the Berlin Wall, and one bound by common attitudes, morals, values and an understanding of democracy. A recent study supports these claims, suggesting that 'East Germans seek solace from the deficits of their social environment in their private relationships with their family, children and partners more so than westerners, whilst neither easterners nor westerners are optimistic that a feeling of community is developing in unified Germany'.[56]

THE PAST, THE PRESENT AND THE FUTURE

One has to consider whether Putnam's terms and concepts introduced in this chapter are applicable to a society in transition or whether they apply only to mature democracies with high employment and income. The evolution of civil society in the east a decade after the collapse of the Berlin Wall presents a paradoxical picture. Remnants of a socialist past mix with reactions to and experiences of the unprecedented transformation process from an authoritarian state to one based on pluralist democracy. Extensive informal networks forged under a repressive system in a dual society have been carried over into the new east German society. Citizens' distrust of institutions and the officials that run them is both a product of the past and the present. East Germans do not feel represented by their imported institutional system, including the political parties and interest associations that go with it; they tend to draw on practices developed before 1989 and which have continued following communism's demise; and they turn to informal networks of immediate family members, friends and close acquaintances for 'mutual aid as a cushion against the shocks of transformation'.[57] Many still meet up on a regular basis with colleagues from pre-1989 collectives and firms to discuss their joint pasts and joint destinies.[58] East German social values still tend to favour collective solutions to societal problems rather than voluntary or individualistic ones;

they favour democracy but with a strong social welfare system. In sum, the informal networks and relations forged in the former cultural context have, to a certain extent, continued into the present all-German context, partly as a buttress and coping strategy against the effects of the unprecedented socio-economic transformation.

Forty years of socialist socialisation and the uncompromising economic, political and psychological transformation have not lent themselves to the creation of a civic community in east Germany. Above all, unemployment remains high and one can reasonably expect that this impacts on the willingness of citizens to participate in society, for the importance of work and social welfare for east German citizens cannot be overstated. The general trend in societal participation among east Germans is downward. Active participation in society – that is wider participatory activities that impact on the community, the public sphere and the organisations within it – is needed to create social cohesion and connectedness.[59] This is especially true in the east German case where the articulation of specific east German interests, that is apart from the regional political party, the PDS, is still underdeveloped.

NOTES

1. For an authoritative assessment of east Germans' attitudes towards the social welfare state see E. Roller, 'Shrinking the Welfare State: Citizens' Attitudes towards Cuts in Social Spending in Germany in the 1990s', in *German Politics,* Vol. 8, No. 1 (April 1999), pp. 21–39.
2. R. Putnam, *Making Democracy Work: Civic Traditions in Modern Italy* (Princeton: Princeton University Press, 1993).
3. Putnam, *Making Democracy Work,* p. 88.
4. Quoted in Putnam, *Making Democracy Work,* p. 167. The following discussion does not employ the Putnam methodology to test civic participation.
5. J. M. Mushaben, 'Auferstanden aus Ruinen: Social Capital and Democratic Identity in the New Länder', in *German Politics and Society*, Vol. 15, No. 4 (winter 1997), pp. 79–101, here p. 82.
6. J. Grix (with J. Smith), 'The German Democratic Republic', in J. Smith and E. Teague (eds), *Democracy in the New Europe: The Politics of Post-Communism* (London: Greycoat Press, 1999), pp. 19–20.
7. G. Gaus, *Wo Deutschland liegt* (Hamburg: Hoffmann & Campe, 1983).
8. A. Almond and S. Verba, *The Civic Culture* (Princeton: Princeton University Press, 1963).
9. Putnam, *Making Democracy Work,* p. 149.
10. K. Schroeder, *Der SED Staat – Geschichte und Strukturen der DDR* (Munich: Landeszentrale für politische Bildung, 1998), p. 515; also A. Pickel and H. Wiesenthal, *The Grand Experiment: Debating Shock Therapy, Transition Theory, and the East German Experience* (Boulder, CO: Westview Press, 1997), p. 27.
11. M. D. Hancock and H. Welsh (eds), *German Unification: Processes and Outcomes* (Boulder/San Francisco/Oxford: Westview Press, 1994), p. 21.
12. M. Fulbrook, *Anatomy of a Dictatorship: Inside the GDR 1949–1989* (Oxford University Press,

1995), p. 12. For a discussion on the meaning of work collectives for women see Bettina Iganski, 'The Meaning of Women's "Second Family" for Current Patterns of Discontinuity in Rural East Germany', in P. Cooke and J. Grix (eds), *Continuity and Change in East Germany* (Amsterdam: Rodopi, 2000).

13. R. Rose *et al.*, 'Getting Real: Social Capital in Post-Communist Societies', in *Studies in Public Policy*, No. 278 (Glasgow: University of Strathclyde Studies in Public Policy, 1997), p. 24.

14. Jürgen Fuchs cited in A. Sa'adah, *Germany's Second Chance: Trust, Justice, and Democratization* (London: Harvard University Press, 1998), p. 62.

15. R. Rose, 'Distrust as an Obstacle to Civil Society', in *Studies in Public Policy*, No. 226 (Glasgow: University of Strathclyde Studies in Public Policy, 1997), p. 8.

16. M. Diewald, 'Informelle Beziehungen und Hilfeleistungen in der DDR: Persönliche Bindung und instrumentelle Nützlichkeit', in B. Nauck, N. F. Schneider and A. Tölke (eds), *Familie und Lebensverlauf im gesellschaftlichen Umbruch* (Stuttgart: Enke, 1995), p. 56.

17. One former teacher in *Bezirk* Schwerin remembers several niches in the school: speaking two types of language, official and unofficial; silence; keeping secrets; refusal; and, finally, family and friends. See the contribution by W. Bratrschovsky in *Landtag Mecklenburg-Vorpommern, Aufarbeitung und Versöhnung*, Vol. III (Schwerin: Stiller & Balewski, 1997), pp. 74–7.

18. Interestingly it was the pastors that filled the power vacuum left by SED officials during the *Wende* of 1989. This anomaly – strong influence of religious figures in political affairs in one of the least religious countries in Europe – could be explained by the fact that many people who were refused the right to study the subject of their choice for whatever reasons were allowed to study theology. Thus many potential dissenters became pastors. Interview with Jörn Mothes (a former carpenter in the GDR and now head of Schwerin's Stasi documentation bureau) who took this route in the GDR, Schwerin, 2 September 1997.

19. V. Havel, 'The Power of the Powerless', in John Keane (ed.), *The Power of the Powerless* (New York: Armonk, 1985), pp. 23–96.

20. S. Wolle, 'Herrschaft und Alltag. Die Zeitgeschichtsforschung auf der Suche nach der wahren DDR', in *Aus Politik und Zeitgeschichte*, B 26, 20 July 1997, p. 33.

21. Putnam, *Making Democracy Work*, p. 178.

22. The social aspect of the workplace was highlighted in several interviews with the author from 7 August 1997–24 March 1998 with, e.g., Thomas Helms (printer), Frank Häusler (mathematician), Paul Dorn (BstU employee), Jörn Mothes (BstU employee), Dr B. Kasten (head of Schwerin City Archive), Ralph Sowart (political scientist, Berlin).

23. J. Grix, *The Collapse of the GDR: The Role of the Masses* (Basingstoke: Macmillan, 2000), pp. 30–1; P. Jackson (ed.), *DDR – Das Ende eines Staates* (Manchester/NY: Manchester University Press, 1994), p. 15.

24. Statistisches Jahrbuch der DDR, 1989, p. 414, cited in A. Staab, *National Identity in Eastern Germany: Inner Unification or Continued Separation* (Westport, CT, London: Praeger, 1988), p. 105.

25. Grix, '*The Collapse of the GDR*', p. 107

26. See J. Grix, 'Competing Approaches to the Collapse of the GDR: "Top Down" vs "Bottom Up"', *Journal of Area Studies*, 13 (autumn 1998) (special issue on revolutions), pp. 121–42, here p. 135.

27. B. Lindner, *Die demokratische Revolution in der DDR 1989/90* (Bonn: Bundeszentrale für politische Bildung, 1998), p. 89.

28. D. Pollack, 'Was ist aus den Bürgerbewegungen und Oppositionsgruppen der DDR geworden?', *Aus Politik und Zeitgeschichte*, B 40-41/95, pp. 34–45, here p. 36.

29. A. Sa'adah, *Germany's Second Chance: Trust, Justice, and Democratization*, p. 79.

30. Putnam, *Making Democracy Work*, p. 167.

31. Rose *et al.*, 'Getting Real: Social Capital', p. 10.

32. K. Hardach, *The Political Economy of Germany* (Berkeley, CA: University of California Press, 1980), p. 15.

33. J. M. Mushaben, 'Auferstanden aus Ruinen', p. 95.

34. C. Seils, *Tageszeitung*, 24 May 1999; also P. Pulzer, 'Political Ideology', in Gordon Smith, William E. Paterson, Peter H. Merkl and Stephen Padgett (eds), *Developments in German Politics* (Basingstoke: Macmillan, 1992), pp. 303–26, here p. 325.

35. *The Times*, 13 July 1998, p. 10.

36. A. Segert, 'Problematic Normalization: East German Workers Eight Years after Unification', *German Politics and Society*, Vol. 16, No. 48 (1998), pp. 105–24, here p. 109.

37. *Vorläufige Angaben: Erwerbstätigenrechnung des Bundes und der Länder* (Schwerin: Statistisches Landesamt Mecklenburg-Vorpommern); for 1989 figures see *Statistisches Jahrbuch, Mecklenburg Vorpommern, 1997* (Schwerin: Statistisches Landesamt Mecklenburg-Vorpommern, 1997), p. 125.
38. Statistisches Landesamt, Mecklenburg-Vorpommern, *Presseinformation*, from 19 May 1999.
39. J. Wielgohs, 'Strategies of West German Corporate Actors in the Creation of Interest Associations in East Germany', in *German Politics*, Vol. 5, No. 2 (August 1996), pp. 201–13, here p. 203.
40. *Sozialreport*, IV. Quartal 1997/Sonderheft 2/1997, p. 54, published by the Sozialwissenschaftliches Forschungszentrum, Berlin-Brandenburg.
41. Taken from *Sozialreport 1995*, p. 350 and IV. Quartal 1997/Sonderheft 2/1997, p. 42, produced by the Sozialwissenschaftliches Forschungszentrum, Berlin-Brandenburg.
42. In Mecklenburg-Vorpommern, for example, membership of sports clubs has risen by some 50,000 over this five-year time period. Statistisches Jahrbuch, Mecklenburg-Vorpommern 1998, p. 101.
43. On this point see A.Staab, *National Identity in Eastern Germany*, p. 70–6.
44. *Sozialreport 1995*, p. 351; *Sozialreport 1997*, p. 42.
45. *Sozialreport 1997*, p. 45.
46. *Sozialreport 1995*, p. 353.
47. W. Seibel, *Nonprofit Organizations in post-1990 East Germany*, paper presented at the conference 'The German Road from Socialism to Capitalism: Eastern Germany Ten Years after the Collapse of the GDR', Harvard University, Center for European Studies, 18–20 June 1999.
48. L. McFalls, 'Eastern Germany Transformed: From Postcommunist to Late Capitalist Political Culture', Montreal University, 1999, unpublished manuscript, p. 27.
49. *Schweriner Volkszeitung*, 17 May 1999, p. 3.
50. Ibid.; p. 3; *Neubrandenburger Zeitung 'Nordkurier'*, p. 2. Gauck's remarks are not dissimilar to those made by Hans-Joachim Maaz in his best-seller on the east German psyche *Der Gefühlsstau* (Munich: Knaur, 1992). For an in-depth discussion of Maaz's views see M. Fulbrook, 'Re-reading Recent (East) German History', *German History*, Vol. 17, No. 2 (1999), pp. 271–84.
51. *Leipziger Volkszeitung*, from 17 May 1999, pp. 1, 3.
52. *Schweriner Volkszeitung*, 17 May 1999, p. 3.
53. *Frankfurter Rundschau*, 13 July 1999.
54. *Schweriner Volkszeitung*, 5 May 1999, p. 4.
55. On the Kosovo war see C. Seils in *Tageszeitung*, 24 May 1999; on east German attitudes to the welfare state see *Politbarometer-Eastern Germany* (1992–1995) at the Zentralarchiv für empirische Sozialforschung der Universität zu Köln.
56. *Frankfurter Rundschau*, 13 July 1999.
57. R. Rose, 'What Does Social Capital Add to Individual Welfare?', in *Studies in Public Policy*, No. 318 (Glasgow: University of Strathclyde Studies in Public Policy, 1999), p. 10.
58. Interview on 23 March 1998 with Karl Schmidt, an employee in the Schwerin office of the Landesbeauftragte für Stasi Unterlagen.
59. See A. L. Seligson, 'Civic Association and Democratic Participation in Central America: A Test of the Putnam Thesis', *Comparative Political Studies*, Vol. 32, No. 3 (May 1999), pp. 342–61.

Index